Teaching Children with Down Syndrome about Their Bodies, Boundaries, and Sexuality

A Guide
for
Parents
and
Professionals

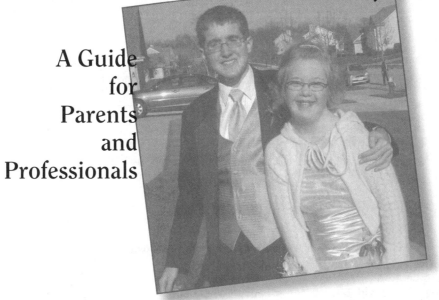

Terri Couwenhoven, M.S.

Woodbine House ◆ 2007

All rights reserved under International and Pan-American copyright conventions. Published in the United States of America by Woodbine House, Inc., 6510 Bells Mill Rd., Bethesda, MD 20817. 800-843-7323. www.woodbinehouse.com

Cover background and non-photo elements © Jeanine Kristy Baechtold, Kristy Valshan™, Inc. www.rakscraps.com

Illustrations on pages 270-87 and 291 by Gary Mohrman

Library of Congress Cataloging-in-Publication Data

Couwenhoven, Terri.
  Teaching children with Down syndrome about their bodies, boundaries, and sexuality : a guide for parents and professionals / Terri Couwenhoven. -- 1st ed.
     p. cm.
  Includes index.
  ISBN 978-1-890627-33-1
  1. Down syndrome--Patients--Sexual behavior. 2. Sex instruction for children with mental disabilities. I. Title.
  RJ506.D68C68 2007
  618.92'858842--dc22

                                                                                      2007025149

Manufactured in the United States of America

10   9   8   7   6   5   4   3   2

Table of Contents

Acknowledgements

My deepest appreciation to:

- The many parents who identified their needs, reviewed and critiqued segments of the book, and volunteered to share their stories and experiences so future generations of parents could benefit from their wisdom.
- My professional colleagues who took time out of their busy schedules to read sections of the book and openly share their thoughts and ideas for changes and improvements—David Smith, Stefi Gratigny, Teresa Prattke, Christine White, Patricia Miles Patterson, Pamela Boyle, Judi Myers, Joan Medlen, Julie Turkoske, Betty Ulanski, Susan Vigg Saucier, and especially my editor, Susan Stokes.
- The women's group of People First Wisconsin, Inc. (and other self-advocates) who helped me modify activities and ideas in this book so they would be more understandable for your sons and daughters—Margie Klar, Daire Keane, Cynthia Bentley, Lisa Cleghorn, Debra Schwalm, Nora Knowlton-Sachner, Nealy Rothe, Cathy Maccani, and Mollie Hanson.
- Mary Clare Carlson, whose overflow of enthusiasm and passion for supporting people with intellectual disabilities spilled over onto me and kept me going during times when I got stuck.
- Joan Medlen, for believing I could write a book and for coaching and mentoring me through the process.
- Planned Parenthood of Wisconsin's librarian, Anne Brosowsky-Roth, who was so helpful at finding, and letting me hold onto resources for extended lengths of time without sending overdue notices.
- Most important, my husband, Jeff, and two beautiful daughters, Anna and Lindy, who were so patient with my slowness and understanding of the time I needed to finish this project.

Introduction

Back in the early 1980s I worked as a sexuality educator for Planned Parenthood of Wisconsin. Early in my career, I was asked to teach a class for adults with cognitive disabilities. A local agency that supported people living in apartments had concerns about one of their clients who had recently been exploited. It started them thinking about ways they could help their other clients be better prepared to keep themselves safe while living in the community. Although I had worked with diverse groups of students, I had never taught people with developmental disabilities about sexuality.

The women turned out to be delightfully refreshing participants. They were honest, welcoming, and hungry for information, so I became determined to teach them whatever they wanted to know. At that time, specialized resources for teaching sexuality education to individuals with cognitive disabilities were just starting to be developed, so I spent much of my time trying to adapt or create materials that could make abstract sexuality concepts more concrete. (These women taught me the meaning of concrete.)

My positive experiences with these women and the many other participants I encountered at conferences and in programs helped me tremendously years later when our first daughter was born with Down syndrome. Admittedly, as anyone would imagine, I became more sensitive and compassionate about helping families teach their children who had cognitive disabilities about their bodies, boundaries, and sexuality issues.

Why This Book?

FROM INTERVENTION TO PREVENTION

I don't like crises. Under intense pressure I don't think very well, I make more than my usual number of mistakes, and later end up regretting my actions. As a result of this aversion, I've learned to becoming a "prevention" thinker. If a crisis emerges, I like to search out root causes and figure out how to work on them so I don't have to repeat the experience. During my early years as an educator, however, I realized that sexuality education for people with developmental disabilities often originates from crises. For example:

■ A 13-year-old boy was suspended from school after touching a girl inappropriately on the bus and now needed help learning appropriate boundaries.

■ A girl who was having her first period would not agree to wear a pad, no matter what her panicked mother said.

■ A woman was sexually assaulted in her sheltered workshop and needed training in self-protection.

All of these individuals had one thing in common: they had very little information about sexuality.

On my prevention quest, I became determined to be proactive with my own daughter from a very early age. I went in search of resources that were understandable, spoke to her at her level, and had good concrete illustrations. I quickly realized the difficulty families faced. Currently, there are only a handful of books designed specifically for families of young people with Down syndrome or other cognitive disabilities and most of them do not include teaching tools or pictures that might be useful. One of my goals for writing this book is to give you some tools that can help you become proactive about sexuality education. Proactive sexuality education means:

■ Introducing basic information about sexuality in childhood so repetition and reinforcement can occur over longer periods of time in a wide variety of real-life situations;

■ Teaching your child about her own and others' rights to privacy;

■ Seeing your child as a sexual person right from the start;

■ Preparing your child for typical stages in sexual development;

■ Initiating conversations before your child asks (if he ever does);

■ Envisioning your child as a sexually healthy adult and identifying ways to prepare him or her for that role over time.

From Why to How

Although many parents have difficulties addressing the issues above with their children, attitudes and awareness have shifted during the past few decades. Twenty years ago, I spent much of my time facing denial and resistance and found myself persuading parents (and professionals) that people with developmental disabilities were, in fact, sexual human beings with sexual needs. These days, parents appear to be more interested and accepting of their children's sexuality and the role they play in helping their children understand it. But they're hungry for the specifics. They want ideas and strategies for educating their children about these issues in ways that are respectful and understandable.

From Powerless to Powerful

Historically, the sexual rights of individuals with cognitive disabilities have been denied and suppressed. Until recently, forced sterilization, segregation of males and females within institutions, laws prohibiting marriage, group home policies and procedures that violate basic rights to privacy and sexual expression were commonplace. The momentum of the self-advocacy movement is changing all that. Self-advocates are assertively banding together to help the rest of the world understand that they have the same rights to information and needs as everyone else does when it comes to sexuality. Increasingly, teens and young adults are asking for information that can help them become knowledgeable about sexuality.

Who Is This Book For?

This book was written first and foremost for parents, since they have the most opportunities to teach their children about their bodies and boundaries, and heavily influence what their children learn about sexuality. More specifically, it was written primarily for parents of children and young adults with Down syndrome, although it will also be useful for families of children with other cognitive disabilities that result in difficulties with abstract thinking. This book includes ideas and stories gathered and collected over my twenty years of teaching and working as a sexuality educator. It is designed to be a guide for addressing sexuality issues across the lifespan. If your child is young, it can help you know what to expect and understand what you can do and say that will contribute to your child's healthy sexuality. If your child is older, you'll be able to gather insights from other parents, as well as determine where you need to begin.

Teachers, paraprofessionals, healthcare professionals, sex educators, and others who enjoy teaching and supporting individuals with Down syndrome or other developmental disabilities will find this book helpful too.

If you regularly live with, teach, or support someone with a developmental disability, you likely have some level of comfort and expertise working with people with developmental disabilities. You may, however, have little information or training on sexuality education. Although this book will help you to some extent, it is not designed to make you a "sexuality expert." If you are a teacher or trainer and are interested in designing and implementing sexuality programs for students with intellectual disabilities, strongly consider additional training and coursework in human sexuality. The resources and contacts listed in the back of the book should provide some helpful options. If you're a sexuality educator with little experience working with individuals with cognitive disabilities, this book can offer insights on teaching techniques that work best, content that may be important, as well as useful language and helpful approaches for sharing information.

Book Overview

Rather than organize this book by age or developmental issues, I've chosen to identify key topics and issues that provide a solid foundation for helping your child learn what it means to be a sexually healthy person. I call these topic areas *foundational concepts* because they act as a base from which to build and repeatedly refer to as more advanced sexuality concepts are introduced. Foundational concepts include:

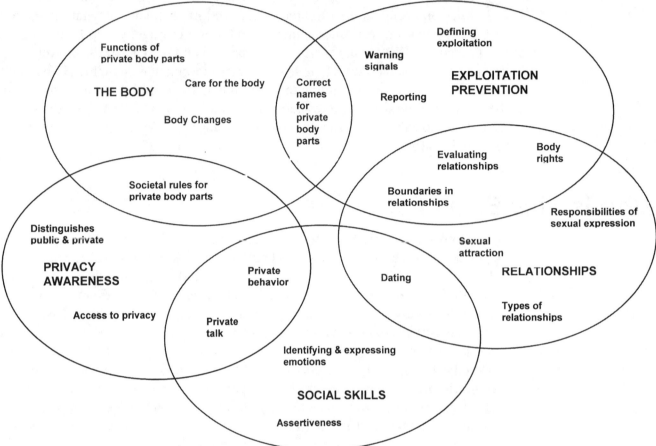

In addition to the above foundational concepts, I have also included detailed content that is specific to predictable developmental stages that are not affected by disability. For example, parents need to prepare their children for puberty and the possibility of marriage and parenting whether or not they have a disability. The last sections provide background information on school sexuality education and introduce strategies for teaching about sexuality, regardless of the age of your child.

HOW TO USE THIS BOOK

Within each chapter, there are segments that are designed to prepare you for teaching. Segments within each chapter include:

PREPARATION OR BACKGROUND INFORMATION

I'm a firm believer that the teacher should have more information than the student. Although you probably have more information than you think, a quick refresher can help you become familiar with the issues and boost confidence. If research exists, the findings will be shared in this section of the chapter.

PARENTAL PAUSES

Sharing information in understandable ways is just one part of educating your child. Being aware of your personal or family values about an issue is another essential component of teaching. *Parental Pauses* are thinking points or breaks that allow you to reflect on your own feelings, values, and attitudes related to a specific topic or issue before working with your child. Being clear about how you feel will influence the words you use and messages you want to communicate. These sections will include questions or other information that can help you clarify your stances.

FRAMEWORKS FOR TEACHING

Sometimes smaller pieces of information are difficult to understand until they can be placed within a larger context. *Framework for Teaching* sheets are designed to be quick overviews or "at-a-glance" summaries of the range of issues covered within each foundational concept chapter, key messages, and how the different concepts relate to the long-term goals of helping your child become a sexually healthy adult. Although there are no rules for the ages when these topics should be covered, the concepts listed on the *Framework for Teaching* sheets do, in most cases, suggest a logical scope and sequence of topics to be addressed as your child matures physically and emotionally. For example, it is helpful for your child to learn basic names for body parts before he learns about functions of those parts, and learning about sexual feelings and crushes is usually a precursor to learning about topics such as dating and sexual relationships.

Framework for Teaching Privacy—Excerpt

Concepts	Key Messages	Goal Behaviors
Privacy at home	■ Private places are rooms where I can go to be by myself ■ At home my private place is _____ ■ I can tell others when I want or need privacy ■ I should knock before entering other people's private spaces	■ Can identify private place(s) at home ■ Moves to private areas when privacy is needed ■ Recognizes violations of own privacy rights ■ Respects the privacy of others
Privacy in the community	■ There are times when I may need privacy when I am in the community ■ In the community, a private place is _____ ■ There are rules when I am using private areas in the community ■ Following the rules will help me stay safe	■ Can identify private place(s) in the community ■ Moves to private areas when privacy is needed ■ Recognizes when privacy rights have been violated ■ Is respectful of privacy rights of others

The range of concepts listed on the Framework for Teaching sheets are of course not mandatory but are meant to help you identify common issues and concerns that often need to be taught. Your own child will dictate the breadth and depth of topics you will teach based on his or her developmental level, interest, and unique mix of life experiences.

TEACHING SECTIONS

After you have read the background information, teaching sections will help you explain and reinforce concepts with your child or student. Each teaching section includes three components: key messages, teaching sheets, and reinforcement activities.

■ Parents often tell me they are unsure how to explain concepts in ways their child can understand. *Key messages* throughout this book suggest ways of saying things or give examples of explanations using simple, unsophisticated language. For many families, vocabulary used to teach about sexuality can feel foreign or unfamiliar because it is used so infrequently and creates significant discomfort. Because you know your child best, you will be more familiar with words and explanations that make sense for your child, and consequently may choose to explain things in different ways. Think of key messages as verbal starting points in the event you get stuck trying to find the right words.

■ It's difficult to find resources that are understandable, realistic, and concrete enough to explain sexuality concepts. Teaching materials at the back of the book include pictures, diagrams, worksheets, or basic summaries that can be used as you work with your child. These sheets will be more effective if they are used at the same time verbal explanations (key messages) are being provided. For example, you can use the key teaching messages to help you define puberty while your child is viewing the puberty progression pictures in Appendices A-9 and A-10. Having a visual example of what you are explaining will improve your child's learning and comprehension.

■ In addition to words and pictures, *learning activities* can be used to introduce information, incorporate repetition and reinforcement, or evaluate learning at home or in the classroom.

PARENT STORIES AND EXPERIENCES

We can learn a lot from other parents. For every issue, situation, or experience you've encountered with your child, there are hundreds of other families who have had similar experiences (honest!). Many families are blazing new trails and their experiences can be a tremendous source of wisdom for families who are not there yet. This book is peppered with these experiences, nuggets of wisdom, and simple thoughts and reflections from families who have accepted their role as their child's primary educators about bodies, boundaries, and sexuality, and are living the journey.

All too often, people with developmental disabilities receive too little information about sexuality. This does not have to be the case for your son or daughter with Down syndrome or other intellectual disability. I'm hoping that the information, activities, and advice in this book will encourage, educate, guide, and support you and your family on your journey. Good luck!

CHAPTER 1

Getting Started

What Is Sexuality?

In our society, being "sexual" is commonly associated with "doing" something that is sexual in nature (usually involving the genitals), when, in fact, sexuality is much broader and complex. Sexuality encompasses fundamental aspects of who we are as humans and is an active and inseparable part of us.

During an education session many years ago, I invited a group of teens to make distinctions between the words *sex* and *sexuality*. One of the participants shared that his mother had taught him that "sex" was between his legs but "sexuality" was between his ears. This teen's mom understood that sexuality is not just about what we do with our bodies but more about "being"—about who we are as men and women.

Sexuality is broad and includes biological, psychological, social, and cultural components. Consider the following examples:

> *Both Andy and Beth, a soon-to-be husband and wife, were deeply saddened when they discovered that Andy was infertile and they were unable to have children. They knew that males with Down syndrome often have lowered fertility and so had undergone testing before the wedding.*
>
> *"I found out about my test results. I thought it was good news that I could father a baby. But I was wrong....he told me I can't father a baby. I told Beth. I was bawling, she was bawling. It was hard but we hung in there together.*
>
> —From *Andy and Beth: A Love Story*

The above story illustrates an example of the biological dimension of sexuality. Biology influences gender, physical development over the lifespan, and reproductive capacity. Sexual drive, aspects of sexual orientation, and our ability to function sexually can also be driven by biological factors.

The psychosocial dimension of sexuality comes into play when our own unique personality traits (thoughts, feelings, and emotions) interface with environment, society, and culture. For example, our understanding about what it means to be a male or female, to be sexual, to be beautiful, or to have a disability influences how we act and respond in different environments. The two stories below illustrate aspects of the psychosocial dimension of sexuality.

David, a young man with Down syndrome, is transitioning from his high school into his district's vocational training program in order to prepare for future employment in the community. At one of his job placements, he develops feelings for an employee and becomes very vocal about his desire to date, marry, and have children with her even though these feelings are not reciprocated.

Monica, a young adult, refuses to associate with other teens who have cognitive disabilities and consequently will not consider the possibility of dating a person with developmental disabilities. Instead, she is insistent on finding a "normal" partner, someone without disabilities.

Myths and Misconceptions about Sexuality and People with Disabilities

During the past few decades, significant progress has been made in helping both parents and professionals recognize that people with developmental disabilities are sexual human beings whose needs are more similar than different from those of

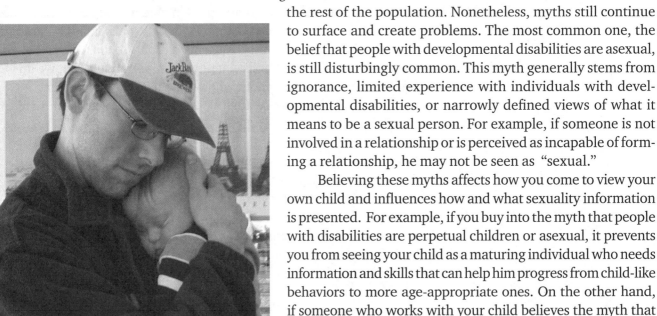

the rest of the population. Nonetheless, myths still continue to surface and create problems. The most common one, the belief that people with developmental disabilities are asexual, is still disturbingly common. This myth generally stems from ignorance, limited experience with individuals with developmental disabilities, or narrowly defined views of what it means to be a sexual person. For example, if someone is not involved in a relationship or is perceived as incapable of forming a relationship, he may not be seen as "sexual."

Believing these myths affects how you come to view your own child and influences how and what sexuality information is presented. For example, if you buy into the myth that people with disabilities are perpetual children or asexual, it prevents you from seeing your child as a maturing individual who needs information and skills that can help him progress from child-like behaviors to more age-appropriate ones. On the other hand, if someone who works with your child believes the myth that people with cognitive disabilities are "oversexed" or "uncontrollable" (meaning their sex drive is somehow more intense than the rest of the population), they may scrutinize or report every sexual behavior, even if they're developmentally appropriate.

One example of a myth I succumbed to is the belief that people with Down syndrome have different and more

Common Myths about Sexuality

MYTH	FACT
People with Down Syndrome:	
Are asexual (do not have sexual thoughts, feelings, needs)	The needs for touch, affection, and meaningful relationships are important for all of us.
Are oversexed or uncontrollable	Just as there are ranges of sex drive in the general community, there are among individuals with Down syndrome as well. Often a lack of information and reduced opportunities for socialization contributes to social inappropriateness.
Have increased needs for touch and affection	The range of touch needs varies much as it does in the general population. Some individuals enjoy affection; others don't due to touch sensitivities. Individuals with Down syndrome can be indiscriminately affectionate as a result of conditioning, lack of socialization training, or stereotyping.
Experience puberty later than their peers (delayed physical development)	Unique patterns of physical development may occur depending on the person's health; however, people with Down syndrome tend to begin puberty at ages very similar to those in the general population
Lack the capacity to form lasting relationships	More and more individuals with developmental disabilities are achieving this goal.
Are sterile	There is reduced fertility in both males and females with Down syndrome, but incidences of reproduction for males and females have been documented (refer to Chapter 11).
Are not capable of maintaining a marriage	Many people with intellectual disabilities marry, but there is little information on long-term outcomes of these marriages. At this time, statistics on successful marriages are expected to be similar to those of successful marriages in the general population.

significant needs for touch and affection than the rest of us ("they are so lovable and affectionate"). I believed this as a result of a volunteer experience I had during my college years in the late 1970s. A good friend recruited me to help with a regional Special Olympics track and field competition. My job was to be a "hugger," which meant I was assigned to embrace runners as they finished their races and crossed the finish line. I was uncomfortable with this directive, but did as I was asked. The experience, however, led me to an inaccurate assumption about people with Down syndrome. I left college believing that they were incapable of learning and understanding how to be appropriate and they hugged everyone. In future interactions with adults with cognitive disabilities, believing this myth prevented me from modeling and teaching more acceptable behaviors and even enrolling my daughter in Special Olympics, even though this hugging practice was eliminated long ago.

How Does Sexual Learning Happen?

INFORMAL
LEARNING

Informal sexual learning happens every day as we live and interact with the world around us. Our earliest lessons are taught without words, usually in infancy. Caring touches, snuggling, cuddling, and gentle caresses help your child know he is loved and valued and lay an important foundation for how your child learns to nurture and touch in his own life. (See Chapter 4 for guidance on helping your child learn about touch and affection.)

Young children also learn about sexuality by observing those around them. For example, children rarely need to attend classes to help them understand gender roles.

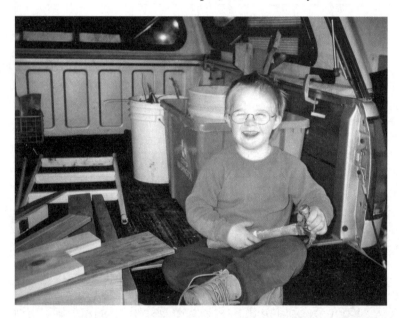

Instead, they learn through watching the men and women in their lives at home, in the workplace, or on television. If females are seen as nurturers and caregivers, a young girl is more likely to believe she will fulfill that role in her adult life. My four-year-old nephew does a comical "dad-as-a-worker" imitation. He puts on his hard hat and big boots, and makes sure he's carrying some type of "tool." He even has a "worker walk" that makes him look more manly and adult-like. A kindergarten teacher once told me how much she learns about gender roles by observing her young students imitate adults in their lives during "house" sessions in the classroom. Young children rarely participate in formal opportunities for learning about sexuality. More often, messages are communicated informally through everyday exposure to the attitudes and behavior of influential people who surround them.

As your child grows and has opportunities to interact with the world, informal sexual learning moves beyond the family to include television, movies, music, the Internet, peers, and culture. Here are some examples of informal sexual learning in typically developing children:

I was a tomboy through junior high and remember feeling like I never quite fit in. The other girls wanted nothing to do with me.

I ended up learning a lot about sexuality when I started reading romance novels. My friend had older sisters and would sneak the books to school so we could read them over the lunch hour.

I received my first kiss during a truth or dare game in my friend's basement during a coed birthday party (her parents were upstairs chaperoning). I still remember how the girl's mouth tasted of Doritos.

During middle school I recall I was silently obsessed with powerful sensations around crushes and sexual attraction. Often my week nights were spent biking to the neighborhood of a favorite boy and circling the block until we (my girlfriends and I) could sneak a bit of innocent conversation.

I learned to figure out what I valued in a partner by experiencing what I didn't like first.

FORMAL LEARNING

Formal learning involves participation in structured programs designed specifically to share information, develop skills, or explore attitudes about sexuality. Schools, institutions, parents, and community organizations typically implement these programs. You may remember the "puberty" programs introduced in elementary school as one of your first formal sexual learning experiences. The onset of puberty or another event may have been the impetus for a formal "talk" with a parent. He or she may have provided specific information about the physical changes that you could anticipate.

Many students today learn about pregnancy, contraception, sexually transmitted diseases, or sexual decision making in Family Life or health classes at school. Some places of worship have created formal programs incorporating religious teachings so families can learn about and discuss sexuality issues together. University courses at colleges or presentations sponsored by community organizations are other examples of ways formal learning about sexuality occurs.

Regardless of whether information comes from formal or informal learning, most experts agree that sexual learning is most effective when it is presented as a positive aspect of life, is understandable, and offered throughout life.

Is Sexual Learning Different for Individuals with Cognitive Disabilities?

Although individuals with cognitive disabilities also learn about sexuality in formal and informal ways, differences have been identified in the literature. I often refer to these differences as *altered scripts*, or the presence of unique circumstances that affect sexual learning. They include:

1. less information,
2. negative attitudes,

3. postponement and delays in when information is taught, and
4. fewer opportunities for socialization.

Studies continually reveal that individuals with developmental disabilities have far less information about sexuality than the general population. Numerous reasons are cited for this. Opportunities for learning, both formally and informally, are typically more limited, resulting in fewer sources for acquiring information in understandable ways. Books or resources with easy text and clear, concrete illustrations, for example, are difficult to find. There is also a tendency to "insulate" or protect individuals with cognitive disabilities from information rather than to "educate" them. When sexuality education is offered in school, many parents choose not to include their child within inclusive classes. They may believe that their child will not understand the information or feel as if it's more than he needs to know. Unfortunately, adapted programs that might be more appropriate are not always offered as an alternative. This frequently results in reduced access to understandable information about sexuality.

Even when information is presented, the cognitive disability itself can affect comprehension and retention. People with intellectual disabilities rely heavily on visual sources for learning, so the media often becomes a primary resource for learning about sexuality. If you are a parent of a child with a cognitive disability, you've probably experienced instances where your child saw improbable things on television and believed they were an accurate depiction of how the world functions. One mom I know attributed her daughter's distorted perceptions about relationship development to watching television shows and movies where people meet, date, and become sexually involved in relatively brief periods of time.

Some people with Down syndrome observe their peers and then attempt to model their behavior without understanding the finer nuances and details of social interactions. One teen with Down syndrome, an incoming freshman at his high school, insisted on touching and kissing girls in the hallway even though the affection was not reciprocated and clearly unwanted. During the teaching process he expressed his frustration with not being able to do what he saw his other peers doing. In this example, the young man was missing critical information related to the process of dating, relationship development, boundaries, and consent.

Retention of learned information is a problem as well. Studies examining retention of sexuality information over a period of time for participants with developmental disabilities have identified repetition as a key and necessary element of effectiveness. Without ongoing repetition and reinforcement, sexuality information may not be retained.

Even among typically developing children in our society there still is much angst and anxiety about sexuality. Among parents and professionals who support individuals with cognitive disabilities, this discomfort is often magnified. Although considerable progress has been made in recognizing and accepting individuals with developmental disabilities as sexual human beings, pejorative attitudes are still prevalent and problematic. When your child is exposed to these attitudes, he will be more likely than other children to learn that sexuality is a negative or unacceptable aspect of who he is. For example, participants in my classes often share experiences involving shame, punishment, or discouragement from talking, learning, or experiencing sexuality. Many of these students have only learned about sexuality within the context of a problem or crisis, making it easier for them to view sexual aspects of who they are as "bad."

Recently, I was teaching a group of adults with cognitive disabilities who were interested in dating about body rights and the importance of respecting boundaries. During a break, I spoke informally with one man about his difficulties with boundaries. He revealed that he had been in trouble a few times for touching other men (without their consent) and then rationalized his behavior by saying he was simply touching these men because he was curious and wanted to know what a penis felt like. When I suggested it would be much more acceptable for him to explore his own body in private, he seemed horrified. "Why would I want to do that? That's disgusting!"

POSTPONEMENT AND DELAYS IN TEACHING SEXUALITY INFORMATION

If and when information is shared, it is often presented much later in life. Children with disabilities are less likely to ask questions or engage their parents in conversations prompted by curiosity. This allows parents and caregivers to postpone teaching. Or parents may feel hesitant and unsure about how to explain or teach sexuality concepts in understandable ways. In many instances, parents do decide to work with their child, but quickly realize that limited resources and support in this arena prevent them from being effective in this role.

FEWER OPPORTUNITIES FOR SOCIALIZATION

Most of us learned about relationships and how to get along with others by encountering a myriad of social situations in our everyday lives. Although parents these days work pretty hard to encourage and facilitate opportunities for their child to socialize, children with cognitive disabilities still experience fewer opportunities to develop and practice social skills.

For individuals with Down syndrome, speech and intelligibility issues can make it harder to casually participate in conversations with peers. Another person (usually a parent or teacher) may be needed to interpret and help relationships along. If a child has an aide or paraprofessional at school, this can affect how peers perceive him. For example, they may see the child as younger than he is or as someone who needs a helper or "buddy" rather than a friend. This can reduce opportunities to develop social skills and form relationships with other peers.

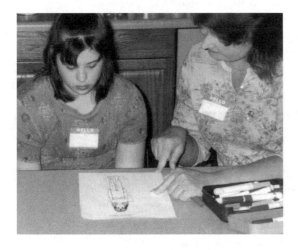

Becoming Your Child's Sexuality Educator—Your Roles

Because of the altered scripts that occur for individuals with cognitive disabilities, parents need to play a more significant role in supporting their children's healthy sexuality. As primary sexuality educator for your child, your involvement will include three key roles:

1. Recognizing sexuality as a healthy and positive aspect of being human,
2. Sharing information,
3. Communicating values.

ROLE #1: RECOGNIZING SEXUALITY AS A HEALTHY AND POSITIVE ASPECT OF BEING HUMAN

Because you're actually reading a book on the subject, you likely recognize and have accepted the fact that your son or daughter is a sexual human being with the same needs for acceptance, information, and understanding that we all have. This book was written for parents who see sexuality as a positive aspect of humanness and are interested in working to help their children become sexually healthy adults.

Parents and caregivers who view sexuality as burdensome and negative will have more difficulty engaging their child and fulfilling the other roles identified below and may need to rely more heavily on outside resources. There are numerous individuals and organizations in your community that already have experience or expertise in the area of sexuality, disability, or both. Take advantage of the knowledge and experience that's out there. If you belong to a parent support group, ask other parents if they are familiar with community resources that may be helpful. Agencies such as United Cerebral Palsy, the ARC, or your local Down syndrome agency may have resource centers, lending libraries, or teaching materials that families can use and check out. Planned Parenthood organizations with education departments may have educators or classes available to address sexuality and disability issues. If you request specific topics or workshops, often these agencies will do what they can to meet your needs.

ROLE #2: INFORMATION SHARER

One characteristic of sexually healthy adults is they have basic information about sexuality that helps them make informed and responsible decisions. Being informed means understanding basic facts about the body, your rights, and the responsibilities of being a sexual person. One of your roles as primary sexuality educator is to *share information* with your child about sexuality issues. Information that is being shared should be:

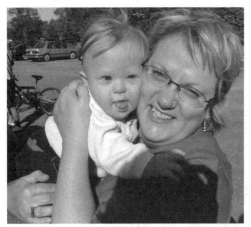

- *Accurate*—Information you are communicating should be true and accurate without distortions. Although parent preparation sections in this book should help with this, there will be times when professionals who are trained and knowledgeable about sexuality can be helpful resources. In these instances, ideas for locating such professionals are included within the chapter.
- *Understandable*— Ensuring that the information you share with your child is understandable is one of the more difficult tasks of teaching. No single teaching strategy will work for every child. Use your own familiarity with your child to identify a plan that will work. See the section below on "Making Information Understandable" for some ideas.
- *Timely and relevant*—Life is full of opportunities for learning and teaching about sexuality. A relative becomes pregnant, you notice your child's body begin to change, your son expresses an interest in dating. Teaching about sexuality will be most effective when new learning can be linked with experiences that are meaningful, relevant, and make sense for your child. In some cases this will be a developmental stage (e.g., puberty), but more often, sexual learning will be situational and associated with moments or experiences that occur throughout life.

MAKING INFORMATION UNDERSTANDABLE

Find Out What Your Child Knows Before Introducing New Information. New learning is more successful if it can be linked to what your child already knows and understands. Before moving into teaching sessions, evaluate what your son or daughter knows about the subject or concept you are interested in teaching. Ask questions like:

"What have you heard about . . .?"

"What did they tell you in school about . . .?"

"Have you heard the word _____? What do you think it means?"

Pay Attention to How Your Child Learns Best. Think of a successful learning experience your child has had. What was it about the experience that worked for your child? What teaching techniques were used? What other factors contributed to your child's success? When I ask parents to identify aspects of the learning experience that contributed to successful learning, they usually come up with similar ideas. For example, they used pictures or visuals with words or incorporated repetition over extended periods of time. Sometimes the child was very excited to learn whatever it was they were teaching and that made new learning easier. Thinking about specific characteristics that helped your child be successful can lead you to strategies that will support sexual learning.

Use Pictures or Other Multi-sensory Techniques. Learning opportunities that engage the senses are more likely to enhance your child's understanding. To make abstract sexuality concepts more concrete, use pictures, slides, demonstration, videos, and role playing. During a puberty workshop for males, one of my participants was intensely curious about semen and wet dreams following a discussion about ejaculation. He asked very detailed questions about color, smell, what semen looked and felt like, etc. I did my best to answer his questions during the workshop, but his mother was the one who really was able to take it to the next level. A few weeks following the workshop she informed me that she had noticed that her liquid stain remover was similar in consistency to semen. She decided to use the product as a concrete way to illustrate for her son the physical characteristics of semen.

Use Simple, Unsophisticated Language. During a national conference a few years back, I wanted parents to practice coming up with simple, factual, and brief explanations for common sexuality vocabulary they would likely need to teach their son or daughter. For some groups, this proved too difficult a task. Finding the right words to explain sexuality concepts is challenging and adults have a natural tendency to use difficult-to-understand words and go into way more detail than is necessary. As a parent you may already be familiar with terms your child will understand. If you're not sure, ask him if he understands the meaning of words you are using. Sometimes slang terms can be helpful as you introduce sexuality concepts. In my experience, the simplest and more basic explanations are most effective.

Check Understanding. As you introduce new vocabulary or concepts, check in often to make sure your child is understanding. Ask questions or use pictures to evaluate learning. Ideas and activities for assessing learning are provided throughout the book.

Repeat, Review, and Reinforce Information. One-shot sex talks don't work for anyone, but are clearly ineffective for people with cognitive disabilities. Parents tell me that it seems like they have had to work on sexuality issues for extensive periods of time, but often it's because there is so much discomfort with the subject. We don't like to repeat experiences that make us feel uncomfortable.

Although most parents understand the important role they play in the learning process, not all will see teaching sexuality as their responsibility. Individuals with Down syndrome and other cognitive disabilities have more difficulty gathering information about sexuality on their own, so it is critical your child have at least one person (ideally two or three) in his life that he can speak with about sexuality issues, concerns, and experiences. Ideally these are individuals your child feels comfortable approaching, are knowledgeable about sexuality issues (or at least have access to resources or can find answers if they need to), and have some understanding of how your child learns best.

ROLE #3: VALUES COMMUNICATOR

A third parental role involves communicating messages that reflect your own views and beliefs about what is okay and not okay. Sometimes these value messages are communicated with actions. For example, value messages are communicated if you give your toddler a look of disgust or a slap upon discovering him fondling his genitals. Value messages are also communicated if you continue to purchase frilly, feminine clothes for your daughter when she has a clear preference for jeans and T-shirts. Other times we communicate our values with words. For example, we identify types of behavior we deem acceptable or not acceptable for a girl or boy or share family values about when it is okay to date and what types of affection are appropriate in public. Personal values and beliefs will influence the words you use to explain sexuality concepts, how much information you share, as well as the boundaries and limits (or rules) you set with your child.

In my work as a sexuality educator, I find that parents and caregivers have not always had time to step back and reflect on their own values about sexuality issues, messages they communicate related to those values, and how those messages influence their child or the people they support. Throughout the book, I therefore include sections that encourage you to proactively explore your feelings about various sexuality topics and determine how to shape value messages that will support and encourage healthy sexuality for your child.

References

Ballan, M. Parents as Sexuality Educators for Their Children with Developmental Disabilities. *SIECUS Report* 29 (3):14-19.

Monat-Haller, R. (1992). *Understanding & Expressing Sexuality: Responsible Choices for Individuals with Developmental Disabilities.* Baltimore: Brookes Publishing.

S. Plunkett, et. al. (2002). An Evaluation of a Community-Based Sexuality Education Program for Individuals with Developmental Disabilities (on-line). *Electronic Journal of Human Sexuality.*

CHAPTER 2

Learning about the Body: Key Information and Ideas for Teaching

In early childhood, it is natural for young children to be curious about their bodies and how they work. Children with Down syndrome are often just as curious but may not have the expressive language abilities to formulate questions and get answers. For this reason, parents who have children with Down syndrome or other cognitive disabilities may need to initiate discussions at the same ages other children would typically be asking and learning about the body. Sharing accurate information early on can eliminate the guilt, shame, and negativity that is often associated with the body and genitals and can set the stage for future discussions with your child as she grows older. This chapter explores body concepts and teaching strategies that can be implemented early in your child's life and continued into adolescence.

Learning about the Body: Teaching Correct Names for Private Body Parts

Teaching accurate terminology for private body parts is important for children with Down syndrome for a number of reasons. First, teaching and talking about *all* body parts is more likely to encourage your child to accept and feel good about her body. If you avoid discussions about the genitals or use other words that are derogatory ("pee-pee," "wee-wee"), or confusing ("down there," "those parts") your child learns that the genitals are not okay to talk about, there is something different or wrong with these parts, or they are bad or shameful. One of the goals of sexuality education is to increase pride, confidence, and self-acceptance so your child can feel good about herself. Teaching accurate vocabulary early is one way to provide a foundation of healthy attitudes about sexuality and help your child know you're approachable.

Key Teaching Messages:

- All body parts have a name.
- Boys have a penis, scrotum, butt.
- Girls have a vulva, clitoris, butt.

Sexual Development and the Body—What's Normal?

Birth – 5	■ Learns to value self through nurturing touch & affection ■ Explores body parts, including genitals ■ Possesses a healthy curiosity about the body & its functions ■ Interested in anatomical differences ■ Tends to need less personal space
Childhood	■ Begins to understand modesty ■ Considerable curiosity about pregnancy and birth ■ Begins to understand responsibility for welfare of own body
Pre-adolescence	■ Physical maturation begins ■ Becomes more modest and private about the body ■ Significant anxiety about body changes associated with puberty
Adolescence	■ Physical maturation almost complete ■ Potential for concerns about body image
Adulthood	■ Physical maturation complete

Second, identifying correct names for body parts in early childhood helps you prepare your child for additional teaching as she gets older. Teaching that you will do involving toilet training, proper hygiene, body changes during puberty, reproductive health procedures, and sexual expression in relationships are just a few examples of moments down the road when an understanding of accurate terms for body parts will be helpful. Teaching correct terminology right from the start prevents your child from having to relearn new words later on.

Third, professional literature suggests that children who have accurate language for private body parts are more likely to report abuse if it occurs, and when they do report it, they are perceived to be more credible when they use accurate vocabulary to describe what happened. Most parents are keenly aware of the increased incidence of exploitation among individuals with disabilities. This fact alone should motivate you to begin to thinking about how you can teach about the body.

Parents are sometimes hesitant to teach accurate terminology. First, we rarely use words like *scrotum* and *vulva* (some people have never used these words) so they can seem particularly strange and unfamiliar. Give yourself time to get used to vocabulary that is difficult for you. Try saying the word repeatedly in front of a mirror out loud. Or, purchase books designed to help you teach your children correct terms for body parts and read them aloud to yourself ahead of time until the words become more comfortable and familiar. Some parents are worried that if they teach their child correct words for body parts they will use these words in inappropriate ways or in public places. Most parents have funny, embarrassing, yet innocent stories of their young children, making social mistakes. This happens with all children and it's realistic to expect that your child will make similar social errors. However, coupling accurate terminology with societal rules about the body and privacy usually reduces the likelihood these social mistakes will occur.

When my daughter was just learning about differences between men's and women's bodies, I experienced quite an embarrassing moment. I had taught her the word penis (although she pronounced it "peanuts") during a book-reading session about differences between girls' and boys' bodies. One of the messages in the book was that "all boys have penises, and all girls have vulvas." Shortly after we had reviewed this concept, we were visiting her grandparents. Out of the blue, she asked, "Grandpa have peanuts?" Grandpa thought she was asking for peanuts so he went in search of some. I knew what she was asking and responded to her question quietly while Grandpa was going through cupboards. It was one time I was grateful my daughter was difficult to understand!

WHEN AND HOW SHOULD I TEACH?

■ *Bathing sessions or diaper-changing times when the genitals are exposed are natural times to introduce correct terminology if your child is young or still requires assistance with self-care.* Most parents engage their children in games that teach names for body parts, but more often than not, they omit labels for genitals. While you're teaching words for eyes, nose, legs, and toes, try adding "penis" or "vulva" to the list. When genitals are free from clothing constrictions, many children will and do touch and explore their genitals. Use this opportunity to give them names for the body parts they're exploring. Statements like "that's your penis" or "here's your vulva" added to "where's your nose?" or "yes, those are your ears" are ways to include private body parts in the conversation.

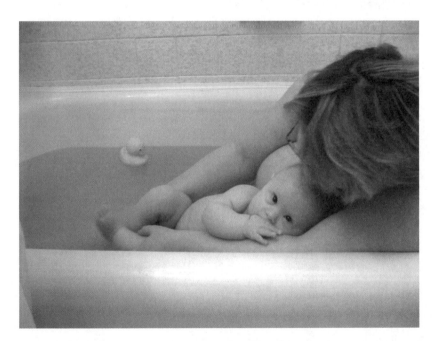

■ *Take advantage of instances when your child may be exposed to private body parts in natural settings to teach.* For example, questions or curiosity may surface during breastfeeding sessions or clothes-changing times at home or at the pool. If your child takes an interest in, or seems curious about a body part (yours or her own), you could say, "Those are breasts; when you grow up you will have them too" (if your child is female) or "That's my breast; I'm feeding your brother." If your child is beyond the age of toddlerhood, consider sharing vocabulary and then introducing boundaries that feel appropriate. For example, "My butt is private, so please don't touch me there."

■ *Exposure to anatomically correct dolls at young ages or around the time a child would normally be playing with these toys can provide a context for talking about male and female body parts and differences and help your child see that the genitals have a place and function on her body, just like her other body parts.* The *Teach-A-Bodies* company carries a line of handmade dolls and puppets that are anatomically complete. For more information, contact the company on the web at www.teach-a-bodies.com.

■ *Read books designed to teach children proper names for male and female body parts. Some good choices for younger children are:*

> **Bellybuttons Are Navels,** by Mark Schoen (Prometheus Books, 1990). A story about two young children naturally discovering their body parts while bathing together. Useful for helping children understand differences between boy and girl bodies and identifying correct names for genitals.
>
> **The Bare Naked Book,** by Kathy Stinson (Firefly Books, 1988). A good introduction to teaching all body parts, including the genitals. Realistic illustrations highlight a specific body part on each page.
>
> **What's the Big Secret: Talking about Sex with Girls and Boys,** by Marc Brown and Laurie Krasny Brown (Little Brown and Company, 2000). An easy-to-read storybook with animated drawings for young children that address how boys and girls are different (come to find out body differences are the only difference). The book discusses societal rules related to talking, looking, touching and being touched, and reproduction.
>
> **What Is a Girl? What Is a Boy?** by Stephanie Waxman (Cromwell, 1989). This book illustrates real differences between men and women; men have a penis and women have a vulva. Photos of a naked boy and girl and adult male and female are included. Great book for learning about gender stereotyping, as well (women are playing basketball, hammering, etc.).

Teaching Activity: "Names for Body Parts"

Teaching about the genitals is always easier if it is taught in the context of learning about the rest of the body. Use the diagrams in Appendix A-1 to A-4 to teach about a wide range of male and female body parts, point out physical differences, and similarities, or to assess knowledge your child may already have. To check comprehension, use the tip of a pencil, point to a body part, and see if your child can give you the name. If your child is nonverbal, name a body part and ask her to point to the appropriate location.

Parental Pause—The Power of Language

The words we use to talk about sexual body parts and functions can be very different based on our personal experiences and culture. In an old but classic book for sexuality profession-als, *Values in Sexuality: A New Approach to Sex Education,* the authors identify four categories of language used to talk about particular body parts:

Scientific/Medical Language—This category of language would be used to communicate with accuracy and precision. I often call this "doctor language," meaning these would be words typically used by a doctor or healthcare provider.

Common Discourse—For many people, scientific language is too sterile or formal and therefore makes people uncomfortable. As a result, sometimes we adapt words to make them reflect our own values, or make them more understandable and comfortable.

Childhood Language—These words are often euphemisms that carry a childish or babyish tone. We normally use these words to hide adult embarrassment or discomfort.

Slang/Street—Language in this category is often meant to be derogatory, demeaning, negative, and sometimes even violent in nature.

Consider the following examples:

Scientific	Childhood	Common discourse	Slang
breasts	boobies	boobs	tits
penis	weewee	dick	cock
scrotum	?	?	?
buttocks	?	?	?
vagina	?	?	?
sexual intercourse	?	?	?
menstruation	?	?	?
ejaculation	?	?	?
erection	?	?	?

If your child is younger and you are just beginning to introduce language for body parts, begin with scientific language and address other vocabulary as it surfaces. If your child is already comfortable using childhood terms, start there but add on. For example, when your son refers to his penis as his "pee pee," let him know that another word he can use is "penis." Then begin using the word from that point on. Your child will begin modeling your use of the words over time.

The older your child is, the more likely it is she has been or will be exposed to (most likely by peers or the media) slang or alternative terms for sexual functions or the genitals. If your child suddenly begins using a term you find unacceptable, explore with her what she knows and understands. For example, "I've never heard you use that word before, do you know what it means?" If she doesn't, define it and give her words you prefer she use. You could say something like:

"_____ is a more negative word for _____, which is a private part of the female/ male body." (Use pictures to point to the part of the body you are talking about.)

OR

"I prefer you use the word _____. It means the same thing but is more positive."

Although experts recommend teaching scientific language, educators find that children with cognitive disabilities frequently have limited knowledge or vocabulary about their bodies, and scientific words can be foreign or unfamiliar. In these situations, educators often introduce a variety of slang or childhood or common language in an effort to begin with a concept that is known and familiar. If your child is a teen or adult, exposing her to a range of vocabulary can also reduce the likelihood of ridicule, embarrassment, or humiliation by more knowledgeable peers.

UNDERSTANDING BODY DIFFERENCES

Becoming aware of the physical differences between male and female bodies is another normal and healthy part of your child's sexual development. A friend of mine told me that when her typically developing son was about ten he asked if she could take her clothes off so he could see her body (she was the only female in the house). Although this disturbed her a bit, I reassured her that his curiosity was normal, that it was completely appropriate for her to say no, and that the request was likely his way of helping her know he had some curiosity about the female body. We discussed appropriate resources she could use to share information.

Your child with Down syndrome may not have the verbal skills to ask questions at young ages but nevertheless will notice body differences. As a young child, my daughter attended an integrated preschool where the bathrooms were used by both girls and boys. Coed toileting helped her become aware of differences in urination styles because at one point I found her in our bathroom at home attempting to urinate standing up. Fortunately, I got to her before she completed her experiment. Needless to say, it was a teachable moment and an opportunity to share information about being a girl and the differences between how boy and girl bodies look and function. Another mother I know had concerns about her six-year-old son who repeatedly stared at her chest and would sometimes touch her breast unexpectedly and at inopportune moments. This may have been his way of expressing curiosity about a body part he realized he did not have. I advised the mom to identify the body part for him, discuss rules related to private parts, and acquire a book that would help him understand how male and female bodies are different.

If you have opposite sex siblings in your household, opportunities for discussing body differences will surface in natural ways. Bathing sessions and swimsuit or diaper changing times when genitals are exposed are moments when children typically notice body differences. Responding to questions or touching can provide teachable moments for addressing these differences. For example, "Yes, you're right. Ethan's body is different than yours. He has a penis because he is a boy. You are a girl, so you have a vulva."

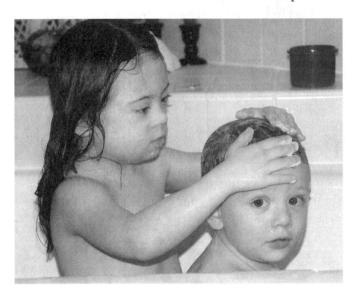

In early childhood, games like "playing doctor" or "you-show-me-I'll-show-you" are common venues for exploring ways the male and female bodies are different. For children with developmental disabilities or speech delays, this same curiosity can lead to similar behaviors at the same age or even a bit later. If you come across your child participating in body exploration with another child or sibling, try not to panic or show alarm (this is hard, I know). Instead, acknowledge what they are doing ("I see you are playing a game"). Then ask them to put their clothes on and invite them to explore body differences through other means such as books or pictures. If they have verbal abilities, encourage question asking. Try to see the behavior from their perspective—a natural and healthy curiosity about the body.

Be conscious of the messages you communicate. Becoming angry, hysterical, or upset will end up making the children feel guilty and ashamed. If you feel as if the behavior violates your value system, acknowledge their curiosity but advise them to come to you with questions or state your values about the behavior. For example, "In our house, bodies are private so we keep our clothes on."

If the child is not your own, speak with the other child's family about the incident and how you handled it. Letting them know how you handled the situation gives them an opportunity to share their own messages with their child. Identify or review clear rules for future playtime experiences such as keeping clothes on, reducing alone time, or keeping doors open. These experiences are usually far more difficult for the adults than they are for the children. For most children, clear information will prevent future occurrences and they will easily move on to other things.

Teaching Activity: "Same and Different"

Show your child the unlabeled boy and girl pictures at the back of the book (Appendix A-1 and A-2). Invite her to point to or tell you what body parts are the same for girls and boys and which ones are different. If she does not know the names for body parts that are different, introduce her to the vocabulary.

HEALTHY SEX PLAY OR EXPLOITATION

When one of the children involved in body exploration has Down syndrome or another developmental disability, there is understandably a heightened concern about the possibility of exploitation. There are differences that help distinguish between healthy child play and exploitation. The behavior is likely age appropriate if:

- The activity is mutually enjoyable and shared between two children who have an ongoing play or school relationship.

- The children are of similar age (within 2 to 3 years), size, and developmental status.
- Body exploration is mutually voluntary and balanced with their curiosity about other things in the world around them.

Sex play that involves threats, violence, painful touching, or oral-genital, anal, or vaginal intercourse are *not* typical behaviors. If either of the children seem fearful, withdrawn, angry, or aggressive, there is reason to be concerned. Speak with the other parent about your concerns.

Functions of Private Body Parts

The idea that all body parts, including the genitals, have a function and purpose is another aspect of teaching about the body. When your child is younger, the three key functions that commonly surface include:

1. elimination,
2. reproduction, and
3. pleasure.

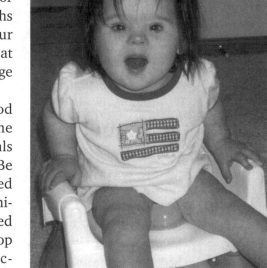

TEACHING ABOUT ELIMINATION

Elimination is often the only purpose people with cognitive disabilities associate with the genitals. This is logical since toilet training occurs quite early in life and for many can extend over a period of months and years. While you are teaching your child how to manage toileting, it is a great opportunity to begin introducing language for the genitals.

Toilet training books offer a good way to help your child understand the natural connection between the genitals and the role they play in elimination. Be aware that the majority of books designed for this purpose do not use accurate terminology for the genitals or include detailed pictures that could help your child develop a more accurate understanding of reproductive anatomy. While teaching your child about the process of toilet training, use the illustrations in Appendix A-7 or A-8 to augment teaching. Other considerations for teaching and supporting healthy sexuality:

 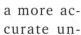

Key Teaching Messages:

- All body parts have a job to do.
- Private body parts have jobs too.

- *Decide on vocabulary for elimination functions*—Take some time to choose vocabulary you will use to describe elimination functions. Although the same categories of language (medical, common discourse, childhood, and slang) exist for elimination functions, the range of words is generally more limited. Select words or signs that:

- are likely to be used and understood consistently by other adults supporting your child,
- improve your child's ability to speak or sign the words clearly (will others be able to understand words your child is using?),
- promote community acceptance. For example, words like "poop" or "pee" are usually a good starting point since they are easy to say and understood in most circumstances. Guidelines discussed earlier in this chapter regarding how to handle situations when your child is using offensive vocabulary to describe elimination functions apply here as well. For example, you can explain words like "piss" or "shit" if your child uses them, then identify preferred vocabulary for her.

- *Introduce accurate terminology for genitals*—Use accurate vocabulary for body parts as you teach toileting hygiene. For example, "After you're done, wipe your vulva like this," or, "When you're done touching your penis, wash your hands" are ways accurate vocabulary can be infused into teaching.

- *Reiterate exploitation prevention messages*—Since toileting involves the private body parts, use it as an opportunity to introduce or review rules about the body. Remind your child, for example, that her body is her own and the only two reasons anyone should ever be touching her private parts is to help with cleaning the body (hygiene) if she needs help or at the doctor's office (health). Encourage her to tell you if anyone is touching or asking her to touch inappropriately for any other reasons.

- *Incorporate privacy principles into toileting routines*—Although it's normal for young children (under age five) to have an undeveloped sense of modesty, that doesn't mean you can't begin to introduce privacy concepts. Examples of ways to introduce concepts include:
  - Having your child close the door after entering the bathroom. Remind her that closing the door makes the room more private.
  - Teach your child to ask for help when she needs it and ask others to back off when help is not needed.
  - Define "going to the bathroom" as private behavior and review what that means. (See Chapter 3 for more information about teaching privacy concepts.)

TEACHING
ABOUT
REPRODUCTION

For some families, discussing reproduction as a function of the private body parts surfaces while their children are quite young. Often teaching is done in relationship to a pregnancy or birth in the family. Even if that has not happened in your family, remember, curiosity about the body and body functions is characteristic of young children, so questions like "Where did I come from?" or "Where do babies come from" are quite common at this age.

Keep in mind that all young children have difficulty understanding ideas that have not been a part of their direct life experience. If your child has not known a family who is expecting, has never had an opportunity to hold a new baby, or has difficulty with expressive language, it's very likely she may not ask these questions and you may have to look for opportunities to share information with her. Look for teachable moments when bringing up the subject seems natural and appropriate—for example, after watching a movie or TV show in which a woman is pregnant or giving birth. The following sections discuss pointers to remember when teaching about reproduction.

FIND OUT WHAT YOUR CHILD ALREADY KNOWS

Even if you have not talked with your child directly about reproduction, she's likely been exposed to notions or ideas (from kids at school or the media) about how pregnancy happens. As bits and pieces of information are presented, children often create stories in their heads that help them make sense of things that may be too hard to conceptualize. For example, during a conversation about her aunt's pregnancy, I asked my youngest daughter, then five or six, how she thought a woman became pregnant. Her thinking was that the person in charge of marrying the man and the woman (minister, preacher, priest) did *something* (she wasn't sure what) to the couple during the wedding that would allow them to have a baby. She obviously had associated the idea of reproduction with marriage, maybe because everyone she knew who had children was also married. Still, she was not sure about the details.

Asking questions can help you assess your child's knowledge and determine where to begin. You can ask, "Where do you think babies come from?" or "What have you heard about how babies are made? or "Do you remember when Mrs. Johnson was having a baby? How do you think that happened?"

If your child is nonverbal but you notice an interest or suspect she is curious about a pregnancy (e.g., she is interested in touching a woman's belly, feeling the baby kicking, etc.), show her pictures from Appendix A-18 so she can at least see an x-ray view of where the baby is located inside the woman.

BE FACTUAL, BRIEF, DIRECT

When considering how you will explain reproduction, it's important to think about your child's level of need. Most children are not looking for long, involved responses. They simply want their questions answered in ways they will be able to understand. If the response you gave them is not enough, they will continue to ask questions. If it is more information than they need, they'll likely take what they can use and mentally discard the rest. Some examples of ways to explain reproduction are provided below. Refer to Appendix A-17 and A-18 for drawings and pictures that can be used to help your child visualize concepts.

Chapter 5 goes into detail about how to teach a child who is entering or in puberty.

Common Questions & Simple Explanations about Reproduction

If your child seems curious about...	You could say:
A pregnant woman's appearance	■ That woman is going to have a baby. That's called being "pregnant." ■ She has a baby growing in her uterus. ■ She's not fat; she's pregnant. That means she has a baby growing inside her uterus. (Appendix A-18)
Where babies come from	■ Babies come from a place inside the woman called a uterus
How the baby gets in the uterus	■ Both a man and woman are needed to make a baby. ■ The man's part of starting a baby is the sperm. ■ The woman's part is the egg. ■ When the man's sperm and the woman's egg join together, a baby begins growing in the uterus.
How the sperm and egg get together	■ When two people love each enough to have children, they show each other in a very special way. When they are together in private, they hug, kiss, and touch each other in ways that feel nice. When they are both ready, the woman helps the man slip his penis inside her vagina. When the penis is inside the woman, the sperm and egg can join together to start a baby. (Appendix A-17)
How the baby gets out	■ When the baby is big enough, it will leave the uterus slowly and move into the vagina. ■ The vagina can stretch (like a balloon) so the baby can pass through. ■ The baby is born when it comes out of the opening between a woman's legs called the vagina. (Appendix A-18)

USE REAL PICTURES AND DIAGRAMS TO EXPLAIN CONCEPTS

To make conversations about reproduction more concrete, use diagrams of the adult male and female body (see Appendix A-11 and A-15) to help your child understand where the sperm and egg come from. When the word "egg" is used, many concrete learners tend to visualize the only type of egg they are familiar with: the hard-shelled kind that come from the grocery store. You could point out that the eggs in the ovary of the woman are different from the ones they have seen and that these eggs don't have shells and are very, very small.

Pamela Wilson, a well-known sexuality educator, suggests making a small dot with a pencil to help your child understand the smallness of the egg. Drawing a tadpole-shaped sperm may be helpful as well. Let your child know that in order to see a real egg and sperm, she would need to use a microscope because they are so small. On the diagrams, you could trace the path of the sperm as it makes its way into the woman's body.

USE TEACHABLE MOMENTS

The subject of reproduction can be brought up more naturally if it's linked to an experience or situation your child is involved in or familiar with. For example, if your child is aware that a friend, teacher, or family member is pregnant, talk about it. Use one of the diagrams in the back of the book to point out where the fetus grows inside the uterus. Discuss the timeframe of a pregnancy and what happens when the baby is ready to come out.

Sexuality programs at school commonly introduce information about reproduction at some point, usually in middle school. (See Chapter 13 for more about sex education programs at school.) Occasionally, the Discovery channel or other science-type TV shows will have programs on human reproduction. If you find one that will work for your child, tape it so you can both watch it together. Taping the show allows you to stop and start the tape when your child has a question or wants to see something again.

> *Toward the end of fifth grade, my daughter with Down syndrome took a one-week class at school called Family Life. It was a general education class that covered the biology of reproduction (the sperm fertilizes the egg and an embryo is formed) but not the mechanics (how the sperm and the egg happen to get together). During this week I kept asking my daughter what she'd discussed in class and whether she had any questions she wanted to ask me. Her main question was HOW does the boy's sperm get to the girl's egg? Swallowing hard, I told her something to the effect that if the girl really loves the boy, she might let him put his penis in her vagina and squirt some sperm in there and then the sperm can swim up to her eggs and maybe make a baby. Her only response was "Oh."*
>
> *Over the next couple of weeks and months, she would periodically say somewhat anxiously. "I don't want to have a baby" or ask, "Do I HAVE to have a baby?" And I would always assure her that it was her decision—if she didn't want a baby, she didn't have to have a baby. I finally found out what was behind her questions when she asked me how she could keep from having a baby if she had eggs inside of her that had babies in them. Although I thought she'd understood my explanation about fertilization, she clearly thought her eggs could spontaneously "hatch" and become babies against her wishes. So I explained again how you can't make a baby without sperm and where THOSE come from. She seemed embarrassed by my explanation this time, so I'm hoping she "gets it" now.*

READ BOOKS TOGETHER

Although there are a variety of books designed to help young children understand reproduction, often they start with discussions about plant or animal reproduction before moving on to human reproduction. For children with developmental disabilities, this can be confusing. Since they have more difficulty generalizing concepts, selecting books that focus on human reproduction are more appropriate. Here are some of my favorites:

Did the Sun Shine Before You Were Born? by Sol and Judith Gordon (Prometheus Books, 1992). A classic that explains the facts about sex, reproduction, and the birth process in clear and concise language within the context of families.

How You Were Born, by Joanne Cole (HarperCollins, 1994). This book includes color photographs that describe how a baby grows and develops in the mother and how it is born.

TEACHING ABOUT PLEASURE

Another function of the genitals not commonly discussed is that the genitals exist to provide pleasure. Babies, for example, explore their genitals almost from birth and continue to engage in genital touching into toddlerhood and beyond. At young ages, genital touching is often not goal oriented, but simply a natural and pleasurable discovery during body exploration. Many parents observe their children engaging in genital touching during bathing or diaper sessions when genitals are exposed. Genital touching can also be calming and relaxing for a child, especially during stressful or emotional times. More information about masturbation is covered in Chapter 6.

Parental Pause—Masturbation

The term masturbation refers to self-stimulation of the genitals or other sensitive areas of the body for pleasure. Your personal experiences with masturbation will directly affect your feelings about genital touching and how you handle situations involving your child. For example, if you were made to feel guilty or ashamed, you may experience anxiety when you observe your own child engaged in self-pleasuring behaviors. If genital touching and masturbation were considered a normal and healthy part of growing up, you're likely to feel it is a natural, healthy, and acceptable part of your child's life as well. Ask yourself:

- What messages (direct or indirect) were communicated about genital touching and masturbation in my childhood?
- How do I feel about my own children experiencing pleasure from genital touching and masturbation?

Body Responsibilities

Generally, infants, toddlers, and many school-aged children rely on adults to help them care for their bodies. As parents, we try to prepare healthy and nutritious meals and snacks, keep track of doctor's appointments, and supervise bath and hygiene routines. At some point, however, you will need to begin thinking about how and

Key Teaching Messages:

- Caring for my body is important.
- Younger children often need help cleaning and caring for their bodies.
- As I get older, I can help take care of my own body.

when you will prepare your child to care for her own body. Children with developmental disabilities take longer and require more direct instruction on how to care for themselves. Beginning early can buy you some time to help your child learn skills that other children learn more quickly. Here are some ideas for teaching self-care skills in early childhood:

TAKE BABY STEPS

Breaking larger tasks into smaller pieces can help your child see progress is being made. Below are a variety of teaching methods commonly used to help your child work towards independence with self-care. (If your child is in or approaching puberty, see Chapter 5 for additional suggestions.)

If your child has fine motor skill delays (and most children with Down syndrome do), consult with your occupational therapist as difficulties related to self-care emerge. Try to be specific about the skills in the task that are difficult for your child to do on her own or that you find yourself consistently doing for your child. Occupational therapists may be able to share good ideas for modifications or adaptations that have worked well for other children.

If your child has sensory issues or is tactually defensive (overly sensitive to touch sensations) *desensitization* techniques will be important as you teach self-care skills that are necessary to stay healthy. This process involves working slowly to help your child tolerate

Common Methods for Teaching Self-Care Skills

Method	How It works
Task Analysis	The skill you are trying to teach is broken down into smaller steps that make sense for your child. The smaller steps are taught one by one until the larger skill is learned.
Chaining	Smaller steps are learned and linked together until larger, more complex skill is learned.
Forward Chaining	Steps in the sequence are taught from beginning to end. For example, step 1 is taught first. After the person can perform step 1, the second step in the sequence is taught. Teaching continues until each step has been mastered and the individual can perform all of the steps
Backward Chaining	In this method, steps of the task are taught backwards beginning with the last step first, then gradually moving forward as each step is learned. For example, if you were trying to teach your child how to take a shower or bath, helping her learn how to "towel dry" the body might be the first skill taught. Once this step is mastered, helping her learn how to turn off the water or drain the tub might be next.
Visual Aids	Use of pictures or visual stimuli to cue memory of order of the tasks that need to be performed. Or picture schedules that aid memory in lists of tasks for hygiene routines.

the presence of sensations that create fear, anxiety, or discomfort. If you need help with this, speak with your child's occupational therapist or a sensory integration specialist.

TRY TO MAKE TEACHING AND LEARNING FUN

Self-care tasks can be mundane. Being creative can help make them more fun and interesting and help motivate your child to be independent. Use music to communicate messages about self-care and hygiene by using familiar kids' songs that address hygiene issues or make them up to help trigger steps in self-care.

When our daughter was younger, we had difficulty getting her to brush her teeth for any length of time. She loved Raffi at the time so we brought her tape player in the bathroom and played "Brush Your Teeth." It became her own little timer for how long she should brush. When the song was over, she was done.

Example: Troubleshooting Tooth Brushing Difficulties

Problem or Barrier to Independence	Examples of Things to Try
Weak grip/difficulty holding toothbrush handle	■ Add rubber (from a bicycle handlebar or garden hose) or rubber foam to toothbrush handle or use wider-handled toothbrushes to make gripping easier
Difficulty getting toothpaste on toothbrush	■ Try pump toothpaste dispensers
Difficulty getting appropriate amount of toothpaste on brush	■ Use visual cues for appropriate amount (e.g., pictures, demonstrations) ■ Repetitive practice
Poor tooth brushing technique	■ Use toothbrushes with smaller heads, angled cuts, or angled handles (create your own angled handles by soaking plastic handle in hot water for a few minutes then bending the handle back about thirty degrees) so access to full mouth is achievable ■ Try battery-operated toothbrush ■ Demonstrate task analysis for tooth brushing process (e.g., front, side, back) at home or by dental hygienist ■ Consider visual aid illustrating proper technique
Too little or too much time brushing	■ Use a timer ■ Buy toothbrush that plays music for an appropriate length of time to brush
Exhibits tactile defensiveness	■ Apply desensitization strategies which require working to decrease resistance to various aspects of the skill over time (desensitization to pressure in mouth, desensitization to toothbrush, desensitization to toothbrush without toothpaste in mouth, etc.)

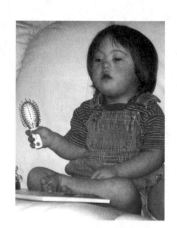

PRAISE YOUR CHILD FOR ANY AND ALL ATTEMPTS AT SELF-CARE

When your child acquires skills that allow her to gain any amount of control over her body, praise her and reinforce the importance of taking responsibility for her body. Try comments like: "You got all the dirt off your feet—wonderful!" or "You brushed your top teeth well; now try doing the same with the bottom" or "Wow, your hair looks so shiny and nice—did you brush it yourself?" Try to focus on her accomplishments rather than criticize her for getting too much water on the bathroom floor or squirting too much toothpaste on the toothbrush (see Chapter 8 for more information on caring for the body).

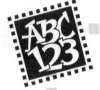

Teaching Activity: "The Amazing Body"

One of my kids' favorite past times in elementary school was to do body tracings on flip chart or easel paper (available at office supply stores). This ended up being a great way to learn about and review vocabulary and functions of all body parts, including the genitals.

If your child is small enough to fit on one sheet of paper, this activity is probably age-appropriate. While your child is lying on the paper, trace around the outside of her body with a crayon or non-permanent marker. When you get to the inside of the legs, stop at the knees (to avoid contact with private body parts), ask your child to get off the paper, and then continue filling in the lines for the genital area. By the time you're done, you should have a full body outline on one sheet of paper. If you want to do front and back, do two tracings and label them FRONT and BACK.

If your child is older, use the diagrams at the back of the book. These diagrams or tracings can be used a variety of ways:

- As a review activity, ask your child to draw in as many body parts on the tracings as she can, both public and private, front and back, male and female (one diagram for each gender). Write in labels for all the parts she can identify. If your child has difficulty with fine motor skills, use the fully illustrated body diagrams in the back of the book and create sticker labels with names of body parts on them. Have your child place the labels next to the appropriate body parts.
- To review functions, after she has identified the appropriate location, ask if she remembers what the body part is for or how it helps us.
- To review social rules, ask if she thinks it's a body part she could show in public (public body part) or would need to keep covered (private body part).
- To review exploitation prevention concepts, ask what she thinks she should do if someone is touching her private parts when she doesn't want them to. (See Chapter 12 for more discussion of exploitation prevention.)

ASSESS SELF-CARE SKILLS REGULARLY

Although it's often faster and easier to do things for your child, it will be important to regularly observe and evaluate her progress. For example, if you notice your child initiating a part of a task, step back and allow her to do it on her own. Or, give her responsibilities for small things so you can evaluate her capacities and identify obstacles to learning. Ask her routinely to try new self-help skills. For example, "Can you get the soap and put some on your body?" or "Do you remember how to do that?" "What do we do next?," etc.

COORDINATE YOUR TEACHING WITH SCHOOL LESSONS

Take advantage of health and "caring for the body" information integrated into the school curriculum to help teach new skills or reinforce skill development at home. Schools understand that children can be influenced early on to take some responsibility for health and hygiene. Having a dental hygienist teach proper teeth brushing techniques or learning how to wash hands correctly are examples of topics frequently introduced in preschool or elementary school. Simultaneously reinforcing the learning going on at school with teaching strategies at home can enhance teaching effectiveness.

References

Baker, B., et al. (2004). *Steps to Independence: Teaching Everyday Skills to Children with Special Needs.* Baltimore: Brookes Publishing.

Brick, P., et al. (1989). *Bodies, Birth and Babies.* Hackensack, NJ: Center for Family Life Education, Planned Parenthood of Bergen County, Inc.

Brick, P., et al. (1993). *Healthy Foundations: The Teacher's Book Responding to Young Children's Questions and Behaviors Regarding Sexuality.* Hackensack, NJ: The Center for Family Life Education, Planned Parenthood of Greater Northern New Jersey.

Cavanagh-Johnson, T. (2000). Sexualized Children and Children Who Molest. *SIECUS 29:* 35-39.

Engel, B. (1997). *Beyond the Birds and the Bees: Fostering Your Child's Healthy Sexual Development in Today's World.* New York, NY: Pocket Books.

Freitas, C. (1998). *Keys to Your Child's Healthy Sexuality.* Hauppauge, New York: Barron's.

Freeman, L. (1982). *It's My Body: A Book to Teach Young Children How to Resist Uncomfortable Touch.* Seattle, WA: Parenting Press.

Gossart, M. (1999). *There's No Place Like Home for Sex Education.* Eugene, OR: Planned Parenthood of Southwestern Oregon.

Haffner, D. (2000). *From Diapers to Dating: A Parent's Guide to Raising Sexually Healthy Children.* New York, NY: New Market Press.

Morrison, E. and Underhill Price, M. (1974). *Values in Sexuality: A New Approach to Sex Education.* New York, NY: Hart Publishing.

Right from the Start: Guidelines for Sexuality Issues: Birth to Five Years. (1995). New York, NY: Early Childhood Sexuality Education Task Force, SIECUS.

Sprung, B. (1999). *Our Whole Lives: Sexuality Education for Grades K-1.* Boston: Unitarian Universalist Association.

Wilson, P. (1991). *When Sex Is the Subject: Attitudes and Answers for Young Children.* Santa Cruz, CA: Network Publications.

Teaching about Privacy

Parent Preparation

In the Disney movie *Freaky Friday*, Jamie Lee Curtis plays a mom/ psychologist who believes that privacy is a privilege rather than a right. Her daughter is expected to *earn* her right to privacy. At one point in the movie, she removes her daughter's door as a form of punishment. This works fine until she *becomes* her daughter and experiences what it's like to live without a door. For many people with Down syndrome and other developmental disabilities, life is a little like that. We figuratively remove their door.

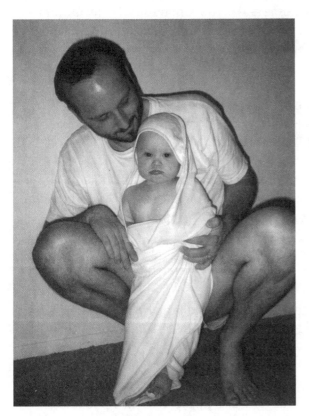

No doubt these door removals are often legitimate and necessary. First, children with developmental disabilities need more time to master toileting, bathing, and dressing skills, requiring you to be in their private spaces for longer periods of time. Sometimes, though, even after these skills are learned, close monitoring continues, more out of habit than need. During a discussion about privacy rules at home, one mother whose preteen had Down syndrome mentioned that she liked to check on her son every five minutes when he was using the bathroom. When I asked her why she did this, she shared that he spent way too much time brushing his teeth! Other parents in the room saw this as an enviable problem and quickly helped her see that her checking routine had become unnecessary.

Second, children with developmental disabilities take longer to develop and learn socialization skills, which means we watch, supervise, and intervene a bit longer. When we can't be there, we have others watch, supervise, and monitor our children, and usually they're watched and supervised more closely at schools than their peers. The increased supervision and ongoing surveillance that is often a part of life for your child creates an altered script that makes learning and understanding privacy

Sexual Development and Privacy—What's Normal?

Early childhood (under 5)	■ Undeveloped sense of modesty
Childhood	■ Emerging sense of modesty about the body and sexual topics ■ Prefer more private discussions about sexuality
Adolescence	■ Increasingly value their right to privacy ■ Increased time spent in private places is common ■ Increased interest in discussing sexual matters with peer vs. parents
Adulthood	■ Privacy is valued aspect of life

concepts more difficult. Many children with Down syndrome or other developmental disabilities become desensitized to the concept of "privacy" and its meaning, and this confusion often leads to difficulties discriminating between public and private.

Almost every topic under the umbrella of sexuality involves an understanding of public vs. private concepts. If your child learns that certain parts of the body are private, he can begin to think about where he needs to be when he is dressing or attending to hygiene issues. When he knows there are designated public and private places in your home, it improves his ability to learn your rules about where certain behaviors can occur. When he understands that there are public and private activities, your child can learn to act more appropriately at home and in the community. If specific topics of conversation are identified as private, your child learns to be discrete about who they talk to about what. In other words, your child needs to learn how privacy concepts apply to at least four areas of life:

1. his body,
2. places at home and in the community,
3. topics of conversation,
4. behaviors (discussed in Chapters 6 and 10)

Much (not all) of the time, this lack of understanding can contribute to inappropriate sexual behaviors. Teaching privacy concepts can help your child understand societal rules, enhancing social appropriateness and acceptance.

Teaching Privacy

There are really only two ways for teaching your child privacy concepts:
1. modeling for your child behaviors that exhibit a respect for privacy, and
2. sharing information.

Both of these strategies are incorporated into recommendations for teaching below. Visual tools that may be helpful for teaching are also included in the Appendices.

Public and Private Body Parts

Key Teaching Messages:

- A boy's private body parts are the penis, scrotum, and butt.
- A girl's private body parts are the breasts, vulva, and butt.

Teaching Activity: "Private Body Parts"

Using the full body pictures in Appendices A-1 to A-4 (the younger picture if your child is younger, the older one if your child is in puberty or beyond), review names for various parts of the body. For example, using the tip of a pencil, point to the different body parts and see if your child can name them. Then explain that parts of the body that are covered by underclothing (bras, underwear, etc.) are considered to be "private body parts." These body parts are "covered up" when we are around other people in public places.

TEACHING MODESTY

Although an undeveloped sense of modesty is common in young children, at some point in elementary school (usually before age nine or ten) most children develop a sense of modesty about their bodies. Often, but not always, this correlates with the beginning of physical development.

The development of modesty in children with cognitive disabilities can be delayed. Although very little research exists on this topic, there are theories for why this happens. Some speculate that individuals who are dependent upon others for intimate care for longer periods of time become desensitized to people seeing their bodies and being in their private spaces (Hingsburger). In other words, they become used to having little or no control over who sees their body. This results in a reduced sense of modesty for themselves and others.

Key Teaching Messages:

- Private body parts stay covered in public places.

I often ask parents to visualize their child at a sleepover, camp, or with peers at older ages. What would modesty look like? How would you know if your child had developed the ability to be modest? Most of the time parents tell me they want their children to use robes or towels to cover their bodies, or they want them to be able to discriminate when rooms are public or private, or notice when other people are present so embarrassing situations can be avoided. Problems with leaving bathroom or bedroom doors open is also a common concern.

I'll be the first to admit my lack of ambition (or perhaps weariness) with teaching this concept until the day my younger daughter had a friend stay overnight. Our

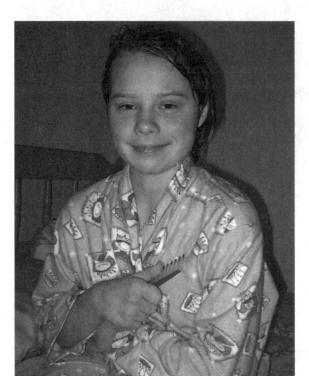

daughter with Down syndrome had taken a shower and was walking from the bathroom to her bedroom (a very short distance, I might add) at *exactly* the same moment my other daughter's friend entered the hallway. Although I didn't notice any obvious embarrassment from my daughter, I could tell the friend was uncomfortable. After this incident, I vowed to be more persistent about robes, closed doors, and rule reviews before we had company.

You can begin teaching the concept of modesty by modeling for your child what it looks like. Use towels or robes (warm ones right out of the dryer are best) to wrap and snuggle them as they walk to a private place to dress or change. En route, verbally identify rooms that are private and appropriate locations for getting dressed. Phrases such as "Let's find a private place to dress" or "Let's dress in your room where it is private" can help your child understand that the body is private and encourage modesty.

Explain to your child reasons why people use robes (to cover their bodies; bodies are private), why you use one ("my body is private too"), and encourage family members to model their use (consistency is important here). Modeling and reinforcing modesty can help your child learn that his body is private and needs to be covered in public areas.

Teaching Activity: "Societal Rules for Private Body Parts"

Once your child understands which parts of the body are private, this activity can help him understand societal rules that apply to the private parts. Explain to your child that *when he is in places where others are around (either at home or in the community),* there are rules. These rules involve two domains:

1. YOUR CHILD'S RESPECT AND MODESTY OF HIS OWN BODY in public places, which means:
   - Private body parts need to be covered
   - No touching private body parts in front of other people
   - Avoid discussions about private parts and functions in public places

2. BEING RESPECTFUL OF OTHER PEOPLE'S BODIES in public. This means:
   - No touching other people's private body parts ("hands to yourself")
   - Avoid staring at another person's private body parts
   - Do not talk about another person's private body parts (e.g., "nice breasts")

Teaching Activity: "Covering Up"

Using diagrams of the naked male and female bodies (again, use the younger pictures if your child is pre-puberty; the mature pictures if your child is close to or beyond puberty). Create bathing suits or underclothing from colored paper that fit the shape of the bodies (they don't have to be perfect or fancy). If your child has good fine motor skills have him do the cutting. Once cut, ask him to use the cut-out clothing to "cover up" parts of the body that need to be covered in public places, rooms of your house, etc.

Review names for the genitals and other private body parts as your child is covering those body parts as a part of the activity. ("Do you remember the name for this body part?…That's right, the penis and scrotum need to be covered if you are in public. Let's cover them up with the clothes.") Then review with him other societal rules for his own body and ways he can be respectful of others (listed above) when in public places.

"DRESSED OR UNDRESSED"

Young children may need to understand basic terminology before this concept can be understood. Decide whether to teach your child the word or sign for naked, nude, undressed, unclothed—whatever word feels most comfortable.

Some children have difficulty applying body rules because they aren't able to discrimi-

Parental Pause—Modesty

1. How do I define "being modest"?
2. What behaviors would reflect that definition?
3. How is modesty modeled in our home?
4. Do these behaviors help or hinder your ability to teach your son or daughter modesty?

nate between when they have clothes on and when they don't, or they are confused with terminology we use as adults. Most children will pick this up naturally with time, but it's worthwhile to make sure your child understands the difference between having clothes on and off. Use teachable moments to introduce words like undressed, naked, nude, or other terms that feel most comfortable for you. Play time with dolls or other toys that come with wardrobes or that can be dressed and undressed is a good

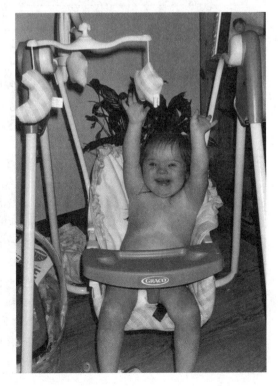

opportunity to assess learning. For example, ask your child to show you (point to) the doll that is naked or undressed.

Once your child can understand these concepts, begin introducing societal rules related to being dressed and undressed. For example, "Look, Molly can't go to school without clothes. Let's dress her." Or use real-life situations to teach vocabulary and modesty rules. For example, "Let's make sure your body is covered before you leave the bathroom."

Troubleshooting—Disrobing in Public

Possible Reasons	Possible Strategies
Physical discomfort	■ Move to private location. ■ Determine physical cause for behavior (allergic reactions to detergents, irritating clothing, rashes, or other health or medical condition). ■ Check with physician for thyroid or other conditions that cause heat sensitivity.
Difficulty differentiating between public and private	■ Teach "private" signs. ■ Use visual strategies to identify private locations okay for disrobing. ■ Communicate education plan and strategy for handling disrobing with people providing care and support. ■ Repeat and reinforce.
Self-stimulation	■ Reeducate (removing clothes is private). ■ Identify private locations. ■ Redirect. ■ Dress child in clothing that's difficult to remove. ■ Analyze environmental triggers. ■ Refer to Chapter 6 (masturbation) for other ideas.
Angry or upset	■ Move to private location. ■ Reeducate (removing clothes is private). ■ Teach about feelings and socially appropriate ways to handle them. ■ Create visual "coping list" to help child identify healthy and safe ways to cope.
Reasons are unclear	■ Request a functional behavior analysis to evaluate disrobing incidents more thoroughly. Consult a behavior specialist or see a book such as Functional Behavior Assessment by Beth Glasberg (Woodbine House, 2006).

Public and Private Places

TEACHING MODESTY

Once your child is able to distinguish between public and private body parts, you can begin helping him apply this concept to other aspects of his life. Explaining that there are public and private places is one example of this.

I think it's important to point out that although everyone has a right to privacy, there are responsibilities that go along with these rights. If there are safety concerns with your child (for example, there is a risk he may injure himself or others), rights to privacy are obviously going to be more limited and restrictive. Likewise, if you are still working on helping your child master independence with morning routines, and he needs significant monitoring and supervision, opportunities for privacy will be more limited. You will need to decide when your child will be ready for the teaching activities I suggest below. Timing can vary greatly for every child and family, but typically at some point during adolescence you can begin to help your son or daughter understand his or her privacy rights and responsibilities.

Key Teaching Messages:

- Private places are spaces I can go to be alone.
- At home my private place(s) is _____.

Some indicators that your child could benefit from more direct instruction about public and private concepts:

- Your child is beginning to develop physically (puberty onset).
- Peers, siblings, or other family members are embarrassed or uncomfortable by your child's lack of modesty.
- Your child is performing private behaviors in public places (at home or in the community).
- Inappropriate behaviors (masturbation, hugging) are interfering with your child's ability to connect and form relationships with others.

When the time is right, you could introduce this concept of privacy by saying, "Now that your body is starting to change" or "You're entering middle school," or "You're 14 now," (or any other statement that represents a transition that has meaning for your child), "you may find that you want to be by yourself and not be bothered."

Next, identify rooms in your home that are private. Most families choose either the child's bedroom (if it is not shared) and/or the bathroom. Explain that these are places he should go if he wants to be alone or do private things (change clothes, masturbate, etc.). Share information with all family members regarding rules you want applied when using or encountering private areas. Let them know that a closed door is a sign a family member wants to be in private. When doors to private spaces are closed, family members should knock and wait for permission before entering. Similarly, if your child wants privacy, he should close his door and expect others to knock and listen for a response before

Parental Pause—Privacy

1. What are examples of privacy issues for my child?
2. How can I support and respect my child's rights to privacy?

entering. People learn to respect the privacy of others when their rights to privacy are observed and respected.

> *When my children were younger, they constantly ignored my attempts at privacy. I know this is common, but difficult when you live in a small house with one bathroom. After thinking about how I could teach privacy, I realized that they had learned many of the behaviors I wanted to eliminate by watching me. I needed to help them understand the importance of privacy for me and for them. I began modeling the behaviors I expected from them: I knocked on doors and waited for a response before entering anyone's room. When they barged into my room, I asked them to knock. When they took a shower, I spoke through the door rather than entering the bathroom. If they needed help, I would help and then let them know I was leaving so they could be in private.*
>
> *Although my younger daughter grasped the concept of respecting a closed door, I often found her peering through the glass windows of her sister's door. I realized that her bedroom was not really private if others could look in whenever they wanted. I sewed some curtains to cover the windows and attempted to help my younger daughter understand the subtle ways she violated her sister's rights to privacy. We still have a long way to go, but my daughter with Down syndrome clearly understands what "privacy" means and regularly lets us know when she wants to be in private—a big step.*

Teaching Activity: "My Private Places at Home"

When your son or daughter is just learning about private places in your home, visual cues can enhance comprehension and help with discrimination. Clearly identify (verbally or with pictures) rooms that have the potential to be private places for your child. Private places are rooms where your child can go if he wants to be alone or have time to himself. Take pictures of these rooms, then label and laminate them. For example, a picture could be labeled "Justin's private place" or "my private place." Place them on a connector ring to use as a routine visual reminder when your child does something in public that he should do in private at home. In the home, public rooms can be defined as those places where other family members can go at any time without knocking. Use the drawing in Appendix B-2 to emphasize that private places are places where one person can be alone.

Teaching Activity: "Public and Private at Home"

After you have explained differences between public and private places (using the definitions above or your own), have your child label various rooms in the house with PUBLIC or PRIVATE labels or symbols. This idea can be used in school settings as well.

Teaching Activity: "Privacy Proofing"

Sometimes we make assumptions about whether a room is public or private without really thinking about the characteristics that are necessary to ensure privacy. Talk with your child about what makes a room private. First, *a private place is a place where no one can see you.* Evaluate with your child things he can do to block others from seeing him in his private place. If he closes the door, but the windows are still open, talk about how others may be able to see him, particularly at night with lights on.

Use a verbal prompt such as "I can still see you . . ." if you suspect your child wants to be private but has omitted taking steps to "privacy proof" his room. (You can do this when any of your family members are forgetting to "privacy proof.") Begin encouraging these "privacy proofing" actions as a routine (e.g., at night) whenever privacy is desirable.

Second, emphasize that *there are rules to follow before entering private spaces.* Teach family members that when a door is closed, knocking is required. Remind them that a closed door means the person or people in the room want privacy.

Teaching Activity: "Knock, Knock—Who's There?"

To enhance ideas about respecting privacy, teach your child that knocking on a closed door to a private space (theirs and anyone else's) is a good idea. You can begin teaching this concept by modeling it for him. Begin by knocking on doors when they are closed. If your child is verbal, teach him appropriate responses to a knock: "who's there?" or "yes?" or "what do you want?" Let him know he has the right to say "don't come in" or "wait," or not to open the door if he is doing something private.

Teaching Activity: "Privacy Please!"

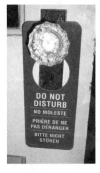

A visual way to help others know you want privacy is to use a doorknob sign. To encourage your child to express a need for privacy, particularly if he is nonverbal, get out the art supplies and have him create a personalized doorknob hanger for his bedroom door. Make one yourself as well. Generic signs can be purchased at craft stores, but your child can still add his personal touch. Messages like "Do Not Disturb," "Stay Out," "Privacy Please," or symbols can communicate clear messages when privacy is desirable. In a pinch, do not disturb signs from hotels work too! Once your child has a sign to hang, review with him what activities are private and encourage sign use during those activities.

Helping your child understand privacy issues out in the community is trickier. Often there are more variables, so your son or daughter may have a harder time generalizing behavior from one situation to another. For these reasons, you need to intentionally teach your child about privacy in specific situations and contexts.

When my daughter was 10 or so, she experienced some regression in her understanding of public and private shortly after she began wearing a Boston brace for scoliosis. She learned very quickly how to remove the brace independently and did so whenever it was convenient. She'd hoist up her shirt on the playground in full view of whoever happened to be watching. This was understandable, since we had not been careful about where and when we removed the brace at home. We revisited the issue of privacy with her and made sure that when we were putting her brace on or when she was removing the brace, we were in the bathroom or in her bedroom with the door closed, which are her private spaces. We made sure the professionals who supported her understood our goals and followed suit. Because she was familiar with the concept of privacy, her understanding of the rules related to brace removal made teaching much easier for all of us.

Teaching Activity: "Favorite Public Places"

Explain that public places are spaces where other people are around, with the help of the drawing in Appendix B-2. To help your child associate the word "public" with "people," create a collage of public places. Label a piece of paper "John's Favorite Public Places" or just "Public Places." Brainstorm with your child places he likes to go (public library, zoo, museums, restaurants, school, sports facilities, etc.) where other people are around. Then, using magazine pictures, family photos, and symbols, create a collage of public places. Remind your child that the places on the page are considered "public" places because other people are around. Hang the artwork on the refrigerator or wall and use it as a tool for reinforcing appropriate behavior in public places (see rules below). Add to the list over time as new places are identified.

Teaching Activity: "Public Restrooms Symbols"

I was recently in a restaurant where the restrooms were simply labeled "Caballeros" and "Caballeras" (no symbols). Because I minored in Spanish, I had no problem figuring out where I should go, but it did make me wonder how individuals with cognitive disabilities 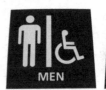 might decide. If you are just starting to help your child learn how to be independent with public restroom use, be sure to review bathroom symbols (they are more universal now) and have him practice choosing the correct one while in public places.

Teaching Activity: "Public Bathroom Rules"

Rules for using restrooms out in the community are very different and more complicated than at home. Because some public restrooms require "sharing the space with others," your child may need additional help and instruction understanding the unwritten rules of bathroom etiquette. Male and female rules are different, so get help or clarification if you're unfamiliar with opposite gender bathroom etiquette. Here are some commonly followed rules:

Male bathroom etiquette
- Go to the urinal that's farthest away from other boys/men
- Keep your eyes down (or stare at the urinal)
- No talking to other boys/men
- Keep your hands to yourself (you should not touch others and they should not touch you)
- Close zipper when done
- Wash hands
- Leave
- If someone touches you in a public restroom, say no, leave, and tell a safe person

When we were trying to teach our son how to use a public restroom independently, we encouraged him to use the stall. It was just easier, safer, and more private.

Female bathroom etiquette
- If there's a line, wait until it is your turn
- Find an empty stall (if unsure, knock before entering)
- Lock door from the inside
- No talking while using the stall
- Zip up, arrange clothing before you open the stall door
- Wash hands
- Leave

Customize instruction based on your child's needs. Social stories or visual task analysis are good tools for teaching appropriate public restroom use. Consider using the process identified in Chapter 7 to teach independence with public restroom use (preparation, practice with supervision, coaching to autonomy).

My daughter often left the door unlocked in bathrooms and people would walk in on her. It took me a while to figure out she couldn't manipulate certain types of locks. Now I show her how to lock the door if it's a type she has never used before.

Teaching Activity: "Locker Room Rules"

Rules can be a bit more confusing in locker room situations since stays are more lengthy and a wider variety of activities may be going on (dressing, showering, grooming, etc.). Teach your child that the locker room is not usually private because it is shared and used by others so "societal rules for private body parts" apply.

Respect Your Own Body
- Cover your private body parts after using the shower. In locker rooms this usually means using a towel to wrap the lower part of the body.
- No touching your own private body parts in front of other people.
- Avoid talking about private parts and functions with others.

Be Respectful of Other People's Bodies
- No touching other people's private body parts ("hands to yourself").
- Avoid staring at another person's private body parts.
- Do not talk about another person's private body parts ("nice breasts," etc.).

Body Rights

Once your child can label body parts and apply societal rules related to body parts, introducing information that can help prevent exploitation is a logical next step. For people with developmental disabilities, the idea that their body is their own is a more difficult concept. The need for assistance with self-care combined with routine violations of privacy by others often contributes to distorted perceptions about body rights.

Key Teaching Messages:
- My body belongs to me.
- No one can touch me if I don't want to be touched.
- No one can make me touch their private parts if I don't want to.
- If someone forces me to share my body when I don't want to, I should tell.

ABC 123

Teaching Activity: "My Body, My Space"

One way to address the concept of body rights is to introduce your child to the idea of personal space and rules that surround it. Explain to your child that everyone has an invisible area around their bodies called "personal space," "bubble," or another word that makes sense for your child.

Help your child visualize his personal space by encouraging him to stand in the center of a hula hoop or a circle of rope or string, or by having him hold his arms out and turning in a circle to create an invisible barrier. Let him know that his body is his own and he gets to decide who to share it with. Explain that sharing his body can mean giving someone a hand, sitting on another person's lap, hugging, or tickling, etc. (If your child is older and dating, more information on this can be found in Chapter 10 on relationships.) Your child gets to decide what feels okay for him. Remind him that nobody can force him to share his body if he doesn't want to.

Identify ways your child can help others know he is not comfortable with a touch or space invasion. He can say, "Stop," "I don't like it," "It's my body," or "Don't touch!" If your child is nonverbal, hand signals such as stop or a straight arm that prevents people from getting any closer work as well.

Your child will more easily grasp body rights concepts if others respect his right to be discriminatory about affection and touch. This means that sharing goals you have with other adults in your child's life (teachers, relatives, therapists, etc.) will be necessary. If you notice, for example, that many adults who work with your child encourage hugging beyond ages that would be considered developmentally appropriate in typically developing children, request their help. You could tell them you are working on ways to help your child understand boundaries so he can be safer and more socially appropriate as a teen (or adult). Remind them that your child is very much a visual learner and consequently modeling by others will be necessary and helpful. Encourage adults to begin giving your child some control by asking permission before touching, or by applying the same rules they use with other kids.

There are various books that can be helpful in teaching about body rights and empowerment. Here are a few:

> **It's My Body,** by Lory Freeman (Seattle, WA: Parenting Press, 1982).
> A good introduction to body rights. Encourages children to recognize touches that feel good and say no to those they don't want. The key message, "your body is special and belongs to you," is emphasized.

> **Just Because I Am: A Child's Book of Affirmation,** by Lauren Murphy Payne (Minneapolis, MN: Free Spirit Publishing, 1994).
> A simple book that encourages appreciation of uniqueness and includes empowering messages about the body, feelings, boundary awareness, touch, and feeling safe.

> **Your Body Belongs to You,** by Cornelia Spelman (Mortons Grove, IL: Albert Whitman & Company, 1997).
> This children's book, written by a social worker, is designed to help children understand their touching rights. The book balances messages regarding the need we all have for healthy affection with our right to determine who touches us. Includes multicultural drawings.

Private Talk

Individuals with cognitive disabilities often have difficulty being discreet, an important component of social appropriateness. For example, a young woman, excited about getting her first period, may want to tell everyone at a family get-together. An adult may share intimate details of what happened on a date last night with the bus driver, or a young teen may feel compelled to share his erection with classmates. A good friend of mine who is a nurse and parent of a daughter with a cognitive disability still remembers how horrified she was when her young daughter asked a man walking by her grocery cart if he had a penis.

In my early years as an educator, I was often told about students who would leave my sessions and share details about what they had learned with anyone who would listen. Shortly thereafter I learned to spend time in my introduction framing sexuality content as a "private" but "discussable" topic. Asking participants to identify specific people they could talk with about things they had learned or had questions about became an important aspect of teaching in sexuality education sessions.

Key Teaching Messages:

- Talking about _____ is private.
- If I want to talk about things that are private I can talk to _____ (list of people in various locations).
- When I want to talk about something that is private I should make sure others cannot hear what I am saying.
- A private place to talk at home is _____.
- A private place to talk at school (or work) is _____.

Helping your child learn to be discreet is often a necessary component of teaching. Once he understands the concepts of public and private, you can begin to label specific topics as either private (inappropriate for discussing with general public) or public (okay to talk about with others), enhancing your child's ability to be socially appropriate.

Often people with cognitive difficulties have difficulty with the concept of discretion related to other issues beyond sexuality. For example, they may ask adults their age, how much money they make, or share details about medical conditions that are usually considered private.

Labeling new information you may be sharing with your child as private right up front can help prevent social mistakes. Try teaching your child a visual or sensory cue that signals a subject is considered private, then use it if you catch your child moving into inappropriate territory. Lowering your voice, putting a hand up, a finger on closed lips, a zipping of the closed mouth, or other cue can help your child know the subject is off limits for this situation. If time allows, remind your child that not all people are comfortable talking about sexuality issues in public places when others are around and that it's best to talk about these things at home, in a classroom, or other program where sexuality is being taught and discussed. Quickly redirect him to other topics more appropriate for conversations. If timing is bad, let your child know you will talk with him later about the issue, and be sure to come back to the subject later.

Our son talks to his pretend friends whenever he gets the chance. His behavior became quite embarrassing in public places and we were never quite sure if he was talking to us or someone else. We explained to him that discussions with his pretend friends needed to happen only in his bedroom, his private place. We explained to him that now that he was older, others would not understand what

Self-Talk and Down Syndrome

Many people with Down syndrome talk to themselves out loud. This phenomenon, deemed "self-talk," is a well-known developmental tool that helps children coordinate actions and thoughts and also helps older people learn new skills and engage in higher level thinking.

We all occasionally talk to ourselves out loud. People with Down syndrome, however, tend to do it more often and with less discretion. In a study conducted at the Adult Down Syndrome Center near Chicago, 83 percent of the adults seen at the clinic engaged in conversations with themselves or imaginary companions. In a European study, 91 percent of a group of 78 young people talked out loud to themselves. Within these studies, self-talk appeared to be used as a coping strategy, to vent frustrations, or as entertainment during times of social isolation.

Although self-talk is not typically harmful, it can be alarming for others who are not familiar with your child or with the frequency of self-talk in people with Down syndrome. Inexperienced observers often misinterpret self-talk as psychosis, mental illness (e.g., schizophrenia), or other severe psychological problems and may consequently advocate for unnecessary use of medications. For these reasons, it is important for your child to view self-talk as a private behavior. When you notice your child engaging in self-talk or conversations with pretend friends in public places, gently and discreetly redirect him to focus on something or someone in their presence.

More information on self-talk in teens and adults is available in **Mental Wellness in Adults with Down Syndrome**, by Drs. Dennis McGuire and Brian Chicoine.

pretend friends were or why he needed them when he had plenty of real friends. We helped him understand that others who did not know him would think he was strange. He still continues to talk to pretend friends when he is in his room, but has stopped this behavior in public.

References

Couwenhoven, T. (1992). *Beginnings: A Parent/Child Sexuality Program for Families with Children who have Developmental Disabilities.* Madison: Wisconsin Council on Developmental Disabilities.

Couwenhoven, T. (May/June 2001). Sexuality Education: Building on the Foundation of Healthy Attitudes. *Disability Solutions 4* (5): 8-9.

Glenn, S.M. & Cunningham, C.C. (2000). Parents' Report of Young People with Down Syndrome Talking Out Loud to Themselves. *Mental Retardation 38* (6): 498-505.

Hingsburger, D. & Harber, M. (1998). *The Ethics of Touch: Establishing and Maintaining Appropriate Boundaries in Service to People with Developmental Disabilities.* Eastman, Quebec: Diverse City Press.

McGuire, D. & Chicoine, B. (July/August 1997). Self-Talk in Adults with Down Syndrome. *Disability Solutions 2* (2): 1-5.

McGuire, D. & Chicoine, B. *Mental Wellness in Adults with Down Syndrome: A Guide to Emotional and Behavioral Strengths and Challenges.* Bethesda, MD: Woodbine House, 2006.

Stangle, J. (1991). *Special Education: Secondary Family Life and Sexual Health: A Curriculum for Grades 7-12.* Seattle-King County Department of Public Health.

Chapter 3—Framework for Teaching Privacy

Concepts	Key Messages	Goal Behaviors
Private	■ When I cannot be seen or heard by others	■ Distinguishes between public and private
Public	■ When others are around and can see me	
Public/private body parts	■ A boy's private body parts are the penis, scrotum, and butt ■ A girl's private body parts are the breasts, vulva, and butt ■ Private body parts stay covered when I'm in public and other people are around	■ Keeps private body parts covered in public places
Privacy at home	■ Private places are rooms where I can go to be by myself ■ At home my private place is _____ ■ I can tell others when I want or need privacy ■ I should knock before entering other people's private spaces	■ Can identify private place(s) at home ■ Moves to private areas when privacy is needed ■ Recognizes violations of own privacy rights ■ Respects the privacy of others
Privacy in the community	■ There are times when I may need privacy when I am in the community ■ In the community, a private place is _____ ■ There are rules when I am using private areas in the community ■ Following the rules will help me stay safe	■ Can identify private place(s) in the community ■ Moves to private areas when privacy is needed ■ Recognizes when privacy rights have been violated ■ Is respectful of privacy rights of others
Private Talk	■ Talking about _____ is private ■ If I want to talk about things that are private, I can talk to _____ ■ When I want to talk about something that is private I should make sure others cannot hear what I am saying ■ A private place to talk at home is _____ ■ A private place to talk at school (or work) is _____	■ Recognizes sexuality topics as private ■ Identifies people who can discuss sexuality issues

CHAPTER 4

Touch and Affection

As parents of kids with Down syndrome, we've all heard it, experienced it, worked hard at fixing it, and sometimes have even perpetuated it: the myth that individuals with Down syndrome are somehow different from the rest of us and require extra doses of affection (usually in the form of hugs because "people with Down syndrome are soooo affectionate").

This myth is still quite prevalent and problematic. First, we know that varying needs for touch and affection are necessary and beneficial for all of us. The difference is that most of us have learned over time how to get these needs met in socially acceptable ways (see ideas at end of chapter). People with Down syndrome are often programmed (by parents, professionals, and sometimes perfect strangers) to express affection indiscriminately simply because they have Down syndrome. On a recent walk to a meeting in our hospital, I noticed a family with a child with Down syndrome running down the hallway. The little girl with Down syndrome couldn't have been more than five years old and already her parents were thinking it was cute that she was trying to hug any and every kid who crossed her path.

Addressing issues of touch and affection in the lives of people with developmental disabilities is not easy and presents a difficult dilemma for professionals in the field of sexuality education. Touch, affection, and intimacy are important and there are proven physical and psychological benefits of touch. Individuals with developmental disabilities, however, often express affection indiscriminately, which can threaten their social acceptance, increase their vulnerability, and at times, violate the rights of others. The dilemma becomes: how do we help people with Down syndrome or other cognitive disabilities express closeness and affection in socially acceptable ways without leading them into touch-deprived lives?

Touch and Affection in Early Childhood

There is no question that touch is essential to human life. Affection in infancy and beyond is critical to physical, social, and emotional development and should be

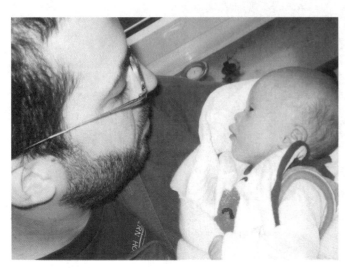

unconditionally shared. In infancy and childhood, children learn to value themselves through nurturing touch and affection. Infant massage classes are frequently offered for families with newborns as a way to facilitate parent-child bonding, increase body awareness, and improve relaxation and sleep.

Not all babies and children enjoy the same kinds of touch, so part of your job as a parent is to figure out what types of touch your child enjoys. Even at an early age, it's important to interpret and respect your child's signals that she doesn't want to be touched. Many children, for example, prefer deep hugs rather than light touch if they are tactilely defensive or have autism. In these instances certain types of brushing protocols (e.g., Willbarger) will be more calming and pleasurable. An occupational therapist can help you learn more about your child's sensory processing needs, as can the book *Fine Motor Skills for Children with Down Syndrome*, by Maryanne Bruni.

My son has autism and Down syndrome and likes different types of touches for different reasons. When he is ill or upset, a very light touch to his arm— almost a tickle—is very calming for him. When he is happy or excited about events, he prefers a very deep touch. Sometimes this means a tight hug while you rub your chin on his shoulders or a firm pat to his back. For him, touch is communication as well as a sensory need.

Touch and Affection: Context Is Everything

The rules for touch and affection are often fuzzy or change based on culture and context, making teaching hard and fast "rules" a difficult task. As a parent I struggle with this on a regular basis. When my daughter entered middle school, I noticed an

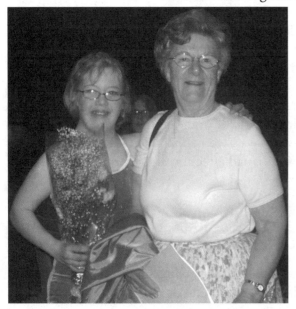

increase in her physical affection toward her female friends. At the same time, like most kids this age, she was struggling to fit in. I stepped in to help her identify what I believed were more socially appropriate ways to let girlfriends know how she felt about them besides hugging. We talked about words and phrases she could use with friends that would reflect her feelings. We brainstormed a list of different types of touch that would work such as high fives, pats on the back, and so on. Imagine my confusion and embarrassment when at Anna's co-ed birthday party, I observed the "nondisabled" girls hanging all over each other. I must say Anna was appropriately distant, yet in this context she looked out of place. It was then that I realized she had been modeling some of the touch and affection she observed in the hallways of her middle school. In the context of middle school culture with females, her expressions of affection had been appropriate.

Marasmus Mystery

During the nineteenth century, babies and young children residing in institutions often died from a disease called marasmus, a Greek word that meant "wasting away." Although death was almost certain for children under two in these facilities, physicians and staff were unable to determine a cause. It wasn't until after World War II that studies analyzing the causes of marasmus revealed a link between "inadequate mothering" and ill health. These early studies illustrated the critical needs for touch in infants and young children residing in institution-like settings. Once this discovery was made, pediatricians were able to reverse the trend by advising staff to implement tender, loving, care (where the term TLC originated). Caregivers were encouraged to pick up, carry, cuddle, stroke, and caress the children—behaviors described as "mothering"—several times per day. At Bellevue Hospital in New York, mortality rates among infants under the age of one dropped from 30-35 percent to under 10 percent by 1938.

Most of the time, touch and affection errors made by children with Down syndrome or other cognitive disabilities occur because they lack information or are unable to generalize information from one relationship, situation, or context to another. For example, a bear hug with a relative you haven't seen in awhile is usually appropriate but the nurse in your physician's office or a teacher at school may find it unwelcome. Putting an arm around a good friend may be fine, but usually is unacceptable with a boss. Thinking about touch within certain contexts and situations can provide insights on what information your child may need and help you develop a plan for improving understanding. Below are examples of common contexts that often create confusion for people with developmental disabilities.

TOUCH AND AFFECTION IN THE CONTEXT OF AGE APPROPRIATENESS

Sometimes touch and affection looks out of place because the behavior does not match what other people would expect from a person without a disability of the same age. Many families I talk to can recall suddenly noticing that their child had "outgrown" a particular behavior and experiencing embarrassment and discomfort.

I never thought much about the influence I had on how my child touched others until we were at a family gathering and I noticed my twelve-year-old playing criss-cross applesauce on her uncle's back. [Criss-cross applesauce is a game with different types of touch performed on the back to generate goose bumps— "Criss cross applesauce, spiders crawling up you back, spiders crawling down your back…."] She and I have played this game for years as a part of her bedtime routine. I do it to her, then she does it to me. With her uncle, it looked strange and completely out of place. That night at bedtime I suggested we try and alter the routine a bit and switch to something else. She suggested a backrub, so that's what we do now. When I envisioned her giving her uncle (or future partner) a backrub, I decided it would be more socially acceptable and age-appropriate.

Key Teaching Messages:

- Touch rules can change as I get older.
- I should ask permission before I touch others.

"Got your nose," tickling, or sitting on laps after your child has completed puberty and looks like an adult are other examples of touch and affection that should prompt parents to explore more socially acceptable ways to touch and connect with others. Children grow up. We just forget how fast it happens. It's also common for parents to think of their children in a developmental context (how old they act) rather than a chronological one (how old they actually are). Observing your child engage in these behaviors should act as a wake-up call to work on more age-appropriate ways for connecting with others. When we as parents ignore age-inappropriate touching, we help others continue to see our children as "child-like" rather than maturing individuals.

If your child is particularly petite or appears to be chronologically younger than she actually is, this presents a different kind of challenge. I know many families who work hard at nudging their child into age-appropriate touch, affection, or behavior and then are routinely sabotaged by family members or others in the community who can't seem to believe that people with Down syndrome or other cognitive disabilities do grow up and develop just like everyone else. At a grocery store we frequent, many of the older cashiers routinely ask my seventeen-year-old daughter if she would like a token for the "prize" machine. (At any given time there are numerous three- and four-year-olds gathered around the gumball-like machine trying to figure out how to get their preferred plastic-encased prize.) I really doubt they ask other seventeen-year-olds this question, but somehow it always comes up. After years of getting asked, my daughter now has a canned response, "No thanks, I'm seventeen and don't do tokens." Sometimes the cashiers are embarrassed, but at least the message is clear.

When dilemmas regarding age-appropriate touch and affection surface here are some things you can do:

USE SAME-AGED PEERS AS A GUIDE

Observe kids or adults as they come out of school, play sports, and interact in typical environments. If your child is in middle or high school where parental involvement is more limited, chaperoning dances, field trips, or other school-sponsored activities can provide opportunities to observe students interacting in natural environments. Speak with other parents you know well who have kids your child's age or get ideas about appropriate touch from older siblings. Staying current with acceptable forms of touch can provide useful information about replacement behaviors that are socially appropriate.

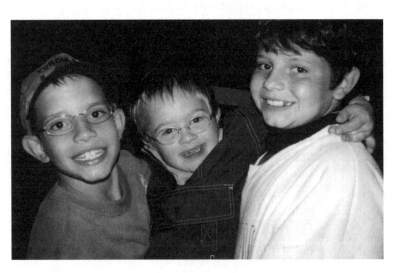

Children with cognitive disabilities are less likely to pick up on nonverbal cues from others and usually require direct instruction and verbal feedback. Peers can act as mirrors for your child, helping her understand more acceptable forms of touch and affection and provide feedback when inappropriate touch occurs.

If your child spends significant amounts of time with peers who are unable to provide age appropriate modeling, consider activities outside of school. Participating in Scouting, church, sports, clubs, or extracurricular activities are good ways to expose your child to age appropriate modeling.

Sometimes the modeling provided within inclusive settings isn't always accept-able or ideal. Students in inclusive settings, with and without disabilities, will model the behavior of those around them. This, in fact, is one of the arguments for inclusion. Children with Down syndrome are great imitators and learn well by watching and following the lead of others.

During gym class in middle school, my son got caught slapping other boys on the butt during gym class, something he had never done before. I reminded him that the butt was private and it was not okay to touch other people there. Later, my older son shared with me some examples of inappropriate locker room behaviors he had observed. It was then I realized my son might be modeling be-haviors he was seeing in the locker room. The other boys, however, just knew how not to get caught.

All children want to be accepted and feel like they're part of the group, and sometimes inappropriate touch becomes a way to interact, join the crowd, or increase peer acceptance. Teens with cognitive disabilities, however, have more difficulty understanding specific circumstances when it's okay and not okay and consequently tend to get "caught" more often than their peers.

If your child has had an experience like this, let her know that you understand how good being part of the group feels, but explain why you don't approve of the behavior. Review body rights and rules (e.g., everyone's body is their own) and that slapping people on the butt without their permission violates those rules. If she expresses a concern about rules being different for other kids, remind her that not all behaviors she sees others doing will be okay for her (e.g., cigarettes, alcohol, or other examples you feel strongly about).

Sometimes explaining why the behavior would be inappropriate in another context can be helpful. For example, using the example above: "If you went to the YMCA and started slapping other boys in the locker room on the butt, what do you think would happen?" Often, discussing your child's feelings about the incident, suggesting more appropriate replacement behaviors, and sharing basic informa-tion in open and nonthreatening ways will be all that is needed. If the behavior continues, explore it further with your child, repeating information if necessary. If your child continues to have trouble making good choices about behavior, consider speaking with key adults to gather additional information and come up with a plan (see Chapter 14).

VISUALIZE YOUR CHILD AS AN ADULT

If you struggle with deciding what types of touch and affection to teach, visualize your child continuing to do the behavior as a teen or adult at high school or in the work environment. How would her peers view the behavior? Her coworkers? Consider the long-term implications of what you allow and remember that changing entrenched behaviors is always more difficult than starting fresh.

BODY CONTEXT AND TOUCH

The intent of the touch and where it occurs on the body is another context to consider. Children with limited verbal abilities tend to use touch more often when communication

Troubleshooting—Touching Others Inappropriately

Suspected or Reported Intent of Touch	Possible Strategies
Desire to connect with others or feel included	■ Teach greeting skills ■ Advocate for social skills instruction ■ Explore use of assistive technology if necessary to interact with others
Attempt to get help or assistance	■ Teach words – "excuse me" or "I need help" or incorporate these phrases into chosen communication system ■ If your child has difficulty with words, identify acceptable and touchable body parts for getting help or attention (e.g., below or above the elbow of the arm). ■ Explore use of augmentative communication
Peer pressure (child was told by peers to touch inappropriately)	■ Review body rights (their own and others') ■ Share family values about expected behavior ■ Role play responses to peer pressure ■ Alert teachers or support staff if this becomes an ongoing problem
Inappropriate modeling by peers	■ Review body rights (their own and others') ■ Share family values about appropriate behavior ■ Identify more socially appropriate replacement behaviors ■ Explore opportunities where child can see appropriate behavior modeled
Attention	■ Avoid exaggerated responses to inappropriate touching ■ Teach greeting skills ■ Advocate for social skills instruction ■ Consider relationship facilitation by teacher or other adult ■ Explore use of assistive technology if needed by child to interact with others ■ Advocate for functional behavior analysis if behavior continues
Curiosity	■ Share information about male or female body (use pictures) ■ Review body rights and responsibilities

is difficult or when others have trouble interpreting their speech. Where a touch occurs on the body, however, can make or break a social interaction. Touching a person's arm usually is acceptable, for example, but a poke on the butt or other private part will (and should) yield a more negative reaction. Below are ideas for addressing inappropriate touch (refer to Chapter 3 for more information on teaching about private body parts).

Teaching Activity: "Body Maps"

If your child is having difficulty understanding social rules for touch, simplify the rules and make them visual. For example, it may be easier to come up with clear rules that are straightforward, reduce ambiguity, and encourage social appropriateness. Use copies of the body outlines in Appendix A-5 and A-6 and shade in specific areas of the front and back of the body that are socially acceptable to touch. Use green marker or crayon to highlight okay-to-touch areas that might be appropriate while out and about in the community. Present a variety of relevant scenarios that illustrate different intents (listed above) to check learning. For example:

- "You need help and want to get your teacher's attention. How could you get her attention? If she didn't hear you, what part of her body would be okay for you to touch to get her to hear you?"
- "Let's pretend you are on the bus and the kids want you to touch Jenny on her butt. Would that be a green or red area of the body? What could you say?"
- "You see the boys from gym class slapping each other on the butt. Is that a green or red area of the body?"

MORE WAYS TO TEACH ABOUT TOUCH AND AFFECTION

Here are additional things to think about when teaching rules related to touch and affection:

GIVE YOUR CHILD THE POWER

Respect your child's right to choose with whom she displays affection. Often young children are born with natural instincts to resist unwanted touch from strangers or people they don't know well, but over time are socialized to be inappropriate. Try not to encourage indiscriminate affection when your child's natural instincts are already the right ones. If you observe adults violating your child's natural resistance, suggest alternative greetings (verbal, or something less invasive) that seem more appropriate (for ways to communicate your concerns to others, see examples below).

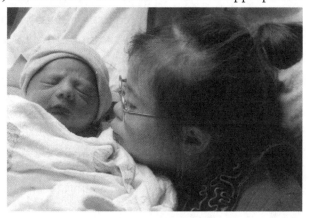

PAY ATTENTION TO MODELING

If your child is really struggling with inappropriate touch issues, pay attention to how you and others around her are modeling touch. Children are great imitators. If people around your child routinely violate her space, she will have a reduced sense of boundaries and experience more difficulty understanding (Hingsburger). If inappropriate modeling is occurring, communicate your goals with key support people and discuss ways they can help you reach them. Work on helping your child become independent with self-care and encourage support people to respect your child's boundaries by asking permission and being respectful of privacy.

One day the guidance counselor called to discuss my daughter's inappropriate affection with a particular boy in one of her classes. Shortly after our discussion, I had to pick her up at school to go to a doctor's appointment. When she was getting ready to leave, the male paraprofessional in her classroom insisted (my daughter had appropriately resisted) on one of those frontal bear hugs. I cringed and was amazed that the other professionals in the room didn't even flinch. I talked with her teacher the next day, reminding her of the difficulties my daughter was having. They hadn't made the connection between the modeling they were providing in the classroom and my daughter's excessive affection with her classmates.

ADOPT A SET OF CONCRETE AND CONSERVATIVE RULES

Once your child enters school, it's appropriate to begin teaching greetings that are socially appropriate to use with authority figures. Introducing information proactively with appropriate repetition and reinforcement over time can prevent confusion right from the start.

For example, teach your child that handshakes, head nods, smiles, and verbal greetings are appropriate ways to greet authority figures such as teachers. If you notice your child demonstrating affection indiscriminately, provide one or two alternatives for a specific inappropriate touch you are attempting to eliminate and have your child pick the one that she like best. Teach your child that when she sees authority figures (or "adult helpers," "paid helpers," or another word that makes sense to your child), she should use the chosen greeting.

Make sure others who support your child know about your goals (see below). Remember, you're not trying to eliminate touch and affection, but simply help your child become socially appropriate. In his *Ethics of Touch* video, David Hingsburger reminds us that individuals with disabilities are already suspect in our society. If you're not sure where to draw the line, he recommends erring on the side of being conservative.

ELICIT HELP FROM OTHERS SUPPORTING YOUR CHILD

In the process of attempting to teach appropriate touch and affection, communicate your goals and expectations with key family members and support people in your child's life. Your child will be more likely to succeed if everyone is consistent in teaching and reinforcing rules related to touch and affection. Use IEP meetings, teacher's conferences, or other natural forums that surface to introduce your goals for social appropriateness or concerns about touch. You could say:

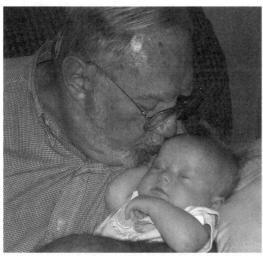

■ "I really want my son to learn how to greet adults in socially acceptable ways. Here is the rule we use at home. Could you help him understand that these rules apply to adults at school (or work) as well?"

■ "How have you helped other students learn appropriate social boundaries with adults? I really want my child to be more appropriate. She has a hard time knowing who she can and cannot hug. This is what we've been doing at home. I think teaching would work more effectively if there was consistency at school as well."

■ "My child is a great imitator and I fear she may be learning to give hugs too often, without considering her relationship with the person. We have started to use this rule about greetings when we're out in the community. How would that work here?"

■ "We have concerns about our son's inappropriate touching and fear for his safety. We want him to learn to be more socially appropriate, so here is what we are doing with him. It would help a lot if you could greet him using _____ rather than a hug . He will need a lot of repetition and reinforcement to be successful."

EXPAND THE TOOLBOX

Provide one or two alternatives for the inappropriate touch you are attempting to change. Too often we assume that the only way to communicate intimacy and closeness within relationships is through touch when, in fact, words can be equally effective. If your child has verbal abilities, help her come up with words that communicate feelings she is conveying through touch. For example, read the statements below:

■ "Great job; keep up the good work."
■ "Take care, see you tomorrow."
■ "Thanks for your help."
■ "It was so nice to see you again. I really enjoy spending time with you."
■ "I missed you while you were gone. I'm glad you're back."
■ "You are very important to me. I'm not sure what I would do without you."
■ "I love you."

Do some of these statements feel more intimate than others? Think about the relationships in your life. Are there people with whom you could share these statements and some you could not? Just like touch, words can be an option for interacting with others in meaningful ways.

ENSURE TOUCH NEEDS ARE MET

In one of the opening scenes of the movie *Life Is a House*, the main character, a divorced man who lives alone and finds himself stricken with cancer, awakens in a hospital room under the care of a nurse. As the nurse caresses his face and forehead with a cloth he immediately relaxes and admits it's the first time he's been touched in years. The nurse doesn't believe him. "No, really? You must have someone in your life who touches you?"

This scene was so powerful for me, mainly because I tried to imagine myself going for years without any sort of human touch and couldn't fathom what it would be like. It also reminded me of the dilemma that sexuality educators and parents struggle over while attempting to address issues of touch and affection in the lives of individuals with developmental disabilities.

As mentioned above, we have a great deal of knowledge and research demonstrating both the physical and psychological benefits of touch. And yet many people I work with have few opportunities to receive and experience caring, nurturing, therapeutic touch and consequently reach out in ways that are not always socially acceptable. Listed below are some ideas for helping individuals get their needs for touch met in socially acceptable ways.

SOCIALLY ACCEPTABLE WAYS PEOPLE GET TOUCH NEEDS MET

Family, Friends, Intimate Partner. Families play an important role in fulfilling their children's needs for touch and affection throughout their lives, but there is wide variability in how touch and affection is expressed within families. Some families are very affectionate, while others rarely express their love in physical ways.

Both my teens still ask for back rubs and foot rubs quite regularly. It really relaxes them. I worry about my daughter with Down syndrome not having anyone to do that for her when she is an adult and living on her own. It is something she really enjoys.

Grooming Services and Paid Therapeutic Touch. In her book *The Power of Touch: The Basis for Survival, Health, Intimacy, and Emotional Well Being,* Phyllis Davis talks about symbolic categories of touch that are recognized as socially acceptable. Quite a few of these categories describe commonly sought-after services in which we pay people to perform a task and get touched in the process. Examples of these services include: chiropractic and health care, massage therapy, manicures, haircuts, pedicures, or other forms of paid therapeutic touch. Some therapeutic touch services (massage, rolfing, reflexology) have proven to have health benefits for patients.

During a recent trip to the salon I observed an elderly man enter the waiting room. My hairdresser greeted him by name and mentioned to me that he was ninety-three years old and came in faithfully for pedicures each month. He was also diabetic, so the foot massage included within the pedicure helped improve circulation in his feet, and, because he could no longer see well, his technician could alert him to subtle changes that might otherwise go unnoticed. Too often we receive messages that young, muscular, smooth-skinned beauties are "touchable," while the elderly and individuals with obvious physical differences might not fit the bill. The sight of the elderly man enjoying a pedicure made me think about how therapeutic this service was for getting touch needs met.

My daughter loves haircuts! I think it all started back in elementary school when there was a head lice outbreak. They did daily lice checks for weeks and she loved them. After the outbreak was done, she would still ask me if I could do a "head check" on her. Ever since then, she has really enjoyed it when her hair is washed, cut, and dried. If she could, she'd go to the salon every week.

During a time when my son was experiencing pain from orthodontia, our dentist recommended we try cranial manipulation, which essentially is a good massage, mostly in the head area. Although it did little to resolve the discomfort associated with his braces, he really enjoyed the sessions and kept asking me when he was going back. Eventually I started doing massages on him at home and he discovered he really enjoyed it. It really helped him relax. For his birthday last year I got him a 30-minute massage from a professional who agreed to focus mainly on the head and neck areas (our son's quite ticklish in other parts of his body). I think as parents we sometimes forget how stressful life can be living with a cognitive disability. Our son is rather hard to understand sometimes and I'm sure that's frustrating. The massage sessions really seemed to help reduce stress.

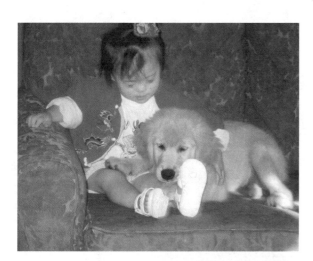

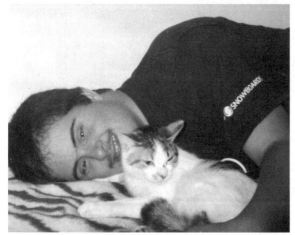

Pets. Did you know that the United States has more pets per capita than any other nation in the world? Pets provide another socially acceptable way to get touch needs met. The therapeutic benefits of pets have been demonstrated repeatedly. For example, individuals who have had difficulty responding to traditional types of therapy have made dramatic therapeutic improvements when pets have been introduced. Some argue that the loving, unconditional acceptance animals can offer creates a safe environment for expressing emotions.

During a recent education session with a client, I was using slides to introduce information about safe sex practices. The woman owned a very curious cat who insisted on being a part of the discussion by climbing up the slide projector and obstructing the view. When my client became uncomfortable, I noticed she reached out for her cat, and stroked it as a way to calm herself down and relax. Following these cat-petting intervals, she seemed better able to continue participating in our discussion.

References

Bruni, M. (2006). *Fine Motor Skills for Children with Down Syndrome: A Guide for Parents and Professionals.* 2nd ed. Bethesda, MD: Woodbine House.

Hingsburger, D., & Harber, M. (1998). *The Ethics of Touch: Establishing and Maintaining Appropriate Boundaries in Service to People with Developmental Disabilities.* Eastman, Quebec: Diverse City Press.

Infant Massage Information Services. Benefits of Infant and Childhood Massage. www.infantmassage-imis.com.au/benefits.

CHAPTER 5

Teaching Your Child about the Physical Changes of Puberty

A mother once told me that puberty was the only aspect of her daughter's development that happened right on schedule. For many families, the onset of puberty becomes a powerful reminder that their child is a sexual human being and will, in fact, develop and mature just like everyone else. In most cases, there are no significant differences between how your son or daughter physically develops compared to his or her peers. What *is* different is the extra time and support needed to help your child understand, accept, and adjust to these changes.

The good news is that the sexual maturation process does not happen overnight, but gradually, over a period of years. The information in this chapter is designed to help you understand typical patterns of physical development so you are prepared to address a range of issues that commonly surface during this phase (see Chapter 7 for information on psychosocial development).

What Is Puberty?

Puberty, technically referred to as *pubescence*, is the biological process of sexual maturation. In humans it occurs sometime between the ages of eight and sixteen. During this time hormones—chemical messengers that can be detected in the bloodstream—are secreted in greater amounts, triggering the appearance of secondary sex characteristics and other physical changes commonly associated with puberty. By the end of puberty, people are generally fully capable of reproducing.

A variety of factors can influence when puberty begins. Genetic factors clearly have a strong influence, which means that the age you began puberty is likely to influence timing for your own child. Other factors can include nutrition, physical activity and exercise, illness, or stress.

Key Players Affecting Puberty Onset in Males and Females

Hypothalamus—a section of the brain that has primary control over the endocrine system, which is the system responsible for secreting (giving off) hormones circulating throughout the body via the bloodstream. One key hormone produced by the hypothalamus is:

- Gonadotropin Releasing Hormone (GnRH), the substance that **controls the production and release** of LH and FSH by the pituitary gland (see below).

Pituitary Gland—This gland is located at the base of the brain and its functions are directed by the hypothalamus. Two hormones associated with puberty and reproduction produced by the pituitary are:

- Follicle Stimulating Hormone (FSH) and
- Luteinizing Hormone (LH).

Both of these hormones trigger activities in the ovaries and testicles and are associated with sexual function and physical maturation in males and females.

Common Questions and Concerns about Puberty

WHEN SHOULD I BEGIN TALKING ABOUT PUBERTY?

Although your child will experience the same physical and emotional changes as his same-aged peers, people with Down syndrome or other cognitive disabilities typically benefit from additional instruction and preparation. This means waiting until the last minute isn't ideal. When deciding on the right time to begin sharing information about puberty, most families I work with choose one of two paths:

1. Some share as much information as they believe their child can understand shortly before physical changes begin. By doing this, they feel they can better prepare their child for body changes before they happen. This frequently stems from a desire to prevent the child from being scared or feeling abnormal. Many parents recall how traumatizing ignorance can be and want their child to have more information than they received.

2. Other families wait until noticeable changes are evident and then begin sharing information. These families have told me that talking about puberty after early changes have begun makes the process more concrete and visible.

You'll have to determine what approach will work best for your own child. The fact is, both of these approaches are proactive. Sharing detailed information about ways to handle bodies and manage feelings reduces anxiety and increases independence and autonomy.

"When I got my period, I thought I was literally hemorrhaging. My mom was embarrassed and I was embarrassed."

—*a self-advocate*

If you have not yet talked about puberty with your child and are not sure how to introduce the information, look for teachable moments that will be meaningful for your child. Consider introducing information if:

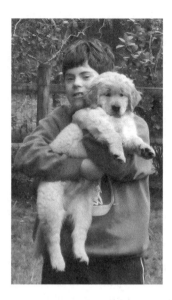

- You begin to notice physical changes.

    "We just bought those pants and they're already too short. You sure are growing. I think you might be starting puberty! Do you know what that is?"

- Your child notices changes or begins asking questions.

    "Yes, that's pubic hair. That happens to all girls your age and is a sign your body is becoming more like mine (or your dad's, or older brother's or sister's). Would you like to hear about other changes that will happen?"

- An opportunity for formal learning arises at school, church, or in the community.

    "At school next month you will be talking about changes that will happen to your body during puberty. I'd like to show you some pictures ahead of time so you will know what to expect."

WHAT IF MY CHILD IS NOT EMOTIONALLY READY?

The start of puberty is not dependent on social and emotional maturity, or many of us would never have matured! It is a biological process that happens, whether we are ready for it or not. Your job is to help your child understand the changes so he can be informed and prepared. My experience has been that individuals who understand what is happening to their bodies are more confident handling the responsibilities associated with growing up.

HOW CAN I EXPLAIN PUBERTY IN A WAY MY CHILD WILL UNDERSTAND?

No single teaching strategy will work well for every child. Throughout this chapter I've presented options for sharing information in different ways. You know your child better than anyone else does, so rely on your personal experiences with him to determine which activities will work or how you can modify information and activities to be more understandable for your child. In general, however, most individuals with Down syndrome benefit from visual strategies and repetition of information over time.

HOW CAN I PREPARE MYSELF FOR DISCUSSIONS ABOUT PUBERTY?

The remainder of this chapter includes information that can prepare you for teaching and handling various issues that commonly surface during puberty and beyond. Suggested resources for both you and your child are also listed in the back of the book. Agencies in your community may also provide classes or have resources that can help you perform in your role as primary sexuality educator (see the Resources for a list of useful organizations). Connecting with other parents who have been through this stage can be helpful as well.

Teaching about Body Changes during Puberty (Males or Females)

Key Teaching Messages:

- Puberty is a time when your body changes from being child-like to adult-like.
- Your body will change on the outside (changes you can see) and on the inside (changes you will not be able to see).
- These changes happen to everyone.
- Your body will change at its own rate. Some kids will change earlier than you; others later.
- Everybody goes through puberty.

Teaching Activity: "Girl to Woman, Boy to Man"

Use this activity to introduce the concept of puberty and identify some of the more obvious ways the outside body changes. With your child, view the puberty progression pictures in Appendix A-9 and A-10. Explain that some time between the ages of 8 to 12 (girls) and 10 to 14 (boys), our bodies change from looking "child-like" to more "adult-like" (choose whatever vocabulary works best). Let your child know that the period of time when the body is changing is called *puberty* and that his or her own body will change in similar ways.

Another way to do this is to have your child stand next to you or the same-gendered parent while facing a full-length mirror (wearing clothing or a swim suit). Focus your child's attention on the mirror and ask him to compare his own body with the body of the parent or adult next to him who has completed puberty. Ask him to point out physical differences (height, shape, breasts if female, or facial hair, arm or leg hair if male, etc.). If he has a hard time doing this on his own, point them out. For example, "See how much taller I am" or "can you see the whiskers on my face? They grow if I don't shave them every morning." If you're a single parent with an opposite gender child, use another relative, other significant adult, or pictures in magazines to point out physical differences between children and adults.

Teaching Activity: "I'm Getting Taller"

Once our children entered first grade, we began tracking their heights on a designated wall in our house. The wall contains many pencil lines with the ages, dates, and weights. The markings became a concrete way of visualizing height changes from one six-month period to the next during pubertal growth spurts. In order to capture the full growth spurt, begin charting your child's height at around age 8 for girls and 9 for boys.

Teaching Activity: "Before Puberty, After Puberty"

Use this activity to introduce specific ways the body will change during puberty or as a review activity when repetition of concepts is necessary. Use the pre-pubertal picture in Appendix A-1 or A-2 that is gender appropriate for your child. While looking at the picture, ask your child to tell you whether he thinks the person in the picture has gone through puberty. If he responds no, ask why. If he answers yes, explore his thinking and remind him that the body changes in very specific ways during puberty.

Use the list below as a way to introduce or review specific physical changes that can be expected. (Or if you've covered this before, ask your child to draw in changes from memory, using the pictures in Appendix A-5 or A-6). As you verbally describe each of the changes, ask your child to illustrate the change on the drawing (whiskers on the face of the male, breasts on the female, drops of blood between the legs for period, etc.). Below is a list of physical changes (not in any particular order) that could be illustrated in some way on the drawing:

Male	Female
Grow taller	Grow taller
More sweat (body odor)	More sweat (body odor)
May get pimples (acne, zits)	May get pimples (acne, zits)
Oilier skin	Oilier skin
Hair will begin to grow	Hair will begin to grow
■ under the arms	■ under the arms
■ pubic area (on & near private areas)	■ pubic area (on & near private areas)
■ longer and thicker on legs & arms	■ longer and thicker on legs
■ face (whiskers)	
■ chest	
Penis & testicles get bigger	Grow breasts
Shape of body changes	Shape of body changes
■ more muscles	■ hips widen
■ gain weight	■ gain weight
Voice gets deeper	Periods begin (menstruation)
Erections are more common	Romantic feelings become stronger
Ejaculation begins	
Romantic feelings become stronger	
Less Obvious Changes	*Less Obvious Changes*
Testicles begin making sperm	Uterus & vagina grow larger
Body produces more sex hormones	Ovaries begin working
Body produces semen	Body produces more sex hormones

If your child has fine motor difficulties, use small printer labels with physical body changes written on them (grow hair, zits, body odor) and encourage him to place them on the area of the body drawing where the changes will occur. For example, a "grow hair" sticker could be placed on the legs, underarms, face, and pubic area on the male drawing. Once the "after puberty" drawing is complete, remind him that his own body will change in similar ways.

Teaching Activity: "Everyone Goes through Puberty"

My daughter loves looking at photographs. During one of her more active growth spurts, I had her peruse old photo albums for pictures of cousins, aunts, uncles, and grandparents in order to compare pictures of family members before and after puberty. This activity naturally led to some interesting discussions about "firsts" (first periods, first shave, etc.) These conversations helped her know these changes happen to everyone.

Another fun way to help your child see how outward appearances change during puberty is to watch long-running TV shows that include child actors. My daughter thought it was pretty cool to see how different the Brady kids looked and sounded in the early shows (first season) compared to later ones (fifth season). Any longer-running show that includes characters your child enjoys can be used (e.g., Disney channel shows, *Full House*, *Leave It to Beaver*).

Teaching Activity: "Early, Late, Somewhere in the Middle"

Rates of growth during puberty vary considerably from person to person. One way to illustrate this change is to point out how kids the same age can all be growing and developing at very different rates. One of my daughter's birthday photos of a group of her same-aged classmates clearly illustrated this point. Some were considerably taller and more obviously developed while others had barely started. Looking at the diversity in the picture became an opportunity to talk about how everyone grows at their own pace.

PARENT PREPARATION FOR MOTHERS AND FATHERS OF BOYS

Signs Your Son Is Approaching Puberty

On average, changes that occur for males during pubescence begin a few years later than for girls—usually between the ages of 10 to 12. Keep in mind that there can be wide variations, however. While body changes may become noticeable for some boys at 11, other boys will not begin these changes until 13 or 14.

Males with Down syndrome have similar patterns of genital development as other males, although there is some evidence that the physical changes typically associated with male sexual development develop more gradually. Health status and genetics also play a role in when puberty begins. Regardless of when the changes begin, the result is similar. The increased production of hormones causes physical changes that tend to follow a somewhat predictable pattern (with some variation). Typically, physicians can monitor your son's progression through puberty using the Tanner Stages. These stages describe specific patterns and characteristics of body changes.

HORMONAL CHANGES

The physical changes occurring during pubescence are caused by hormones, or chemical messengers, that are sent throughout the body and provide instructions for specific parts of the body to "do" something. There have been few studies examining hormonal differences between males with Down syndrome and males in the general population. In one study, however, the hormone levels associated with pubertal development in 46 males with Down syndrome were reported to be similar to those in boys without Down syndrome.

ENLARGEMENT OF TESTES AND SCROTUM

The testes are the two oval-shaped structures that hang behind the penis and are protected by the sac of skin called the scrotum. Inside the testes, clusters of tiny tubules (called *seminiferous tubules*) begin producing sperm sometime during puberty. In contrast to females, who are born with a set amount of eggs in the ovaries, males don't *begin* producing sperm until sometime during puberty.

The sperm-making process that occurs in the testes actually produces testosterone, the hormone responsible for the secondary sex characteristics that become apparent during puberty. This means that one of the earliest signs that your son is entering puberty might be an increase in testicular size (although this may go unnoticed, particularly if your son is independent with showering and self-care). In fact, during routine check-ups, physicians will visually "size" the testicles to estimate what stage of puberty your son may be in. Testicular growth occurs gradually over a period of two to three years. One study found that testicular volume in males with Down syndrome was smaller when compared to males without Down syndrome, so enlargement may be less noticeable in your son (Pueschel, 1985).

Just as it is common for female breasts to grow unevenly, testicular growth and eventual size can be uneven as well. In many grown men, for example, the right testicle can be larger than the left, or sometimes the left testicle hangs lower than the right.

The incidence of undescended testicles (*cryptorchidism*) is reported to be more common in males with Down syndrome. Normally, shortly before or after a boy's birth, his testicles move from the abdominal area down through a canal into the scrotal sac. Sometimes, one or both testicles do not make it to the correct location. Physicians usually check for this early during routine well-baby exams and can inform you if there is a problem.

TANNER STAGES—Male Physical Development

Stage 1
- preadolescent body
- reproductive organs are beginning to mature
- considerable growth in height and weight
- increases in body fat

Stage 2
- early growth of testes and scrotum (without pubic hair)
- height spurt
- increases in fat and muscle
- areola (area around the nipple) increases in size and darkens

Stage 3
- further enlargement of the testes and scrotum
- lengthening of penis
- spreading and darkening of pubic hair
- height spurt accelerates
- broadening of shoulders
- increase in muscle mass
- facial features appear more adult
- larnyx enlarges and voice may deepen

Stage 4
- continued growth of genitals (mostly in breadth)
- pubic hair pattern resembles adult's but sparser
- scrotal skin darkens
- axillary hair appears (underarms, facial hair on upper lip and chin)
- first ejaculation, indicating growth of prostate gland, occurs early in this stage
- deepening of voice
- breast enlargement (gynecomastia)
- oil glands approaching adult size and function

Stage 5
- adult-sized penis & testicles
- pubic hair denser and fully distributed in genital area
- maximum height almost complete
- body shape resembles that of mature male

If a testicle has not descended on its own during your son's first year of life, surgical intervention is recommended. This is because there is a strong association between undescended testicles and poorer testicular function and testicular cancer. Although surgically moving the testicle to the scrotum does not prevent testicular cancer, it does allow the testicle to be monitored more easily.

Testes that are present in infancy rarely ascend later in life. Regardless, testicles should be monitored as a part of annual medical checkups. During the teen years, ask your son's physician to speak with your son about testicular self exams. Ask for teaching materials (brochures or pamphlets) that include pictures of steps for performing a Testicular Self Exam (TSE) so your son can learn how to routinely check for unusual lumps or bumps.

PUBIC HAIR

The growth of pubic hair may be the first sign of puberty that your son notices. Some boys may notice tiny little bumps that appear on the surface of the skin just prior to hair growth. This is normal and results from pubic hairs pushing through the skin. Early pubic hair is light, long, and feathery in the beginning and usually grows around the area where the penis joins the body. As growth continues, hair becomes darker and coarser, and expands into areas above the penis towards the lower abdomen and thighs.

HEIGHT, WEIGHT, AND BODY CHANGES

Other obvious signs that your son has begun puberty are noticeable changes in height and weight and overall body growth (including shoe size). Just like other adolescent boys, boys with Down syndrome will have height growth spurts, but typically the growth is less dramatic.

Age	Average height (50th percentile) of Boys with Down syndrome*	Average height of Boys without Down syndrome**
10—beginning of puberty	49.5 inches 125.7 cm	54 inches 137.2 cm
17—end of puberty	59.5 inches 151.1 cm	68 inches 172.7 cm
Total average growth	10 inches 25.4 cm	14 inches 35.56 cm

* Down syndrome growth charts
** National Center for Health Statistics (NCHS) percentiles

Weight is often a significant concern for families of teens with Down syndrome. Keep in mind that the natural growth spurts that occur during this time can be uneven. For example, weight gains may occur before height changes, creating a sense of temporary "chubbiness." This creates anxiety for families who may have a heightened awareness of weight changes in their children with Down syndrome. If your child is on the chubby side, puberty can be an opportunity for him to slim down as a result of height changes. Consult your physician and/or a nutritionist to discuss dietary and exercise changes that can be beneficial during this time.

HEALTH CONDITIONS THAT AFFECT GROWTH

You may be so busy helping your child adjust to all the changes that puberty brings that preventative health care moves to the bottom of your list. There are, however, a handful of health medical conditions that occur more often in people with Down syndrome that can affect health and growth during puberty.

Scoliosis. Scoliosis is a curvature of the spine (right to left, or front to back). Although the presence of this condition does not affect growth, it often develops during periods of rapid growth associated with puberty. My daughter was about ten when we discovered her scoliosis during a routine cardiology visit. It was a year in which a chest x-ray was scheduled. During the visit, we were all able to see a significant lateral curve in her spine. Up until this time, my daughter had had regular checkups with our pediatrician as well as other specialists. Scoliosis is commonly identified in many kids during puberty, but our cardiologist mentioned it seems to occur more often in children who have had open heart surgery. He theorized that the manipulation of the rib cage during open heart surgery combined with the low muscle tone commonly found in individuals with Down syndrome may contribute to an increased susceptibility. Scoliosis can also be hereditary.

There are varying levels of severity of scoliosis. Mild curvatures are usually monitored over time, moderate curves may require bracing, and severe curvatures require surgery. Untreated, severe curvatures can lead to reduced cardiac and respiratory function, pain, and in severe cases, physical disability. Yearly exams before, during, and after puberty should include a screen for scoliosis. If your child has had open heart surgery, be aware of and ask questions about the spine during annual checkups.

Thyroid Problems. Hypothyroidism, or an inadequate production of thyroid hormone, occurs in 10 to 15 percent of people with Down syndrome. Undiagnosed hypothyroidism during puberty will slow or delay growth, and, in females, can delay menstruation. Hyperthyroidism, a condition in which an overabundance of thyroid hormone is produced, can also alter physical development, onset of menstruation, or disturb menstrual flow patterns. The health care guidelines for people with Down syndrome recommend yearly screens (blood tests) to monitor for changes in thyroid function.

Celiac Disease. Celiac disease is a genetic condition that results in an intolerance to gluten, a common protein found in wheat, barley, rye, and possibly oats. The incidence of celiac disease among individuals with Down syndrome is estimated to be around 4 or 5 percent, which is slightly higher than in the general population. If a person has celiac disease, exposure to gluten over time damages the lining of the intestine, making it difficult to absorb nutrients needed for growth and nutrition. Although celiac disease can develop at any age, when it goes undetected during puberty, it can result in reduced rates of growth, shorter stature, and delayed onset of puberty.

The Health Care Guidelines for people with Down syndrome recommend celiac screening (blood test) between the ages of 2 and 3 years old. Since this recommendation is a more recent addition to the guidelines, it's possible older children may have missed being screened as a toddler. Ask your physician if you're unsure whether your child has been tested. If screening has not been done, include it as a part of your child's next physical exam.

All of the above conditions illustrate the importance of preventive healthcare using the Health Care Guidelines for People with Down Syndrome. If you're not familiar with these guidelines, they can be downloaded in narrative or flow sheet form (so healthcare providers can place them directly in your child's chart) by going to www. ds-health.com. Regular checkups with a physician who is knowledgeable about Down syndrome can ensure that your child is developing to his maximum potential.

PENIS GROWTH

After a boy's pubic hair begins to appear, and scrotum and testicles begin growing, his penis will thicken, then grow in length. Although parents of baby boys and young boys with Down syndrome often express concerns regarding the smallness of the penis in childhood, data evaluating males with Down syndrome (Pueschel, 1985) during puberty suggests that there are no distinct differences in genital size of adolescent or adult males with Down syndrome, when compared to similar-aged peers.

As your son's penis grows and his sexual feelings become more intense, erections will become more common. This is due to the increased amounts of hormones flowing through the body during this time.

VOICE CHANGES

Eventually, voice changes will become more noticeable as well. You may notice your son's voice quality becoming inconsistent—for example—changing from high to low, or periodically crackling or squeaking. For others, voice changes will be hardly noticeable. When you are teaching your son about the variety of changes he can anticipate during this period, be sure to identify voice changes as one possible change. Once the larynx is fully grown, your son's voice will begin to sound lower and deeper, and the larnyx will push the Adam's apple forward, causing it to show more.

FACIAL AND BODY HAIR

A year or two after pubic hair initially appears, hair will become more noticeable on other parts of your son's body as well. Typically, hair in the chest and underarm area that may have been present before becomes more noticeable. Early facial hair (usually on the upper lip area) will have a soft appearance, but over the next few years, this hair will become thicker and coarser. Because testosterone continues to be produced throughout a male's life, facial and chest hair will continue to become more apparent beyond 20 years of age.

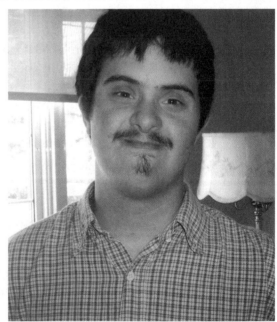

The amount of hair a male ends up with is largely determined by genetics. If other men in your family tend to have lots of body hair, chances are your son will as well. If males in your family are smoother and less hairy, your son will end up looking similar.

Alopecia areata, a condition that causes hair loss, is a bit more common in individuals with Down syndrome. If your son or daughter has this diagnosis, it can affect hair growth and distribution anywhere on the body.

OIL AND SWEAT PRODUCING GLANDS AND ACNE

The skin contains millions of sweat glands that become more active during puberty. In addition, glands near the genitals and under the arms begin working for the first time during puberty, resulting in more sweat produced in more places. Many parents attending my workshops tell me that these new "scents" are most noticeable with increased activity. Sweat itself is mostly water and doesn't, on its own, create an odor. The combination of sweat and bacteria together creates the new for good hygiene routines.

Skin problems, specifically acne, are a fact of life for almost everyone going through puberty. Oil glands located on the face, neck, chest, and back begin working overtime, resulting in more oil than the skin needs. This clogs pores and often leads to acne. Even though teens with Down syndrome have drier skin than most, acne can still be a problem.

Recurrent boils (different from acne) in the genital and buttock area also seem to be more common in teens and adults with Down syndrome and may require more than good hygiene skills to control. Often these conditions require use of antibiotics or special skin washes over longer periods of time, so be sure to see your physician or dermatologist if you have questions or concerns.

GROWTH AND MATURATION OF INTERNAL REPRODUCTIVE ORGANS

Much like menstruation is a sign that a female's internal reproductive organs have reached physical maturity, ejaculation is an indicator that the male reproductive organs are developed and functioning. Although fertility is reduced in males with Down syndrome, there is no evidence to suggest that the ability to ejaculate in boys with Down syndrome is any different than in the general population (see Chapter 11 for more information about fertility). On average, most boys experience their first ejaculation around 13 or 14 years of age.

Erections are not a new phenomenon for your son. Since birth (and even in utero) erections have been occurring. During puberty, however, increased testosterone levels in the bloodstream can cause the penis to be more sensitive to touch, thoughts, or sexual feelings, resulting in more frequent erections. Erections may be triggered by seeing someone who is attractive, experiencing feelings of happiness or excitement, seeing something on television, or having a pleasurable dream. *Spontaneous erections*, or erections that occur for what seems to be no apparent reason, are common as well.

TEACHING YOUR SON ABOUT ERECTIONS AND EJACULATIONS

Helping your son understand what an erection is and how to handle them in socially appropriate ways is another aspect of teaching. If the subject hasn't come up before now, use one of the puberty activities early in this chapter to identify or review the full range of changes he will experience, including erections.

You could explain that most of the time the penis is soft and floppy but sometimes it will get harder and longer. Use the picture in Appendix A-12 to help him see and compare differences between an erect and non-erect penis. It's quite possible your son may not be familiar with the term erection, but may have heard people use other slang terms. For example, words like "hard-on" or "boner" or "woody" may be familiar and can serve as a starting point for teaching new vocabulary. (See Chapter 2 for more information about teaching about the body).

Key Teaching Messages:

- An erection is when the penis gets hard.
- Erections are more common during puberty.
- Erections are normal and happen to all males.
- Erections are private.

Remind your son that during puberty, erections are more common and can happen for no reason at all. Touching, rubbing, or playing with the penis will make an erection more likely to happen, so advise against touching the penis in public places (school or work) and instead encourage him to wait until he is in his private place at home.

HANDLING SPONTANEOUS ERECTIONS

When erections happen in public, your son should have some ideas on how to handle them. During my puberty workshops, fathers often share stories about their own experiences with erections. This discussion usually generates a good list of ideas for "hiding" erections when they occur in public places (even though they are normal, they are still private). Here are some of the ideas dads have shared during my workshops:

■ If you can get to a bathroom, readjust your penis to the side.

If you can't be in private:

■ Try sitting down; the erection will become less noticeable.

■ Place your books, clothes, backpack, or whatever you're carrying on your lap to cover up the erection.

■ Hide your erection with books, notebooks, etc. as you walk.

■ Tie a sweatshirt or jacket around your waist so your front is covered

■ Wear longer, baggier shirts and let them hang out so the crotch area is covered.

■ Wear pants or shorts made from stiffer materials like denim rather than baggy sweats or thin meshes which allow erections to be more noticeable.

■ Exercise.

Reassure your son that erections are normal and all boys experience them, but remind him they are private. He should not tell or show others when an erection occurs but, instead, use one of the strategies above. Explain that as he gets older and moves out of puberty, spontaneous erections generally subside or become less frequent.

Some boys with Down syndrome have more difficulty understanding or are less aware of the implications a visible erection (even with clothes on) can have on others. They will need respectful support and assistance. A friend of mine whose son has Down syndrome told me how angry she became one day while reading her son's school-to-home communication book. The inexperienced male aide who supported her son had written comments in the notebook about her son's erections (how many he had observed on that particular day). The mother was not sure how she was supposed to use this information, but was keenly aware of how many people read his book in a typical school day and felt her son's privacy had been violated.

If your son relies on helpers to get him through his day and he is struggling with handling erections, offer them some strategies for redirecting, preventing erections from being noticeable, or teaching or reinforcing privacy concepts. Seasoned staff are more likely to have useful ideas for handling these situations in healthy and supportive ways.

TEACHING ABOUT EJACULATIONS

Just as menstruation is the benchmark for physical maturity in females, ejaculation is the signal for males that they are reaching the end of puberty, producing sperm

Key Teaching Messages:

■ Ejaculation is when white or yellowish liquid comes out of the penis after rubbing the penis (masturbation).
■ Ejaculations that happen at night while you sleep are called wet dreams. Wet dreams are normal and happen to all boys.
■ Ejaculations are private.
■ My private place for masturbating/ejaculating is _____.

and are potentially capable of producing a child. Ejaculation is technically the release of semen, the fluid that contains sperm, from the body. Initial ejaculations occur most often during masturbation. If your son does not masturbate (this is completely normal as well), his first ejaculation will more likely occur during sleep (nocturnal emissions or wet dreams). Just like many other aspects of puberty, there is a wide variation in age at which first ejaculation can occur. On average, boys begin ejaculating between the ages of thirteen and fourteen.

Use the pictures in Appendix A-13 while you share the teaching messages above. Teach your son that because fluid comes out during ejaculation, he will need to clean the genital area following masturbation or after a wet dream (see Chapter 6 for more information about masturbation in puberty). Keeping a supply of wipes near the bed can be a handy and private way for your son to handle clean up. If your son is fairly independent with showering and bathing, you could suggest he masturbate at these times. This eliminates the need for clean up. If you believe your son may have difficulty distinguishing between the shower at home and showers at school or at the gym, this may not be a good idea.

Teaching about erections and ejaculation can be a natural lead-in to more in-depth discussions about reproduction and pregnancy. If your son seems interested, add on information and move to the next level. You could begin a discussion about reproduction by saying: "The white stuff (fluid) that comes out of the penis during masturbation (when you rub the penis) or during a wet dream will have sperm in it. Sperm is one of the parts needed to make a baby. Do you know what else is needed?"

Use the pictures of fertilization and reproduction in Appendix A-17 as you provide explanations. Let your child be your guide for how much detail you provide. If he loses interest, seems bored, or is insistent on doing something else, choose another time to share information. If he seems interested, curious, or continues to ask questions, keep going. The concepts of intercourse, fertilization, and reproduction are abstract and usually require multiple discussions and clarification over time. If you have not introduced these ideas prior to puberty, linking physical changes with the capacity to reproduce is a natural time to begin teaching.

Teaching Activity: "Male Decision Clouds"

Use the decision cloud template in Appendix B-1 and apply it to common situations your child is likely to experience during puberty. (See page 128 in Chapter 7 for instructions on using decision clouds.) Use this activity to introduce ideas for social appropriateness, review information, or evaluate learning. Write any of the problem situations listed below (or one not listed that your son encounters) at the top of the cloud and help him come up with some possible solutions. This will work with individuals who have question-answering abilities. Some examples of usable situations are:

1. You get an erection in the hallway at school. What do you do?
2. You are getting pimples (zits) on your face. What could you do?
3. Your penis itches during class. What could you do?
4. You notice wet spots on your sheets when you wake up. What might have happened? What could you do?
5. You want to masturbate (or touch your private parts) but you are in public. What could you do?
6. A classmate says you have BO. What do you do?
7. You have a question about puberty. Who can you talk to?
8. A student at school touches your penis. What should you do?
9. You get sexually aroused at work (school). What could you do?

Teaching Activity: "Public or Private Behaviors"

Use this activity to evaluate learning and to review and reinforce public and private concepts and appropriate behavior during puberty. Write the behaviors listed below (or illustrate if you need to) on index cards. Use the public and private symbols in the back of the book to create two piles. Read or hand your child one card at a time and ask him to decide if the behavior would be public or private and then place it in the appropriate pile.

- Ask where the restroom is
- Shave
- Touch my private parts (masturbate)
- Ask a question about my body or sexuality
- Talk about sexual feelings
- Get dressed
- Put on deodorant
- Buy deodorant
- Take a shower
- Use good manners
- Have a physical by a doctor

PARENT PREPARATION FOR MOTHERS AND FATHERS OF GIRLS

Signs Your Daughter Is Approaching Puberty

Researchers have found there are no significant differences in the progression of puberty in girls with Down syndrome compared to girls without Down syndrome. Just as there are wide variations in how physical development occurs with all girls, there will be differences among girls with Down syndrome as well. Weight, overall health, and genetic factors will help determine the timing of puberty and onset of menstruation for your daughter. For a large majority of girls, however, the physical changes that occur during puberty do tend to follow a pattern. Being aware of the sequence can help you know what to expect and when to begin sharing information with your child.

The increased production of hormones causes physical changes that tend to follow a somewhat predictable pattern (with some variation). Typically, physicians can monitor your daughter's progression through puberty using the Tanner Stages. These stages can describe specific patterns and characteristics of body changes.

BREAST DEVELOPMENT

One of the first signs of physical maturation in girls are changes in the breast (*thelarche*). Early breast changes can be subtle and may appear simply as raised areas around the nipples. These slight elevations in tissue are called "breast buds." A large majority (about 95 percent) of girls begin developing breast buds sometime between the ages of 9 and 13. If your daughter does not experience breast changes by the age of 13, speak with your physician.

A general rule of thumb I often share with parents is that once breast development begins, expect menstruation to begin within two years. Uneven growth (one breast growing faster that the other), pain or tenderness, or swelling as the breasts are growing are normal and common experiences for many girls. If you have questions about your daughter's stage of development speak with your physician. Medical professionals use rating scales for breast maturity to help them determine the stage of development your daughter may be in. The rating scales (also called Tanner stages) for breast development include five stages (see the chart on page 73).

When breast development falls within stages 2 and 3 in the maturity ratings or you can see your daughter's developing breast buds through clothing, it's time to think about getting your daughter's first bra. Although bras are not actually necessary to keep breasts healthy, they can provide breast support during exercise or activity. Bras come in a variety of styles, colors, and fabric, so make sure your daughter goes shopping with you and is an active part of the decision-making process.

Because little support is actually needed in the early stages of breast development *training bras* are a popular choice for young girls. These bras are designed for girls who are just beginning to develop breasts (A to AAA cup), and are easy to put on, much like a T-shirt. Styles are generally made of comfortable cottons with no seams, reducing the chances of chafing, itching, and irritation. For girls with Down syndrome

TANNER STAGES—Female Physical Development

Stage 1
- preadolescent body
- enlargement of uterus and ovaries

Stage 2
- breast budding begins (small raised areas)
- areola (area around nipple) darkens and diameter increases
- presence of pubic hair
- adolescent height spurt begins
- hips widen
- increases in fat

Stage 3
- breast enlargement continues
- spreading, darkening, and thickening of pubic hair
- ancillary hair growth (underarm)
- vaginal growth, mucous production
- height spurt peaks

Stage 4
- breast growth close to complete
- pubic hair pattern resembles adult but sparser
- menarche (menstruation begins)
- oil glands approaching adult size and function

Stage 5
- breast growth complete
- adult-sized reproductive organs
- pubic hair denser and fully distributed in genital area
- maximum height almost complete
- body shape resembles that of mature female

who have difficulty with small closures and fasteners, training or sports bras are a less complicated option initially. Nowadays, there are many varieties and styles that don't require advanced fine motor skills.

If your daughter experiences sensory issues, she may need to adjust gradually to wearing a bra. Involve her in the trying-on and buying process to ensure maximum comfort and fit and let her be your guide for what feels most comfortable. Washing the bras a few times before wearing, removing any tags, or having your daughter wear the bra for gradually increasing increments of time (with rewards, as necessary) may help.

As your daughter adjusts to wearing a bra, you may notice her hands venturing up her shirt to fidget, adjust, or itch. Some girls and women do experience increased "nipple itchiness" at certain times during the menstrual cycle (often around the time of ovulation), so feel the need to get relief. Other girls may develop a new interest and understanding of the pleasures of nipple stimulation. Whatever the reason, teach your daughter that touching her breasts or bra are private behaviors. Help her iden- tify appropriate places at home, school, and in the community where she can make adjustments. Other things to consider:

- Have your physician check for skin conditions that might be present.
- Ensure the bra fits properly.
- Provide non-drying soaps with moisturizers (e.g., Dove) to use in the shower or bath.
- Encourage use of moisturizers following baths or showers since skin under the bra can get chafed and irritated, especially during winter months.
- Use milder, less irritating laundry detergents to wash underclothing.

PUBIC AND AXILLARY HAIR

Around the same time breast development begins, hair in the pubic area, vulva (the folds of skin and tissue between the legs), and under the arms will begin to ap- pear (*adrenarche*). In the early stages, this hair is almost unnoticeable and can appear very light in color. Over time, these hairs increase in numbers, and become thicker, curlier, and usually darker.

HEIGHT AND WEIGHT CHANGES

Among the most obvious changes associated with puberty are increases in height and weight. Females with Down syndrome experience growth spurts similar to their peers but with slightly less dramatic results:

Age	Average height (50th percentile) of Girls with Down syndrome*	Average height of Girls without Down syndrome**
9—beginning of puberty	47.5 inches 120.6 cm	52 inches 132.1 cm
16—end of puberty	56.5 inches 143.5 cm	64 inches 162.6 cm
Total average growth	9 inches 22.86 cm	12 inches 30.48 cm

* Down syndrome growth charts
** National Center for Health Statistics (NCHS) percentiles

Keep in mind that the growth spurts that occur during puberty can be uneven. For example, weight gains may occur before height changes do, creating a sense of temporary "chubbiness." This often creates anxiety for families who may have a heightened awareness of weight changes in their children with Down syndrome. If your child is on the chubby side, puberty can be an opportunity for her to slim down as a result of height changes. Consult your physician and/or a nutritionist to discuss dietary and exercise changes that can be beneficial during this time.

When both of my daughters stopped growing (after a year of no increases on the measuring wall) I talked with them about paying close attention to their body and hunger so they could be sure they weren't eating more than they needed.

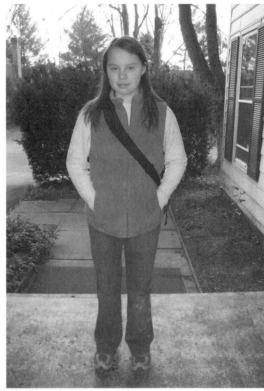

In order for menstruation to occur, fat percentages in the body must be adequate. This explains why chubbier, larger girls may menstruate earlier, and very small, petite girls later. It also explains why female athletes who have lowered fat percentages may not menstruate at all. Since menstruation is one of the last changes during puberty, your daughter will likely be close to her full height once she gets her first period.

Girls with Down syndrome, like boys, may also be susceptible to various health problems that can affect growth. See the section on "Health Changes That Affect Growth" on pages 66-67.

PERSPIRATION, BODY ODOR, AND ACNE

*S*weat glands become more active during this time, which means odors that are new and unfamiliar become more common. For all kids these changes require the development of good self-care and hygiene routines. Showering more frequently, using deodorant, grooming, and the development of self-care routines become especially important during this time (see Chapter 8, page 137). Also see the section on Oil and Sweat Producing Glands on page 68.

GROWTH AND MATURATION OF INTERNAL REPRODUCTIVE ORGANS

A girl's internal reproductive organs develop throughout puberty but the official sign that physical maturation is nearly complete is *menarche,* or the onset of menstruation. Although there is considerable variation, the large majority (over 90 percent) of girls begin menstruating sometime between the ages of 10½ and 14½ . The average age that menstruation begins in the United States is at 12½ years of age for Caucasian females, and younger for African-American and Hispanic girls. The most important factors that will determine when your daughter begins to menstruate include genetic factors, ethnicity, health, and nutrition.

Studies have found that girls with Down syndrome begin menstruation at ages similar to girls without Down syndrome. For example, Sigmund Pueschel found in a study of 51 females with Down syndrome that their average onset of menstruation was 12 years, 6 months.

Girls (with and without Down syndrome) who begin menstruating early are commonly irregular and often do not ovulate at first. Over time, however, many girls with Down syndrome do become regular and do experience ovulatory cycles (Pueschel and Scola). Based on data collected thus far on girls and women with Down syndrome and the cases of pregnancies that have been documented, you should presume that your daughter is fertile once she begins to menstruate.

MENSTRUATION BASICS

It's likely been a few years since you studied the mechanics of menstruation. A review of the four phases of the menstrual cycle can increase your awareness of what your daughter is experiencing throughout the month as well as help you understand basic physiology behind the symptoms.

The cyclical nature of the menstrual cycle is created by an intricate communication and feedback system involving the ovaries, hormones, and the brain. The phases of the cycle look like this:

Pre-ovulatory Phase (or Proliferative Phase). Immediately following menstruation (sloughing of the endometrial lining), low levels of estrogen in the bloodstream trigger the hypothalamus (situated right next to the pituitary gland in the brain) to send GnRH (Gonadotropin Releasing Hormone) to the pituitary gland. This message triggers the pituitary gland to release *FSH (Follicle Stimulating Hormone)*, which does exactly that. It stimulates follicles, or egg sacs, inside the ovaries, to begin to mature and ripen. Multiple follicles are usually affected by FSH, so numerous egg sacs can begin maturing simultaneously. This ripening process inside the ovary produces the hormone *estrogen*. Eventually, one follicle will dominate (*Graafian follicle*) and produce higher levels of estrogen in the bloodstream. This triggers the pituitary gland to stop releasing FSH and begin producing Luteinizing Hormone (LH).

Ovulatory Phase. A rise in LH causes the mature follicle or egg to be released from the ovary. The actual release of the egg is called *ovulation*. This is the shortest (24 to 49 hours) and most fertile phase of a woman's menstrual cycle. Common symptoms experienced by women during this phase include:

- Mittelschmertz (German for "middle pain")—mild to severe pain on alternating sides of the lower abdomen around the time of ovulation
- Softening and opening of the cervical os (entry to the uterus)
- Increases in vaginal discharge (usually clear, more watery) or feelings of wetness
- Abdominal bloating
- Breast sensitivity (different from breast tenderness)
- Itchy nipples

Post-Ovulatory Phase (Secretory Phase). After the egg has been released, the remaining matter in the ovary (referred to as the *corpus luteum*) occupies a large portion of the ovary and acts as a temporary gland by producing and secreting the hormone *progesterone*. Increases in progesterone (and smaller levels of estrogen) cause blood and other tissue to build the endometrial lining in the uterus. In the event the egg that has just been released is fertilized, the uterine lining will remain intact so the developing embryo can be nourished and protected. More often, the lining will not be needed and the corpus luteum inside the ovary will disintegrate, progesterone levels will drop, the uterine lining will begin to break down, and menstruation (or the release of the endometrial lining) will begin. During the post-ovulatory phase, hormone levels in body are at their highest levels which is why many women experience premenstrual symptoms a week or so prior to menstruation. Common physical symptoms associated with this phase include:

- Fatigue
- Breast tenderness/fullness
- Abdominal cramping
- Thicker, stickier vaginal discharge
- Mood swings
- Irritability

Menstrual Phase. The first day of bleeding is considered to be day one of a woman's menstrual cycle. During this time, the female hormones estrogen and progesterone are at erratic levels in the bloodstream as the blood-rich uterine lining begins to break down and be expelled. The average length of time of the menstrual phase is three to five days. By the time a woman is finished menstruating, hormone levels in the bloodstream are at their lowest. This is not coincidentally a point in time when many women have fewest symptoms and feel their best.

Are Girls Starting Puberty Earlier?

There is no disputing that the average age of menarche, the initial onset of menstruation, in this country has dropped significantly over the past few centuries. Back in the mid-1800s, the average age of the onset of menstruation was 16. Today, girls in North America are likely to get their first period sometime between the ages of 12 and 13 years of age. Most experts attribute the shift to better nutrition.

Although this trend is showing signs of slowing, some professionals advocate lowering the average "normal" age for the appearance of secondary sex characteristics. Endocrinologists, however, argue that lowering the prevailing standards can interfere with the ability to assess conditions that, when diagnosed early, respond effectively to treatment (e.g., precocious puberty). If you notice initial signs of puberty (breast development, pubic hair) *before* the age of 8 in your daughter or 9 in your son, speak with your physician.

Teaching Your Daughter about Menstruation

Your own attitudes about menstruation will be the single most important factor in how your daughter comes to view her own menstrual cycles. Many mothers I speak with had few discussions and very little information about puberty or menstruation as a teen. Realize that these experiences will affect how you view puberty and menstruation in your own daughter. Presenting menstruation as a normal, healthy, and natural process can help your daughter feel more positive about the experience.

It's easy to feel overwhelmed with the tasks associated with helping your daughter learn how to handle menstruation. The level of detail you decide to include in your explanation will depend on several things. First, your timing. If your daughter is now

Key Teaching Messages:

- Menstruation (having a period) is one of the changes that happens during puberty.
- Getting a period means blood from inside the body comes out from an opening between your legs (vagina).
- The blood that you see during your period is a sign your body is healthy and working as it should.

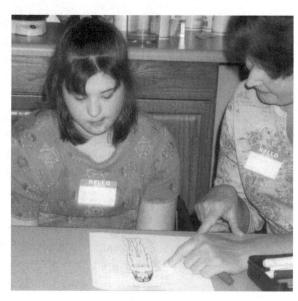

experiencing her first period but has had little preparation, be positive and frame menstruation as normal and healthy. Your goal in this situation is to help your daughter master the use of pads while alleviating fear and anxiety. Second, your daughter's level of understanding will determine how much detail you provide. Begin with more basic messages and add on over time as goals are reaching.

As your daughter becomes more comfortable with using a pad, offer a simple explanation of menstruation. Talk to her (or remind her if you've covered this in the past) about the reproductive organs inside her body that have been growing and changing since she began puberty. Spend time becoming familiar with the illustrations at the back of the book (Appendix A-15 and A-16) so you can feel comfortable using them to teach your daughter about menstruation. The drawings include what I call "x-ray" pictures (pictures that show the full body, but also illustrate proportional-sized reproductive organs in their natural locations) so your daughter can view pictures as you talk. You could have your daughter use her finger or pencil to trace the path of the blood from the uterus, down the vagina, and into the air space between legs to illustrate blood flow and why a pad is needed.

Let your daughter know that getting her period is a sign that her inside body parts are working as they should and that her body is normal and healthy and that all woman have periods. If your daughter understands those concepts, you can add on the role menstruation plays in reproduction. Use the pictures of fertilization and reproduction in Appendix A-16 and A-17 (or other suggested resources) as you provide explanations. Let your child be your guide for how much detail you provide. If she seems interested, add information and move to the next level. If she seems bored or is insistent on doing something else, choose another time to share information. You could begin a discussion about reproduction by saying:

- *"Now that you have started your period, let me show you what happens inside your body every month."* (use pictures to illustrate ovulation)
- *"Even though you can't see it, once a month your ovary will release an egg and it will move through the tube. If the egg joins together with sperm from a man, a woman can get pregnant. Do you know ways the sperm and egg get together…how this happens?"*
- *"The egg inside a woman is one of the parts needed to make a baby. Do you know what else is needed?"*

How Much Information Is Enough?

The Scarborough Model, developed by Willie Scarborough and made popular by Winifred Kempton, a pioneer in the field of sexuality education for people with developmental disabilities, can be used to help you match and prioritize information about sexuality with your child's cognitive level. Begin with most important information and add on over time.

EXAMPLE: Teaching about Menstruation

Level 1—Self-care, hygiene, and socially appropriate behavior.
  Examples of attitudes, information, or skills taught at this level:
  - Normalizing menstruation (reducing fear & anxiety)
  - Correct use of feminine hygiene products
  - Hygiene skills (hand-washing, handling accidents, etc.)
  - Social appropriateness during menstruation (private nature of menstruation and pad changes, appropriate people to talk to if your daughter needs help or has questions)

Level 2—Health and biological aspects of menstruation
  Examples of attitudes, information, or skills taught at this level:
  - The biology of menstruation (menstrual cycle, length of period, etc.)
  - Common symptoms of menstruation (mood swings, cramps,etc.)
  - Strategies for alleviating menstrual symptoms

Level 3—Social and psychological implications of menstruation
  Examples of attitudes, information, or skills taught at this level:
  - The role menstruation plays in reproduction
  - Birth control

This chapter focuses primarily on teaching content in Levels 1 and 2; advanced information focusing on Level 3 is shared in Chapter 11.

The concept of intercourse, fertilization, and reproduction are abstract concepts that usually require multiple discussions and clarification over time. If you have not introduced these ideas prior to puberty, linking physical changes with the capacity to reproduce is a natural time to begin teaching.

TRACKING PERIODS

If your daughter does not have a calendar, purchase one. Show her how to mark the start date of her period and each consecutive day she menstruates. This can be done with symbols, or a code that makes sense for her. Let her know that at some point she will get her periods around the same time every month and that it will usually last 4 to 7 days. (You can inform her that it is very common for girls her age to have irregular periods or missed periods during the first year, but that some girls have regular menstrual patterns right away.)

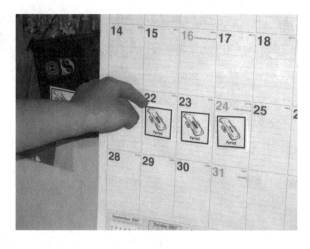

Key Teaching Messages:

■ Periods will come once a month and last 4 to 7 days.

Encourage your daughter to mark the estimated start date on the following month as well. A few days before her period is scheduled to begin again, remind and prepare her. Review pad use with her and restock pad supplies if necessary. Charting periods with her until she's familiar with her own unique cycle can help her anticipate and plan for her period and achieve independence more rapidly. If the calendar approach is too abstract, help her learn to identify physical signs and symptoms that, for her, indicate her period is about to begin (see box on menstrual cycle and common symptoms).

PERIODS ARE PRIVATE

Once your daughter has started menstruating, teach her about privacy rules associated with menstruation. Point out that menstruation is a function of the private parts of the body and therefore needs to be discussed and talked about in private. Identify designated people (parents, teacher, school nurse, etc.) she can speak with if she has questions or needs assistance.

If you're a single father raising a daughter with Down syndrome, ask a female relative or friend to be a resource when your daughter has questions or to help teach these concepts. It's important for all girls (and boys) to have a person they can go to with questions or concerns.

Key Teaching Messages:

■ Menstruation is private.
■ At home, you can talk to _____ if you have questions or concerns.
■ At school, you can talk to _____ if you have questions or concerns.

ALWAYS CHECK FOR UNDERSTANDING

All girls who have not started menstruating or have little experience have difficulty understanding the finer details of how the body works and implications for self-care. I remember an eight-year-old girl (without a cognitive disability) who left one of my puberty workshops thinking that once she started her period, she'd be bleeding every day until menopause.

When my daughter first started having periods in sixth grade, she ruined a lot of underwear. I discovered later that she would stop wearing pads before her cycle was over. Even though I would remind her each morning of her period that she should still be wearing a pad because her period wasn't over, she would sometimes lie to me about having a pad on and then go off to school without one. Several times I got called to the nurse's office to bring her changes of clothes. Finally, I got a clue as to why she wasn't wearing her pads—she told me that she'd decided she was NOT going to have any babies, so she didn't need to have a period. She apparently thought that the blood flow was under her control, like urine, and that she would be able to keep it from coming out if she wanted to. I told her in so many words that she couldn't hold the blood in, and I could tell by her reaction that this is what she'd been thinking.

The first time my daughter had her period, she thought it was a one-time deal. She said something to me like, "Megan said she got her period when she was eleven. Do you think she still has it?" She seemed to think that after you "got" your period, you were done with the whole affair. Even though I told her right then that girls and women "got" their periods every month for years and years, it didn't sink in. She was quite dismayed when she got another period the next month.

Presenting lots of information about menstruation (or any topic for that matter) all at once can be overwhelming. Many girls will give you cues that will help you assess their level of comprehension and determine whether additional teaching is needed. All of these examples point to the need of ongoing communication, open discussions, and the need to reinforce and clarify information over time.

TEACHING FEMININE HYGIENE PRODUCT USAGE

With advance preparation, concrete instruction, and ongoing review and repetition, most girls with cognitive disabilities do quite well learning to use a pad and manage their periods. As with anything else, girls with Down syndrome often need more time to adjust to the idea of menstruation (one reason proactive education is so important) and develop menstrual hygiene skills over longer periods of time. Eventually, though, most girls with Down syndrome do learn how to manage their periods appropriately. In a survey of twenty-nine menstruating women with Down syndrome, the large majority did not require help with menstrual hygiene. Six of the twenty-nine needed assistance at times with changing pads (Pueschel). Anecdotal information shared by mothers of daughters in my workshops supports this finding.

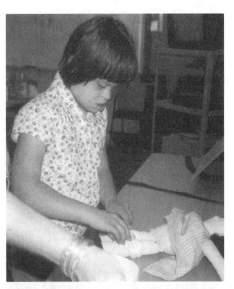

A task analysis for teaching pad usage is listed below. Keep in mind that this process can be made more or less detailed depending on your daughter's individual needs.

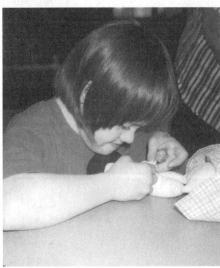

Key Teaching Messages:

- When you get your period (or notice blood) you will need to use a pad.
- Using a pad stops the blood from getting on your clothes.
- Changing a pad is private.

TASK ANALYSIS—TEACHING FEMININE HYGIENE PRODUCT USAGE

SKILL #1—RECOGNIZE BLOOD AS BEGINNING OF MENSTRUATION

The initial introduction of the blood-comes-out-of-your-body idea can be alarming and scary. Many girls with and without disabilities have significant aversions to blood, associating it with pain (blood draws), illness, or injury. As a result, thinking about or seeing blood coming from a part of the body that doesn't normally bleed can seem unnatural. Framing menstruation in a "normal and healthy" context right from the start can help alleviate some of these fears.

Key Teaching Messages:

■ Getting a period means blood from inside the body comes out from an opening between your legs (vagina).
■ The blood you see during your period is a sign your body is healthy and working like it should.
■ When you get your period (or notice blood) you will need to put on a pad.

If your daughter has not started menstruating, it will be helpful to talk with her about ways she will know her period has started. For example, spots of blood that appear on her underwear or on toilet paper may not be red, but more brownish in color initially. Assure her that periods generally start slow and gradually and that she will have time to find a pad or get help if needed. The important message is that if she notices spotting, she needs to take action. If you're not sure your daughter can handle this on her own, especially in the beginning, role play with her how to ask for help and identify specific people she can go to for help.

I remember the day my daughter came home from school and told me she got her period at school (this was after about four years of menstruating regularly). I was all ready to do the wash but she told me she put on a pad right away and that she didn't wait. When I asked her how she knew she had her period, she told me "she just felt it." It was clearly a breakthrough for us with independence.

SKILL #2—LOCATE PADS

Your daughter should know where feminine hygiene products are located in your home. Identify a place in the bathroom that's within her reach and easily accessible. If you suspect your daughter is nearing the time when she will begin menstruating, create a plan for what to do if she begins her period when she is not at home. At school girls often carry an extra pad in their pencil pouch (opaque ones work best), purses, or backpacks. Speak with your daughter's teacher to see how these situations are typically handled. Whatever your plan, share it with your child so she understands what to do. Review the plan often.

During community outings to public places, look for portable pad dispensers located in public restrooms. Explain what they are and encourage your daughter to try them. Knowing where these boxes are and how to use them is another option for her in an emergency.

SKILL #3—IDENTIFY PRIVATE LOCATION

Whether at home or in public, explain to your daughter that changing a pad is a private behavior. No matter where she is, pad changes should occur in the bathroom behind closed doors.

Buying Pads

Once your daughter has started menstruating, show her where feminine hygiene products are located at your local grocery or drugstore. Encourage her to be an active participant in selecting which pads might work best for her. Plan to purchase a few different types of pads initially so she can experiment and find one she likes. Let her know that most women choose pads based on what feels most comfortable, how much protection will be needed, or how easy it is to use. If you haven't used pads yourself in a while, you may want to buy a few different kinds in order to become familiar with unique pad features (e.g., ultra thins, winged).

Pay close attention to packaging or other characteristics that may make it easier or harder for your daughter to use the pads. For example, some pads are enclosed in difficult-to-open wrapping, have complicated "wings," or are so large that discreetly carrying them or disposing of them is difficult.

Three factors to bear in mind when selecting products:

1. **Pad Size**—If your daughter is small and petite, pads designed for adult women will seem cumbersome and too large. Many companies have developed petite-sized products that are narrower in width and shorter in length, improving fit for younger girls. As your daughter's body continues to grow and develop, traditional-sized pads will fit more appropriately.

2. **Deodorant**—Television ads targeted at menstruating women work hard to convince us that deodorized feminine hygiene products are important for optimal hygiene. In reality, the vagina is a self-cleaning organ so douches, sprays, or other products marketed to "clean" the vagina are unnecessary. In fact, using these products can cause irritation or allergic reactions. Proper hygiene and frequent showers during menstruation should be all that is required.

3. **Absorbency Rates**—Feminine hygiene products include package adjectives such as light, regular, super, super plus. These words are designed to help women match the level of protection that is needed with absorbency characteristics of the product. For example, products labeled "super" or "super plus" are designed to be used during times when menstrual flow is heaviest. Products described as "lite" are designed for lighter flow. It will take time for your daughter to become familiar with her own unique menstrual flow pattern and then adjust to the type of pad that is needed. Some parents encourage the use of a more absorbent pad than necessary, just to be safe, until their daughter's pattern is well established. Usually after a year, your daughter's menstrual pattern will become more regular. Once this happens, health experts recommend using feminine hygiene products that most closely match menstrual flow patterns.

Skill #4—Use a Pad Correctly

One of your goals during this time will be to help your daughter learn how to use a pad correctly. There are a variety of teaching strategies that work well. Here are some ideas:

Demonstration. If you feel comfortable, encourage your daughter to watch you manage your periods before she begins her own. For some girls this can be a great way to understand that periods are normal and that all women have them and manage them. While you're demonstrating the steps for pad use, make sure you are in the bathroom

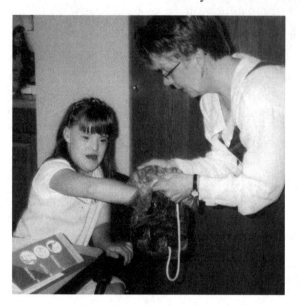

with the door closed in order to reinforce the idea that pad changing is a private activity. Not all mothers feel comfortable modeling this and some may no longer be menstruating, so using alternative teaching strategies is certainly okay.

Following demonstrations, your daughter *will still need* hands-on opportunities to get comfortable touching and handling pads. During my puberty workshops, girls practice pad-changing skills with me modeling alongside them using a sample pair of underwear and their own bag of supplies (various pads and some toilet paper). I am their guide as we move through the steps together. These demonstrations are an opportunity to go over some of the finer points of pad use (e.g., correct positioning of pad in crotch of underwear or amount of pressure it actually takes to make sure your pad is on firmly), to practice fine motor skills associated with using a pad, and to address individual questions and concerns

Visual Aids. There are a handful of resources designed specifically to teach girls and women with cognitive disabilities how to use pads correctly (see below). Unfortunately, many of them are too costly for families. Contact your local Down syndrome group, ARC, UCP, Planned Parenthood or other resource centers to check lending availability. Detailed information on where to purchase these resources can be found in the bibliography.

Visual aids can be useful if retaining information from month to month is a problem for your daughter or if modeling with verbal instruction seems ineffective. If your daughter reads, a simply written step-by-step task list for changing a pad might be helpful. If she prefers pictures, create your own visual task analysis tool (red food coloring can be used to create soiled pads) for teaching steps involved in changing a pad. Digital cameras work well for this. Start by breaking down the task of learning to use a pad into smaller steps. You can decide if your daughter needs more or fewer steps. Some examples of task breakdowns are listed below:

Using a pad (starting period)
1. Close bathroom door
2. Get new pad out of package
3. Sit on toilet (and use if necessary)
4. Open new pad
5. Stick pad in panties
6. Pull up panties (and pants)
7. Wash hands

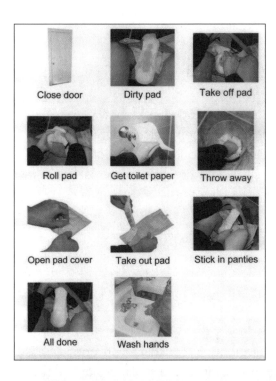

Close door | Dirty pad | Take off pad
Roll pad | Get toilet paper | Throw away
Open pad cover | Take out pad | Stick in panties
All done | Wash hands

Changing a used pad
1. Close bathroom door
2. Get new pad out of package
3. Sit on toilet (and use if necessary)
4. Remove used pad
5. Fold pad in half
6. Wrap used pad in toilet paper
7. Throw wrapped pad in trash can
8. Open new pad
9. Stick clean pad in panties
10. Pull up underwear (and pants)
11. Wash hands

If you don't want to develop your own teaching tools, there are programs available that can help with this. For example, Picture This® or Boardmaker® software companies both contain pictures for teaching correct pad use.

Visual Aids for Teaching Pad Usage

Resource	Description
Janet's Got Her Period	An Australian book and video for teaching self-care during menstruation. The curriculum and ideas for teaching and problem solving are excellent. The video highlights an Australian mom and her adult daughter with Down syndrome learning about pad changes mostly from her sister. Although the content is good, the Australian accents are thick and some of their vocabulary is regional and not understood by participants in my workshops.
A Girl's Guide to Growing Up	An ethnically diverse, animated video that addresses physical (and psychological) changes during puberty. One of the sections includes instructions on how to use, change, and dispose of pads. The teaching guide that accompanies the video includes a nicely done task analysis (with pictures) for pad changes.
Life Horizons I	This comprehensive slide series includes sections on pad and tampon usage. Actual pictures of women changing pads or tampons are used.
Sexuality Education for People with Severe Developmental Disabilities	Another more limited slide series that includes a section on changing and disposing of menstrual pads

Teaching Activity: "Pretend Periods"

Once you have taught your daughter how to use a pad, encourage her to show you her skills before she actually has a period, or, if she's started, between cycles. Ask her if she'd like to pretend she is having her period and practice using pads. This simulation can help reinforce steps involved in pad changes, desensitize your daughter to the feel of the pad, and allow her to gain confidence with self-care skills.

Teaching Activity: "Using Metal Boxes"

While helping your child become proficient at pad changes, coach her on pad disposal etiquette in public restrooms. If there are metal boxes inside the stalls, explain what they are and why women use them (they are a private way to throw away used pads). If no boxes are present, explain that she will need to fold the pad, wrap it in toilet paper, and carry it unobtrusively to the nearest garbage can.

Skill #5—Know When to Change a Used Pad

If your daughter has just started having periods, she will need considerable time to become familiar with menstrual flow patterns and understand how they affect the need for pad changes. The difficulty in understanding this concept can be reflected at both ends of the extreme. For example, one mother told me that her daughter changed her pad no matter the amount of blood (even a drop) every hour on the hour. Others have complained that their daughters' pad changes are too infrequent, resulting in regular leakage.

Early on, it's quite all right to ask an aide or teacher at school to provide gentle and discreet reminders. If your daughter has a good sense of time, linking pad changes with clock reading or schedules may work. For example, identify specific times throughout the day (noon, 2:00, 4:00) or events (during lunch, science, gym, before you leave the house) for pad changing. If your daughter uses visual schedules, introducing a picture symbol that can be included on her schedule can help her remember to make pad changes part of her routine.

Skill #6—Stop Using a Pad When Bleeding Stops

Deciding when to discontinue pad use can be tricky. Often clear patterns take time to become established. If your daughter's pattern is for the flow to gradually diminish and eventually stop, remind her that when she no longer sees spots of blood on her pad or after she wipes with toilet paper, she is done with her period and can discontinue pad use. If your daughter's flow is more erratic—for example, she bleeds a few days, stops for a day, then starts up again—encourage mini-pad use in the interim so she can shift to a regular pad when needed.

Teaching Activity: "Time to Change"

One way to help your daughter learn when a pad should be changed is by allowing her to look at and compare pads with different degrees of saturation. To produce samples, drop red food coloring (medicine droppers work well for this) on several pads (ideally the same brand she will be using). One pad should be obviously saturated, and another barely saturated. If you want, add a third or fourth one that is somewhere in the middle to clarify your own standards for when pad changes should occur. You could create samples with panty liners as well. Ask your daughter to examine the pads and point to the one(s) that should be changed.

SKILL #7—USE HYGIENE SKILLS DURING PERIOD

Often when teaching about menstruation and pad usage, it's helpful to review and reinforce hygiene skills. For example, proper hand-washing techniques can be reinforced and reviewed as one of the steps for changing a pad. Emphasizing the importance of cleaning the genital area during menstruation can be revisited as a part of learning how to shower or bathe. Other hygiene issues that will likely come up:

Bathing during Menstruation. If your daughter has particularly heavy periods, inform her of the possibility of dripping when a pad is not in place. This may occur, for example, as she moves into the shower or bath. If your daughter becomes anxious about menstrual blood (usually anxiety decreases over time), consider baths as opposed to showers. Menstrual flow *will* stop once the genital area is submerged in water. Let her know that when she emerges from the water, however, her flow will resume.

Clothing Accidents. Leaks and accidents are inevitable as your daughter is learning how to manage her periods. When you notice blood on your daughter's clothing, be gentle but direct: "I see you have blood on your pants. That happens to me sometimes too. Let me show you what to do when that happens." Or, "It looks like there is blood on your clothes. That happens when there is too much blood on the pad (or too much time has gone by since the pad was changed, or periods are really heavy, or a person stops wearing a pad before their period is done"—whatever the issue may be for you daughter). "Can you think of things you could do to stop the blood from getting on your clothes next time?"

Communicate a clear message that any soiled clothing should be changed before going into public again. Find out how your daughter's school would like to handle clothing changes. Would they prefer your daughter leave an extra set of clothes in her locker? In the health room? Make sure she knows where her spare clothes are kept at school and how to let teachers know she needs them.

Come up with a designated (ideally discreet) place at home where your daughter could at least get the soiled clothes in water when you're not around. Remind her to always use cold water since hot water will set the stain, making it more difficult to remove. Involve her in all other aspects of handling the clean up after she has had some initial training. This is not for punishment purposes, but rather to help her understand that prevention is a more efficient way of handling self-care responsibilities (for more information about accidents, see below).

IF YOUR DAUGHTER STILL WEARS PULL-UPS

Many families wonder what to do if their daughter is approaching puberty and is not yet toilet trained. Diapers or pull-ups alone will not provide the protection that is needed once menstruation begins, so use of a pad with the diaper will still be necessary. The teaching process will be similar but instead of inserting the pad in underwear, your daughter will place the pad inside the crotch area of the diaper or pull-up. Pad changes should occur regularly, usually every two to three hours. Generally, girls with more significant needs are more likely to need physical assistance along with verbal instructions (see Chapter 8 for levels of physical prompts).

TEACHING TAMPON USE

Although few girls I know (or mothers, for that matter) have been comfortable attempting to use tampons initially, I do include instructions on how to use tampons during my workshops. This is done primarily through the use of slides, pictures, and other visuals. Most parents are more interested in helping their daughters master the use of pads before moving to tampons, but even if your daughter doesn't use tampons on a regular basis, she may be interested in trying them periodically for swimming.

Because the tampon is placed inside the body, learning how to insert and remove one is less concrete and more difficult for inexperienced girls. If your daughter wants to try using tampons at some point, here are some tips:

- Using tampons requires a clear understanding of external female anatomy. Use the diagram in Appendix A-14 to help your daughter identify the vaginal opening. Since vulvas can look different in real life than they do in pictures, encourage your daughter to also view the openings between her legs using a handheld mirror. After she has washed her hands, have her touch and feel the vaginal opening so she understands where tampons are inserted. See if she can insert a clean finger into her vaginal opening. If she struggles with this, use a hand-over-hand prompt to guide her in the right direction. Obviously, this should be done in a private place, preferably when you are not rushed for time.
- Let her take apart a tampon. Explain that the cotton part is what is inserted into the vagina and is the part that actually absorbs the blood and prevents the blood from getting on her underwear. The cardboard or plastic part is there to help get the cotton part into the vagina. It does not stay in the body!!
- Make sure your daughter understands that tampons, when inserted correctly, cannot get lost or travel inside the body, but sometimes can be hard to reach. Show her the diagram of the internal organs in Appendix A-15. With a pencil, draw a tampon in the vagina so she has some perspective of where the tampon sits

after insertion. If the string is not visible, direct her to squat on her legs and bear down (like she's having a bowel movement) in order to bring the tampon closer to the vaginal opening. Usually the tampon can then be felt and easily removed.

- Slim or junior tampons can make early use easier. These products are smaller, thinner, and tend to be easier to insert.
- Tampons with the rounded tip applicators seem to work best, and plastic is typically easier to insert than cardboard brands.
- Rubbing a small amount of water-based lubricant such as KY Jelly around the tip of the applicator can facilitate insertion. Be careful, though—too much lubricant can make the tampon applicator slippery and difficult to manipulate.
- If your daughter is comfortable touching her vagina but has difficulty working the applicator, try tampon brands that can be inserted directly into the vagina without an applicator.

When my daughter was learning to use tampons, I bought a few boxes and had her simply practice getting the tampon out of the wrapper and then pushing it to get the cotton part out. The repetitiveness of opening and pushing, opening and pushing, opening and pushing helped her master one of the fine motor skills necessary for tampon use. After that we worked on vaginal insertion.

- Knowing when it's time to change a tampon is a little trickier since it can't be seen like a pad. It takes considerably more practice than knowing when to change a pad. Help your daughter pay attention to sensory or visual cues that could indicate a tampon is ready to be changed. Blood on the string, spotting in her underwear, or a feeling of "fullness" inside her vagina are examples. I encourage consistent mini-pad use in conjunction with tampon use in case some leakage occurs. Scheduled changes based on individual menstrual flow patterns (e.g., every two hours during the first few days of period) are critical.
- Let your daughter know that tampons, when inserted correctly, should *not* feel uncomfortable (advice many moms wish they had received). If wearing a tampon seems too uncomfortable for your daughter even though it appears to be inserted correctly, speak with your healthcare provider.

WHAT IS A HYMEN?

The hymen is a thin sheath of membrane-like tissue that can completely or partially cover the opening to the vagina. Historically, the presence of an intact hymen was used to confirm virginity. Today we know that the absence of a hymen is not an accurate indication of prior sexual activity. Physical activity, stretching exercises, or masturbation are common ways a hymen, if present, can break or stretch. If tampon insertion seems difficult, your daughter has significant discomfort or pain during insertion, or the tampon gets stuck often, it may mean her hymen is partially or fully intact and tampon use will be more difficult. Speak with your physician or nurse practitioner if you have concerns.

Menstrual Hygiene—Common Issues Among Inexperienced Learners

The need to teach and reinforce rules of social etiquette related to menstruation is fairly common. Sometimes social inappropriateness is due to lack of awareness of public and private concepts or inexperience with applying these concepts to the many new situations that surface during puberty. Other times your daughter may be unclear about who she can talk to about private matters. It's difficult to predict and plan for all possible problems, but it is common for girls with Down syndrome to need ongoing coaching and support as new experiences and situations arise.

Teaching Activity: "Female Puberty Decision Clouds"

Use the decision cloud template in Appendix B-1 and apply it to common situations your daughter is likely to experience during puberty. (See page 128 in Chapter 7 for instructions on using Decision Clouds.) Use this activity to introduce ideas for social appropriateness, review information, or to evaluate learning. Write any of the problem situations listed below (or one not listed that your daughter encounters) at the top of the cloud and help her come up with some possible solutions. Depending on your daughter's question-answering abilities, you may be able to ask her an open-ended questions such as "What would you do if" or you may want to suggest several possible solutions and let her indicate which she thinks is a good one. Some examples of usable situations are:

- You get your *first* period during school.
- You are getting pimples (zits) on your face.
- Your breast itches during class (work).
- You start your period at school (or work) and weren't expecting it.
- Someone asks you to go swimming and you have your period.
- It's time to change your pad but you don't have one.
- Your private parts itch during class (work).
- You notice blood on your underwear and pants while changing your pad.
- You notice a strong odor while you are changing your pad.
- You get sexually aroused at work.
- A classmate says you have BO.
- You have a question about your period. Who can you talk to?
- You have a question about your body. Who can you ask?
- You run out of pads at home.
- A student at school touches your breast.
- Your friend asks you to go to the movies but you have cramps from your period.

Teaching Activity: "Public or Private Behaviors"

Use this activity to teach social appropriateness, review and reinforce public and private concepts during puberty, or evaluate learning. Write the behaviors listed below (or illustrate if you need to) on index cards. Use the public and private illustration in Appendix B-2 to create two piles. Read or hand your child one card at a time and ask her to decide which pile (public or private) is appropriate.

- Ask where the restroom is
- Shave
- Touch my private parts
- Ask a question about my body
- Talk about sexual feelings
- Get dressed
- Put on deodorant
- Buy deodorant
- Take a shower
- Use good manners
- Be examined by a doctor
- Change my pad (or tampon)
- Buy a bra
- Buy menstrual pads or tampons
- Fix my bra strap
- Scratch my vulva

ACCIDENTS

As a puberty education instructor, I frequently speak with families about the difficulties their daughters with Down syndrome may have managing menstruation. (I should point out that they don't tend to call me when things are fine. More often I'm a magnet for problems.) Accidentally getting blood on the underwear is one of the most common ones. Accidents will happen, but when they occur repeatedly over long periods of time, you may have to play detective to identify potential causes.

One common cause of accidents is incorrect pad placement. Sometimes pads are placed too high or low in the panties, other times pads have different looking tops and bottoms creating confusion, or sometimes pads move with activity or improper fit. Putting underwear on backwards can also affect how well the pad fits. If pad placement is the problem, use a laundry pen (so it doesn't wash off) to trace lines at the top and/or bottom of the pad in your daughter's underwear. This becomes a visual cue for where to line up the pad in the underwear. Make sure the pads are not huge or too small; this affects pad movement as well.

Some girls place the pad correctly, but pad saturation occurs. One obvious solution is to switch to a higher absorbency pad. When your daughter is first starting her period, it is trickier to predict what her flow patterns will be like. Over time, however, her periods will become more individualized and familiar. Using a higher absorbency pad during heaviest flow days or at night can prevent saturation. If your daughter is just learning how to manage her period and/or you know there are limited opportunities for pad changes during the school day, you may want to purchase heavier absorbency pads for use at school, then resume more regular pad changes at home. If your daughter showers or bathes daily during her menstrual cycle, this shouldn't pose a problem and may work well, especially after the first few days of the cycle (usually the heaviest flow days).

Encouraging more frequent pad changes during the day is another solution, but figuring out how to help your child do this isn't always easy. If your child is included in regular classes, for example, students have only a few minutes to move from one classroom to the next. With multiple class changes throughout the day, sometimes getting to a bathroom to change a pad is a challenge. Or, if your daughter brings supplies to school in backpacks, they may not be accessible when an opportunity to change presents itself. You may have to help your daughter identify clever and discreet ways to stash pads. Opaque pencil pouches, zippered pockets in pants or vests, freezer pouch areas in lunch containers, or purses (if carried regularly) are some ways to keep supplies readily available.

> *When my daughter was having accidents, I sat down and talked to her about the importance of changing pads more often during the school day. Once we began talking, I realized that leaving a classroom to go to the bathroom was not an option for her. She hated to miss anything going on in class or enter a classroom late after things had started, which is why she rarely changed her pad. Identifying natural times in her day when she could get to the bathroom without interfering with school seemed really important to her independence and autonomy, so that's where we started. After talking about times in her day when she could change, it became obvious she wouldn't have her backpack or supplies with her. I encouraged her to wear her cargo pants, or pants that had pockets that could discreetly hold one pad in a pocket further down the pant leg. If an opportunity to stop at the bathroom presented itself, she would have a pad with her.*

Reviewing school schedules with your daughter to identify ideal "change pad" times throughout the day can also be helpful. Find out when natural bathroom breaks occur during her day and encourage pad changes during those times. Speak with support staff or designated teachers about providing discreet cues or reminders, either verbally or visually until pad changing becomes more automatic.

If your daughter has an aide or support person, work out ways to communicate with them when reminders for pad changes are necessary. One mother whose daughter has difficulty communicating sends in a special black bag with supplies to school in her daughter's backpack when she is menstruating. When the aide sees the bag, she automatically understands that reminders for pad changes will be needed. Other families bring in supplies at the beginning of the school year and communicate via e-mail or voice mail to let support people know when reminders or assistance is necessary. Speak with key people who will be supporting your daughter. It's very likely experienced support staff have procedures in place or creative ideas for helping your daughter manage her periods.

If pad saturation seems to be caused by heavier than normal menstrual flow, switch to a heavier absorbency pad. If heavy flow lasts longer than seven days or is accompanied by disruptive symptoms such as extreme mood changes or aggression, talk with your physician.

All girls who are just learning to manage their periods will make mistakes. To minimize the impact on your daughter, encourage her to wear dark-colored clothing during her period so when accidents do occur they are less noticeable. Also, as a part of the celebration of puberty, invite your daughter to help you purchase five or six darker colored, roomy underwear (to allow for a pad) that she can use during the times she is menstruating. When accidents do occur, stains will be restricted to just a few pair, and the extra roominess may make wearing a pad a bit more comfortable. If visual cues are needed for pad placement, the markings will be limited to a few pair of underwear rather than her entire supply. Keeping extra clothes and underwear at her school or in your car can be helpful as well, especially during the first year when periods may be unpredictable.

Troubleshooting—Blood in Underwear

Potential Problems	Possible Strategies
Incorrect pad placement	■ Use laundry marker to insert markings that can be used as reference points for lining up pad. ■ Make sure underwear is on correctly. ■ Check pad size. Pads that are too large or small will affect movement.
Incorrect pad type	■ Make sure pad choice matches flow. ■ Winged pads can provide fuller coverage. ■ Ultra thin pads may make it harder to detect saturation (because there is less bulky wetness against body).
Infrequent pad changes	■ Review when pad changes are necessary. ■ Have her demonstrate her understanding of how and when to change a pad. Incorporate visual strategies if she has difficulty remembering. ■ Identify natural pad-changing times in her schedule or ask helper to provide discreet reminders. ■ Explore ways to carry supplies so pad changes can occur when opportunity arises. ■ Identify appropriate helper until she becomes independent
Heavy menstrual flow	■ Monitor frequency of menstrual pad changes and level of saturation (you could check discarded pads to gauge this). ■ Discuss unusually heavy flow patterns with physician.

My daughter was very blasé about accidents at school in the beginning. The first time her pad soaked through onto her pants and the nurse called me to tell me she needed new pants, she was mad. She thought that since her pants were purple, nobody would even notice the stain. I had to impress upon her that other kids would think poorly of her or make fun of her if they noticed blood on her clothes.

When my daughter first started having periods, they were pretty irregular. Often she went two or three months without a period. Because we could never predict when the next one would come, we just kept an extra set of clothes, underwear, and pads handy in the trunk of each car, at school, and anywhere else we went. These supplies came in handy when my daughter got her period when we were away from home at my son's baseball tournament.

ODOR Although blood itself is odorless, when menstrual blood is exposed to air it can become smelly. Odor during menstruation is usually the result of poor hygiene or infrequent pad changes, so revisiting proper hygiene and/or identifying ways pads can be changed more often are common solutions. Some women use deodorized feminine hygiene products. These products contain deodorant that can cause irritation, so be alert for redness, itching, or discomfort. These symptoms could signal an allergic reaction or sensitivity. Extreme odors during menstruation are unusual and should not be ignored. If your daughter is experiencing an unusual discharge, itching, or burning, she could have an infection. Speak with your healthcare provider if you have concerns.

Troubleshooting—Odor during Menstruation

Potential Causes	Possible Strategies
Infrequent pad changes	■ Review when pad changes are necessary. ■ Have her demonstrate her understanding of how to change a pad by watching her go through the steps using a sample pair of underwear and pad. Use visual strategies (written or picture cues) if she has difficulty remembering. ■ Help her identify natural pad-changing times in her schedule. ■ Explore ways to discreetly carry supplies so pad changes can occur when opportunity arises. ■ Identify helper who can provide discreet reminders until she becomes independent.
Poor Hygiene	■ Review cleansing techniques for vulva area. ■ Encourage daily showers or baths during period. ■ Consider use of moist wipes during periods.
Suspect Infection	■ See your physician.

REFUSAL TO
WEAR PADS

There may be times when your daughter is resistant to wearing a pad or removes pads prematurely or at inappropriate times and places. Reasons for this can be numerous, but all should be explored. If your daughter has verbal skills, encourage her to discuss her feelings and concerns with you.

Troubleshooting—Resistance to Wearing Pads

Problem	Possible Strategies
Refusal to wear pads	■ Check for possible underlying physical problem such as boils, broken skin, that may make pad usage uncomfortable. ■ If you suspect discomfort (from a particular pad or perhaps the adhesive) review pad placement or try another brand. ■ Reeducate about purpose of pad use. ■ Verbally or physically help her put on pad. ■ Reeducate on where to find pads and how to use. ■ Use positive reinforcement (praise, rewards, or other appropriate incentives) at designated intervals for continued pad use. ■ Consider instructing her on tampon use (see tampon instruction section).
Removal of pad in inappropriate places	■ Remind her pad changing is a private activity. ■ Escort her to the bathroom and help put on pad. ■ Remind her that the bathroom is the appropriate private place for removing pads. ■ Explore other pad options if you suspect discomfort. ■ Dress her in clothes that are more difficult to remove.
Discontinuing pad use before period is done	■ Reeducate her about purpose of pad use. ■ Mark on a calendar the typical length of her period so she knows how long she will be expected to wear pads (average length of her periods during the past year). Have her keep track of days. If she responds better to visual calendars, create a "period calendar" and have her remove days each night until period is over (see picture on page 80). ■ Have her demonstrate her understanding of how to change a pad. Incorporate visual strategies if she has difficulty remembering. ■ Explore other pad options if you suspect discomfort.
Persistent refusal to wear pad	■ Consult behavioral specialist for possible functional behavior assessment to determine what your daughter is communicating. ■ If sensory issues are possible, consult OT. ■ Speak with physician about menstrual management options (see pages 98-100).

Although my daughter is fairly independent with managing her periods now, at one point she regressed and was having more accidents. When I talked with her, she told me that she didn't like wearing pads and seemed to think that if she stopped wearing pads, her period would stop. We reviewed the lengths of her periods and talked about the consequences of not wearing pads. We also experimented with other pads. She told me she didn't like the kind with wings.

Although my daughter is toilet trained, she has pretty significant behavioral challenges and continued to refuse to wear pads during her period. We ended up trying Depends® with good success. Her period is not very heavy so that works fine.

Other Concerns

FEAR OF EXPLOITATION AND PREGNANCY

Parents' anxieties and fears about exploitation and pregnancy often become magnified once their daughter's periods begin. The start of menstruation can act as a visual reminder for parents that their daughter is now physically capable of becoming pregnant. One of my first career experiences at a Planned Parenthood clinic involved working with a mom and her twelve-year-old daughter with Down syndrome. The mother brought her daughter in for a pelvic exam so she could start her on birth control pills before leaving for camp. This mother was genuinely fearful about the possibility of exploitation. Another mother recently told me that she finally broke down and had a frank educational session about intercourse with her daughter after her period was a few weeks late. Although her daughter was not in a relationship, the mother still had ongoing concerns that her daughter could be exploited.

It's important to remember that although birth control methods will prevent pregnancy, they do not prevent exploitation. Sexuality education that includes exploitation prevention information is still a necessary step toward encouraging and supporting your daughter's healthy sexuality and safety. (See Chapter 12 for information on abuse prevention.) If your daughter is in a relationship and you have concerns about pregnancy risk, concerns regarding contraception are discussed in Chapter 10.

MANAGING MENSTRUAL SYMPTOMS

If your daughter experiences milder, more common menstrual symptoms (mild abdominal cramping or lower back pain) standard treatments should be offered. Strategies known to reduce milder menstrual symptoms include a healthy and nutritious diet (see, for example, *The Down Syndrome Nutrition Handbook,* by Joan Medlen); stretching or exercise; use of heat (heating pads or warm baths) for cramps; relaxation techniques; or use of a non-steroidal anti-inflammatory drug (e.g., Aleve) during the first day or two of the menstrual cycle.

Although there is no evidence that having Down syndrome means periods will be more difficult, it is true that females with cognitive disabilities often have a harder time verbalizing or expressing discomfort and pain in traditional ways. This can make diagnosis of problems or abnormalities more difficult. Commonly reported behavioral symptoms associated with premenstrual syndrome (PMS) for females with cognitive disabilities include:

- increased violence and aggression,
- changes in behavior,

- seizures or exacerbation of seizure disorders,
- temper tantrums,
- crying spells,
- irritability,
- mood changes,
- restlessness, and
- self-abusive behaviors.

In addition to the list above, other symptoms that warrant a discussion with your healthcare provider include heavier than normal menstrual flow (*menorrhagia*), or extreme pain or discomfort during menses (*dysmenorrhea*). Charting symptoms listed above as well as the start and dissipation of symptoms can help your physician determine if these changes are cyclic and related to menstrual cycles or potentially caused by other health issues. If your daughter is less verbal, consider visual pain scales typically used with children to help her communicate discomfort associated with menstruation. These types of scales typically use graphics such as happy or increasingly sad faces to indicate the degree of discomfort.

Indicators of Menstrual Pain in Girls with Down Syndrome

In an unpublished study, Margaret Kyrkou interviewed seventy-five menstruating women and girls with Down syndrome and their mothers regarding pain associated with menstruation. Eighty-five percent of the females with Down syndrome in this study reported experiencing pain with menstruation (much higher than the percentage reported by their mothers). In this study, the majority of women with Down syndrome communicated pain in the following ways:
- verbal reporting of pain symptoms,
- vocalizations (e.g., moaning),
- reductions in activity levels (becoming less physically active),
- facial grimaces,
- reduction in socialization (desire to be alone).

The females reported successfully managing pain associated with menstruation through use of: over-the-counter meds (e.g., ibuprofen), hot baths or water bottles for cramps, rest, distraction, exercise, and alone or private time.

PREMENSTRUAL SYNDROME OR PREMENSTRUAL DYSPHORIC DISORDER—WHAT'S THE DIFFERENCE?

Many women experience physical symptoms associated with menstruation a week or so before menstruating, but for some, symptoms can be more debilitating and interfere with an ability to participate in everyday activities. Premenstrual Syndrome (PMS) and Premenstrual Dysphoric Disorder (PMDD) can be characterized by moderate (PMS) to severe episodes (PMDD) of depression, sadness, mood fluctuations, anxiety and tension, fatigue, discomfort, or anger and irritability *that worsen during the post-ovulatory phase of the menstrual cycle and then disappear after menstruation starts.*

Although there is still much to learn about PMDD, treatments that have shown promise include healthy lifestyle changes (regular exercise, regular sleep, diet modifications, etc.); nutritional supplementation; non-pharmacological treatments such as stress management, patient education, or behavioral therapy; and pharmacological treatment with birth control pills, NSAIDs (ibuprofen), or SSRI's (Selective Serotonin Reuptake Inhibitors), a specific class of antidepressants. Differentiating between PMS and PMDD and other mental health problems can be complicated and requires tracking of symptoms over time. Speak with your daughter's physician if you have concerns.

Menstrual Management Options

Evidence suggests that most girls with mild and moderate cognitive disabilities do quite well handling their periods with advance preparation, understandable instruction, and, sometimes, behavioral management techniques. Others, just as in the general population, experience more severe symptoms or have a more difficult time with self-care, reducing the quality of life for them and perhaps also their parents or other caregivers. In these instances the hormonal or surgical methods described below are sometimes used to help reduce symptoms or the frequency of menses or to eliminate menstruation altogether. Common reasons for suppressing menstruation include:

■ Challenging behaviors that jeopardize the individual's safety or the safety of others;

■ Health conditions that seem to be exacerbated (e.g., seizures, diabetes) by the hormonal cycle;

■ Presence of gynecological conditions that have remained unresponsive to other, less invasive treatments;

■ Difficulties managing periods even with good training and support;

■ Informed choice by the girl or woman herself to suppress or eliminate menstruation.

It's important to remember that physicians generally follow a set of rules that encourage least restrictive practices or approaches to medical interventions. For example, asking your physician to consider any of the options discussed below after your daughter has experienced only one period is probably unrealistic. At this stage, a more logical and appropriate intervention might be to refer your daughter to resources or individualized instruction for self-care. Similarly, your doctor is more likely to suggest a trial of OCP's (oral contraceptive pills) to reduce painful cramping or heavier menstrual flow before considering a surgical option. Your physician's priority is to assist and support you in making decisions that minimize risks for your daughter and maximize self-determination.

HORMONAL OPTIONS

Hormonal methods are a common initial intervention for attempting to reduce certain problematic menstrual symptoms when a woman is otherwise healthy. Some of the more common options are listed below. Most of these methods work in similar ways by suppressing or stopping ovulation. Although these methods were originally developed to prevent pregnancy, they are also commonly used to reduce certain menstrual symptoms.

Hormonal Methods

Hormonal Method	What It Is and Why It Is Used	Other Considerations
Oral Contraceptives (OC's)	Pills containing varying levels of synthetic estrogen or progesterone are taken around the same time daily for 21 days followed by 7 days off. OR certain regimes (e.g., Seasonale®) can be taken continuously in order to reduce number of periods to 4 per year. Often used to regulate periods or reduce painful cramping or menstrual flow with heavier periods.	■ Caregivers may have to assist in making sure pill is taken daily although many women can be reliable pill takers if concrete, complete instruction is provided. ■ Bleeding can be irregular. ■ Improves bone density. ■ Patient may have difficulty verbalizing common adverse side effects (nausea, moodiness, breast tenderness, headaches). ■ Weight gain can be an issue.
Contraceptive Patch (Ortho-Evra®)	Patch placed on the lower abdomen, upper outer arm, buttocks, or upper torso and replaced weekly. Used to regulate periods or reduce painful cramping or menstrual flow with heavier periods.	■ Long-term health effects not studied in women with developmental disabilities. ■ Increased risk of Deep Vein Thrombosis (a form of blood clot); symptoms may be more difficult to report by women with DS. ■ Reduced effectiveness in women over 198 lbs. ■ Anecdotal reports of patients with DS removing patch prematurely, so may need to monitor. ■ Those with sensitive skin may have site reactions. ■ May not be appropriate for females with anxieties about bandages or who engage in chronic picking
Levonorgestrel IUD (Mirena)	Hormone-releasing IUD (intrauterine device) that is inserted into uterus and is effective for 5 years Can be used to reduce blood loss and pain associated with menstruation.	■ May need to be sedated for gynecological exam and insertion. ■ Insertion may be more difficult and painful in women who have not had children ■ Risk of infection in women who are sexually active. ■ Regular string checking may be more difficult.
Depo-Provera	Injection of progestin in buttocks or arm by health care professional once every 3 months. Often periods diminish and eventually cease (reducing symptoms) within a year. May be used if self-care and hygiene are difficult or difficult symptoms accompany menses.	■ Can cause heavy, unpredictable bleeding initially. ■ Weight gain often more significant in women with DS. ■ Reduces bone density; there is already a known increased risk of osteoporosis in women w/DS, so many physicians avoid its use. ■ Long-term health effects not studied in women with developmental disabilities.

SURGICAL METHODS

When hormonal methods aren't effective or health reasons prevent their use, surgical options may be considered. Below are examples of surgical options and reasons they're used.

Surgical Methods

Method	What It Is and Why It Is Used	Other Considerations
Endometrial ablation	Outpatient procedure in which endometrial lining of the uterus (the part that builds up and sloughs off each month) is purposely removed or destroyed. May be used to treat heavy bleeding (menorrhagia) or eliminate menses altogether.	■ May affect reproductive capacity. ■ Considered permanent since can cause sterility. ■ May require similar legal consent procedures as sterilization. ■ Amenorrhea (absence of periods) is not guaranteed and sometimes procedure needs to be repeated.
Hysterectomy	Surgical removal of uterus (and sometimes Fallopian tubes) stops menstrual flow. Sometimes used to treat heavy bleeding (menorrhagia) when other methods have failed to produce results.	■ Major surgical procedure. ■ Irreversible and causes sterility. ■ Check state laws for consent procedures. ■ May be difficult to find physician who will perform the procedure. ■ May not affect symptoms associated with PMS/PMDD.
Myomectomy	Surgical removal of fibroids from uterus. Reduces pelvic pain and excessive bleeding caused by presence of fibroids.	■ Can preserve fertility

GYNECOLOGICAL EXAMS

Before making recommendations, your healthcare provider will want to evaluate or update your daughter's health history and possibly conduct a thorough physical examination. When reproductive health concerns surface, questions regarding gynecological exams often surface. Below are some common questions and concerns.

DOES YOUR DAUGHTER NEED A GYNECOLOGICAL EXAM?

There is disagreement among professionals in the disability community regarding conditions that warrant the need for a gynecological exam. Some professionals advocate that young women with Down syndrome start having gynecological exams at the same time as other young women do—at age 18 or once sexual activity is initiated. Other professionals recognize there are unique circumstances among individuals with Down syndrome and other cognitive disabilities and consequently may use a different set of guidelines when deciding when and if a gynecological exam would be beneficial. For example, there is evidence that the overall incidence of abnormal pap smears is much lower in women with developmental disabilities, presumably due to lowered rates of sexual activity. In addition, breast cancer and other solid tumor cancers that commonly affect the general population seem to appear less often in women with Down syndrome.

Here are some key considerations a healthcare provider might use to determine whether a pelvic exam is advantageous:

- Is the person sexually active?
- Are there immediate problems or concerns that indicate a more thorough examination would be beneficial?
- Is there an unknown or known history of sexual abuse or trauma?
- Are there physical disabilities or mobility issues?
- Will the information gained from a reproductive health/gynecological exam add to what is already known?
- Can the person use relaxation techniques effectively?

PREPARING YOUR DAUGHTER FOR A GYNECOLOGICAL EXAM

One way to introduce the idea of reproductive healthcare is to explain that specialists are people who are specially trained to take care of certain parts of the body. If your child has a cardiologist, for example, you could explain that her "heart" doctor is trained to know about and take care of her heart. Her "eye" doctor, her eyes, and her ear doctor, her ears, nose, and throat. Let her know that just like the other parts of the body need care, private body parts need care as well. Emphasize the fact that all women have this type of care in order to make sure they are healthy. Use the pictures in Appendix A-14 and A-15 to remind her about private body parts (breasts, vulva, and internal reproductive organs) that need care, how that care is typically provided, and why it is needed.

Beyond specialized audiovisual resources, other ideas for preparation include:

- *Guest speakers*—Encourage your local DD or Down syndrome agency to invite a health or sexuality educator to speak with teens, young adults, or self-advocates (males benefit from this type of information as well) about reproductive healthcare and how to take care of their genitals. Reproductive health information can be easily incorporated into a more comprehensive health, hygiene, or sexuality series. Professionals often have access to anatomical models or audiovisuals that can make learning concrete and relevant. A mother I know arranged for a local female gynecologist in the community to come speak with a group of young women from their ARC. The girls received a tour of the doctor's office and exam room, and were well prepared for their first exam.
- *Desensitization visits*—Some providers are willing to help prepare patients by scheduling a series of visits rather than trying to fit ev-

erything in during one appointment. An initial visit could involve a tour of the exam room, an introduction to equipment that will be used, a discussion about why the exam is being performed, and a demonstration of what will be done. Including time to practice getting on and off the table and lying down in the correct position (with clothes on) can be helpful as well. For some women, desensitization visits can reduce anxiety and fear, give them a better sense of control, and allow time for individual questions and concerns.

■ *Separate gynecological exam from routine health care procedures*— Many individuals already experience considerable anxiety with routine healthcare visits. Consequently, some experts recommend the gynecological exam occur at a separate appointment time.

Directly before the visit:

■ *Anticipate questions the provider is likely to ask during the gynecological exam and help your daughter come up with accurate responses.* For example, have her identify the first day of her last menstrual period by checking her calendar and writing it down so she will have the information when asked. Other information that will be important:

- a description of what her cycles are usually like (duration, flow),
- a copy of charts used for symptom documentation,
- questions your daughter may have for the provider.

Resources for Teaching about Reproductive Health

Resource	Description
The GYN Exam Handbook: An Illustrated Guide to Gynecologic Examination for Women with Special Needs	A video and picture series that walks women through steps for scheduling and obtaining a reproductive health exam. Components of the exam include both the breast and pelvic exam.
Looking After My Breasts (BSE/ mammogram) *Looking After My Balls (testicular self-exam)* *Keeping Healthy "Down Below" (pap smear)*	A series of colorfully illustrated stories (no words) from the Books Beyond Words series that address reproductive health issues in both males and females (separate books). Sample narratives for explaining the process are included in the back of these books.
Anatomically Correct Dolls	Dolls can be useful in explaining internal and external anatomy and demonstrating parts of the exam and how they are performed.

■ *Ask your provider whether a support person is allowed in the room while a pelvic exam is being performed.* If he or she seems uncomfortable with this request, explain your reasons and advocate for this practice, particularly for females with developmental disabilities. This allows you to reassure your daughter you will accompany her to the visit and stay in the room with her so she is not alone—especially if a new provider relationship is being established. If your daughter indicates she wants you to leave the room so she can speak with the provider alone, respect her right to privacy and leave.

■ *Teach or review relaxation strategies that can be used during the exam.* All women understand the important role relaxation plays in reducing discomfort. If your daughter is unfamiliar with relaxation techniques, work on deep breathing or helping her understand the difference between tight muscles and relaxed muscles through clenching and then relaxing various parts of the body. Then explain that muscles in her vagina can be clenched and relaxed as well (she can practice during urination) and that the exam will be more comfortable if she can try to relax these muscles.

WHAT IF YOUR DAUGHTER RESISTS A TRADITIONAL PELVIC EXAM?

Physicians or nurse practitioners who have experience providing care to women with disabilities will likely have ideas for alternative positions and techniques they have used to make the exam more comfortable. Well-known modifications include:

Finger-Guided Pap. When a pap smear is necessary, the speculum is traditionally inserted into the vagina so the cervix (the lower part of the uterus) can be viewed and samples of cells can be removed and screened for changes and abnormalities that might be indicators of cervical cancer. In women who are not sexually active, the opening to the vagina can be tight, making the use of a speculum particularly uncomfortable even with the smallest size speculum. One alternative is to avoid the use of a speculum altogether and instead use the finger. The finger-guided pap method allows the cervix to be palpated by the examiner and then, while the finger is still inserted, a pap stick, swab, or brush is guided into the vagina to the cervical os (small opening to the uterus) where a sample of cells is taken. Although views of the cervix using this method are usually minimized, this technique can reduce discomfort for the patient.

Ultrasound. If the healthcare provider feels there is a specific problem (uterine fibroids, ovarian cysts, other pelvic masses) that needs to be explored further and the pelvic exam provides inadequate information or would be viewed as traumatic, an ultrasound is sometimes ordered. Although some level of cooperation is still required (the patient must remain still with her bladder full) it is a less invasive option. It's important to note that the use of ultrasound as a screening tool for reproductive health problems is not an established practice in the general population and therefore is viewed as controversial by some professionals.

Sedation. Performing gynecological exams while the patient is sedated is generally viewed as a last resort by most health practitioners. Again, most providers will opt for least restrictive practices for gathering necessary information. Use of sedation is higher risk and usually requires outpatient facilities and closer monitoring, making it a more expensive option. When sedation is used, ethical issues often surface for providers. Is the patient actually consenting to the procedure if medications are necessary for compliance? Even with oral sedation, patients can resist the exam, which interferes with the operating principle of "do no harm." Still, performing an exam under sedation may be necessary if there is a problem that needs to be addressed and all other attempts have failed. If sedation is necessary, your daughter should be given adequate information ahead of time and attempts should be made to coordinate sedation with other healthcare procedures that are needed.

References

Angelopoulou, N., Souftas, V., et al. (1999). Gonadal Function in Young Women with Down Syndrome. *International Journal of Gynecology and Obstetrics 67* (1): 15-21.

Anderson, S. E. & Must, A. (2005). Interpreting the Continued Decline in the Average Age of Menarche: Results from Two Nationally Representative Surveys of US Girls Studied 10 Years Apart. *Journal of Pediatrics 147* (6): 753-60.

Bahtia, S. & Bahtia, S. (2002). Diagnosis and Treatment of Premenstrual Dysphoric Disorder. *American Family Physician 66* (7): 1239-1248.

Caring for Individuals with Down Syndrome and Their Families (1995). Third Ross Roundtable on Critical Issues in Family Medicine. Columbus, OH: Society of Teachers of Family Medicine & Ross Laboratories.

Cento, R. M., Ragusa, L., et al. (1996). Basal Body Temperature Curves and Endocrine Pattern of Menstrual Cycles in Down syndrome, *Gynecological Endocrinology 10* (2): 133-7.

Chew, G. & Hutson, J. (2004). Incidence of Cryptorchidism and Ascending Testes in Trisomy 21: A 10 Year Retrospective Review. *Pediatric Surgery International 20*: 744-747.

Couwenhoven, T. (1992). *Beginnings: A Parent/Child Sexuality Program for Families with Children Who Have Developmental Disabilities*. Madison, WI: Wisconsin Council on Developmental Disabilities.

Cunningham, C. (1996). *Understanding Down Syndrome: An Introduction for Parents.* Cambridge, MA: Brookline Books.

Elkins, T.E. et al. (1988). A Clinical Observation of a Program to Accomplish Pelvic Exams in Difficult-to-Manage Patients with Mental Retardation. *Adolescent Pediatric Gynecology 1*: 195-197.

Elkins, T.E. et al. (1997). Integration of a Sexuality Counseling Service into a Reproductive Health Program for Persons with Mental Retardation. *Journal of Pediatric Adolescent Gynecology 10*: 24-27.

Elkins, T. E. (1997). Reproductive Health Care for the Mentally Handicapped, *The Contraception Report 8* (4): 4-11.

Gillooly, J.B. (1998). *Before She Gets Her Period: Talking with your Daughter about Menstruation.* Los Angeles: Perspectives Publishing.

Goldstein, H. (1988). Menarche, Menstruation, Sexual Relations and Contraception of Adolescent Females with Down syndrome. *European Journal of Obstetrics and Gynecology, and Reproductive Biology 27* (4): 343-9.

Hasen, J., Boyar, R. et. al. (1980). Gonadal Function in Trisomy 21. *Hormone Research 12* (6): 345-50.

Hasle, H. et al. (2000). Occurrence of Cancer in Individuals with Down Syndrome. *Ugeskr Laeger* [Danish journal] *162* (34): 4535-39.

Hsiang, Y. & Berkovitz, G. (1987). Gonadal Function in Patients with Down Syndrome. *American Journal of Medical Genetics 27* (2): 449-58.

Janet's Got Her Period. (1990). Santa Barbara, CA: James Stanfield Publishing Co.

Kaur, H., Butler, J., & Trumble, S. (2003). *Menstrual Management and Women with an Intellectual*

Disability: A Guide for GP's. Oakleigh, Victoria, Australia: Monash University. www.cddh.monash. org/assets/menstrual-management-guide-gp.pdf

Kopac, C. (2002). Gynecological and Reproductive Services for Teenage and Adult Women with Special Needs. *Exceptional Parent Magazine* (Feb.): 54-82.

Kyrkou, M. Women with Disability: Knowledge and Understanding of Psychosocial and Management Issues from Menarche to Menopause. Adelaide: Flinders University (unpublished thesis).

Mangan, S, et al. (2002). Overweight Teens at Increased Risk for Weight Gain While using Depot Medroxyprogesterion Acetate. *Journal of Pediatric Adolescent Gynecology 15*: 79-82.

Nofziger, M. (1988). *Signs of Fertility: The Personal Science of Natural Birth Control.* Nashville, TN: MND Publishing.

Paransky, O. & Zurawin, R. (2003). Management of Menstrual Problems and Contraception in Adolescents with Mental Retardation: A Medical, Legal, and Ethical Review with Suggested Guidelines. *Journal of Pediatric Adolescent Gynecology 16*: 223-235.

Pravatt, B. (1998). Gynecologic Care for Women with Mental Retardation. *Journal of Obstetric Gynecological Nursing 27* (3): 251-255.

Pueschel, S. (1988). *The Young Person with Down Syndrome: Transition from Adolescence to Adulthood.* Baltimore: Brookes Publishing.

Pueschel, S., Orson, J., et al. (1985). Adolescent Development in Males with Down syndrome. *American Journal of Diseases of Children 139* (3): 236-8

Rondal, J., Perera, J., et al. (1996). *Down's Syndrome: Psychological, Psychobiological, and Socio-Educational Perspectives.* San Diego: Singular Publishing Group.

Sakadamis, A. et al. (2002). Bone Mass, Gonadal Function and Biochemical Assessment in Young Men with Trisomy 21. *European Journal of Obstetrics & Gynecology and Reproductive Biology 100* (2): 208-212.

Satge, D. et al. (2001). Breast Cancer in Women with Trisomy 21. *Bulletin of Academic National Medicine 185* (7): 1239-52.

Satge, D. (2002). Breast Screening Guidelines Should be Adapted in Down's Syndrome (Editorial). *British Medical Journal 324* (7246): 1155.

Siegel, P. (1991). *Changes in You.* Richmond, VA: Family Life Education Associates.

Scola, P., & Pueschel, S. (1992). Menstrual Cycles Basal Body Temperature Curves in Women with Down syndrome. *Obstetrics & Gynecology 79* (1): 91-94.

Steiner, M., et al. (2006). Expert Guidelines for the Treatment of Severe PMS, PMDD, and Comorbidities: The Role of SSRI's. *Journal of Women's Health 15* (1): 57-69.

Van Dyke, D. et al. (1995). *Medical & Surgical Care for Children with Down Syndrome: A Guide for Parents.* Bethesda, MD: Woodbine House.

Wingfield, M. et al. (1994). Endomentrial Ablation: An Option for the Management of Menstrual Problems in the Intellectually Disabled. *Medical Journal of Australia 161* (8): 533-36.

Wu, T., Mendola, P., et al. (2002). Ethnic Differences in the Presence of Secondary Sex Characteristics and Menarche among U.S. Girls: The Third National Health and Nutrition Examination Survey 1988-1994. *Pediatrics 110*: 752-757.

CHAPTER 6

Masturbation

Most infants and children (with and without disabilities) discover quite early (and without help from anyone, mind you) the pleasure and comfort that comes from touching and exploring the genitals. Genital touching in infants and children is now widely recognized as a normal and healthy stage of sexual development. Although there are people who use the term "masturbation" to describe any sort of genital exploration across the lifespan, most sexuality experts understand there are clear distinctions between childhood body exploration and masturbation in adulthood (see the table below). This chapter is aimed at helping you understand the distinctions, as well as the normalcy and benefits of both, and will give you strategies you can use in teaching your child when and where these behaviors are appropriate.

Genital Touching in Infants, Toddlers, and Young Children

In young children, genital touching is often used as a way to relax, handle stressful situations, or just explore the body and figure out what feels good. Here are other general facts about masturbation in children:

- Because genitals in males are more accessible, boys tend to masturbate earlier and more often than girls.
- There is a wider variation in when masturbatory behaviors begin occurring in girls. Some explore their body early; others inadvertently discover genital pleasure through life experiences such as biking, horseback riding, or monkey bars; others may be introduced by other children; and some later when they become involved in sexual relationships.

Young children with Down syndrome generally follow similar developmental patterns in discovering the genitals. However, there are unique circumstances that

Masturbation—What's Normal?

Infancy & childhood	■ Healthy curiosity about body parts and their functions ■ Exploration and touching of genitals common ■ Begin to associate genital touching with pleasure ■ Often lack understanding of appropriate social contexts for touching or talking about masturbation
Preadolescence & Adolescence	■ Masturbation occurs with increased frequency ■ Private nature of masturbation understood ■ Enhanced awareness of own unique responses to touch and self-stimulation (erotic potential) ■ Sexual fantasy emerges as a component of masturbation ■ Can be increased anxiety regarding "normalness" of behavior (is this normal and something others do?)
Adulthood	■ Sexual fantasy routinely a component of masturbation ■ Masturbation functions as rehearsal for mature, adult sex play with partners ■ Common source of pleasure, relaxation, sexual release, and fulfillment in presence or absence of sexual partner

should be considered as you think about how you will handle masturbation and genital touching in your child with Down syndrome:

- For individuals with developmental disabilities who may have more limited abilities to develop and form relationships with others, masturbation may be a primary form of sexual expression in adolescence and adulthood.
- Individuals with Down syndrome often have less privacy. When limited opportunities for privacy exist, your son or daughter will likely choose alternative, less appropriate places to masturbate.
- Children with Down syndrome and other cognitive disabilities often require more time and direct instruction on privacy rules associated with masturbation, so repetition and reinforcement over time is typically necessary.

RESPONDING TO GENITAL STIMULATION IN YOUNG CHILDREN

Not all episodes of genital touching need to be "handled." You may notice, for example, that your child routinely touches her genitals during bathing sessions or diaper changing. This is normal and doesn't really require any action on your part—except, perhaps, some introduction to genital vocabulary. Body exploration does tend to occur more often when genitals are exposed and accessible. Bathing sessions are a popular time to touch and explore the body. If your child is young and requires supervision, allow the exploration to happen as you wash the rest of her body. It is also common for children to engage in genital touching at bedtime as a way to relax and calm themselves. As your child grows, the bathroom and bedroom will continue to be appropriate places to explore the body.

How you respond verbally and nonverbally to these behaviors will influence your child's feelings about masturbation and the genitals. Avoid negative remarks, hand slapping, or escalated responses. These actions often result in guilt and shame over the body and communicate early messages that the body and its functions are somehow taboo and not okay to talk about. Evidence suggests that repeated exposure to punitive attitudes and punishment related to masturbation often contributes to feelings of guilt, shame, and, in more severe cases, psychological problems or sexual dysfunction in adulthood.

Redirection is commonly used when young children explore their genitals in less acceptable, public places. For example, if you notice your child stimulating her genitals in the grocery store, redirect her behavior by engaging her in an activity. Have her help pick items off shelves, unload the cart, or play with a favorite toy or book while sitting in the cart. Often boredom or inactivity are triggers for genital touching and self-stimulating behavior in children (of all ages and ability levels!).

ENCOURAGING SOCIAL APPROPRIATENESS

The most common parental concern associated with genital touching involves the behavior occurring in public places or at appropriate times. As your child's receptive language ability grows and/or she becomes more mobile, you can begin communicating basic messages about the private nature of genital touching.

Clear, calm, and direct messages should be communicated. For example, remind your child that touching her vulva (or his penis) is a private behavior. If you've previously identified her private space, ask her to tell or show you where it is and remind her she needs to be in private (ideally the bedroom or bathroom with the door closed). If your child does not respond to a verbal prompt, physically move her to her bedroom, avoiding negative or punishing remarks in the process. When genital touching occurs in public, repetitive, gentle, and discreet reminders about the inappropriateness of the behavior when others are around or in public places is usually all that is needed.

If you have identified the bathroom as a designated private space for your child, be sure to specify the bathroom "at home." This advice stems from my own experiences with individuals who may think that what's okay in one bathroom is okay in all bathrooms and then do private activities like masturbation in public bathrooms—which, of course, has undesirable consequences. You can determine how specific your teaching should be based on your child's abilities and unique family circumstances. The important thing is that your child knows that masturbation is private and understands where to go when privacy is desired.

If your child is touching her genitals in a rather public arena, calmly acknowledge the behavior ("I know it feels good to touch/rub your penis/vulva"), explain the behavior is private ("but touching your penis/vulva is private"), and suggest she move

Key Teaching Messages in Childhood:

- Touching my private body parts (or penis, vulva) feels good but is private.
- If I want to touch my private parts, I should move to my private place.

to a private place ("so you need to go to a place where you can be safe and no one can see you"). This action communicates acceptance about the behavior, but also teaches rules about safety and appropriate behavior.

Remember that many children, with and without Down syndrome, need consistent repetition and reinforcement over time before they understand that touching private parts is a private behavior. Discuss your plan with your partner to ensure your approaches remain consistent. If your child spends time with other caregivers, share your goals, expectations, techniques, prompts, and cues and encourage them to address genital touching in similar ways. Rule out potential physical causes that may be causing discomfort. For example, chafing, uncomfortable clothing, urinary/penile/vaginal infections, or irritation from soaps or detergents are possible contributors.

Also remember that children fixate on things that feel good when they are bored or uninvolved. Make sure your child has opportunities to participate in meaningful and age appropriate activities wherever she is. As children get older, many families I know develop simple verbal or visual cues as prompts when inappropriate touching occurs in public places. Statements like "that's private" or "we're in public" serve as quick reminders when your child is just beginning to understand societal rules in public places. If verbal prompts don't seem to work, redirecting or engaging her in an activity can help.

Masturbation Is Private: A Social Story

Writing a Social Story, individualized to your child's situation, can be a good way to teach appropriate behavior. For example:

- All people have body parts that are private.
- My private body parts are the penis, testicles, scrotum, and butt (vulva, breasts, butt, if female).
- Sometimes it feels good to touch my private body parts.
- Many boys and men (girls and women) touch their own private body parts. It is okay. Touching my private body parts to feel good is called masturbation.
- Touching or rubbing my own private body parts (masturbation) is private so no one should see me.
- If I want to touch or rub my private parts, I need to be alone in my private space (identify the space) with the door closed so no one can see me.
- People get upset if I touch or rub my private body parts in front of them, even if I have my clothes on. It is not okay to touch or rub between my legs when I am at _____ (school, work) where others can see me.
- If I am not in my private place I can keep my hands at my side, fold my arms, or place them on my lap. It is not okay to put my hands in my pants or between my legs when others can see me.
- I will remember that touching my private body parts is private. I will only touch my private parts when I am in my private place where no one can see me.

Common Questions and Concerns about Masturbation in Adolescence

Key Teaching Messages in Preadolescence/Adolescence:

■ Touching or rubbing your private parts (penis or vulva) feels good and is called masturbation.
■ If done safely and in private, masturbation cannot hurt you.
■ My private place for masturbating is _____.

The hormones released during puberty can create more powerful sensations that spark the discovery of, or a renewed interest in, genital touching, masturbation, and pleasure. Many parents find that once puberty begins, the messages about masturbation they shared during childhood need to be repeated, reinforced, or expanded upon. Other parents find themselves dealing with this issue for the first time. It's easy to be tongue-tied and at a loss for words.

HOW MUCH MASTURBATION IS NORMAL?

Although there is a perception that individuals with cognitive disabilities masturbate more or less often (depending on who you talk to) than the general population, research exploring the frequency of masturbation in individuals with cognitive disabilities is limited. We do know that a lack of understanding of privacy rules and limited access to private places may contribute to being "caught" more often. Research related to frequency of masturbation conducted on the general population tells us:

■ Among boys, there are dramatic increases in frequency of masturbation between the ages of 12 and 15, with 82 percent of males initiating masturbation by the time they are 15. Although many girls begin masturbating around this same time, the increase is more gradual over time, with initiation of masturbation continuing into adulthood (Kinsey, Janus).
■ There is a strong correlation between testosterone levels and frequency of sexual activity (either masturbation or sexual intercourse). This correlation is more dramatic in males than females, however (Udry, 1988).
■ There is a broader variation in frequency and onset of masturbation among females compared to males. Some girls begin masturbating as early and sometimes earlier than males do, but some begin much later, and some not at all (Janus, Kinsey).
■ Masturbation is the most frequent type of sexual activity for most young people until they begin forming stable relationships in late adolescence.

The bottom line is increased frequency and interest in masturbation, especially during puberty and adolescence, is common and perfectly normal. Some individuals, just as in the general population, will not be as interested in the activity and that's okay as well.

BEYOND NORMAL AND TYPICAL

For some young people, an increased interest in masturbation in adolescence or adulthood becomes problematic, resulting in considerable anxiety and discomfort for their families. Masturbation is usually considered problematic when:

■ It interferes with your son's or daughter's ability to participate in everyday life or to fulfill commitments and responsibilities.

■ It results in injury.

■ It is performed at the wrong time or place.

When young people with cognitive disabilities who have limited communication abilities are engaging in problematic masturbation, a variety of factors need to be considered. They include:

■ *Rule out physical causes*—Sometimes what looks like masturbation is actually an attempt by the person to communicate discomfort. Improper or poor hygiene (e.g., penile infections, improper cleansing of foreskin), irritating or tight clothing, chafing, reactions to soaps and detergents, or uncomfortable erections are examples. The behavior may also signal more serious health issues such as rashes, urinary tract infections, prostate problems, or vaginal or sexually transmitted infections. As a first step, all possible physical causes should be ruled out by your physician.

■ *Evaluate medications*—Certain medications can affect sexual urges and desires or the ability to feel and experience sensation. Ask your physician about known sexual side effects of medications that might be affecting your child.

■ *Assess lifestyle*—People with Down syndrome or other disabilities are often less physically active and have fewer opportunities for socialization than their peers without disabilities. Ensuring that your child is involved in interesting activities prevents boredom and inactivity, two common triggers for masturbation. Encouraging physical activity, specifically aerobic activity, can also reduce incidences of masturbation that may be caused by boredom or anxieties associated with sexual maturation or everyday life. On the other end of the spectrum, some individuals have few opportunities for privacy, or their schedules are so structured and rigid that there really is no time to relax, unwind, or make personal choices on how to spend down time. In these instances, scheduled private time may be beneficial in eliminating public masturbation.

■ *Analyze private space*—It is well known that individuals with developmental disabilities are more closely supervised when it comes to sexual behaviors and often have less privacy (Hingsburger). It is essential for your adolescent to have a private place to go where she can have uninterrupted time. That means if you have not been adamant about respecting your child's privacy up to this point, now is the time to start. Remember, like all adolescents, your maturing son or daughter will have a growing need and desire for privacy, even if that need has not been communicated.

Evaluating Your Child's Private Space

If your teen can accurately identify (by telling or showing) her private place but continues to masturbate in public areas, take a moment to view your child's bedroom from her perspective. Things to consider:

- Are doors always open?
- Do other family members go into and out of the bedroom without permission?
- Is the bedroom shared?
- Is your child allowed extended periods of uninterrupted time?

Examining traffic and behavior patterns of family members or housemates may provide insight on what prevents your child from moving to or remaining in her designated private space. If she shares a bedroom with a sibling (or roommate) consider developing a schedule so each person has designated times they can be in private. Use a concrete signal, such as a privacy sign, during these times to ensure that private time is respected and uninterrupted. Keep in mind that if a sibling or parent walks in on your child when she is masturbating in her private space, it is not **her** problem but rather a reminder for you, other family members, or roommates to have a new respect for a closed door. If you or a sib knocked and your child gave permission to enter even though she was engaged in private behaviors, apologize, close the door, and later review with your child how she should respond to door knocks. Remind her that masturbation is private and that she has a right to let people know they cannot come in when she is doing something private (see Chapter 3).

- *Improper Technique*—Parents sometimes express concerns about whether their child is masturbating correctly. These concerns may be related to the use of objects they fear will cause damage (edges of furniture, sharp objects, etc.). Other times parents are concerned that their child is not sure how to "finish" masturbating or reach orgasm (she may throw herself on the floor), resulting in anxiety, frustration, and/or perpetual states of arousal. In these situations, it would be appropriate to seek help from a professional sex educator, sex counselor, or sex therapist (see "Getting Help with Teaching Advanced Topics" in Chapter 10). During the past decade or so, specialized resources have been created to help individuals with developmental disabilities learn to masturbate in safe and healthy ways.

■ *Environment*—It's important to remember that sexual behaviors can be used to communicate unhappiness, boredom, or frustration, or to get attention in a particular environment or circumstance. People with cognitive disabilities often learn quickly that these sexual behaviors elicit a more immediate and powerful reaction than other behaviors do. A functional behavior analysis can provide insights on reasons for inappropriate sexual behaviors (attention seeking, task avoidance, sexual arousal when the cute aide/student helper begins working with your child or enters the room, etc.). Once triggers have been identified, a more appropriate strategy targeting those triggers can be implemented.

References

Cornog, M. (2003). *BIG Book of Masturbation: From Angst to Zeal.* San Francisco: Down There Press.

Couwenhoven, T. (May/June 2001). Sexuality Education: Building on the Foundation of Healthy Attitudes. *Disability Solutions 4* (5): 8-9.

Hingsburger, D. (1998). *The Ethics of Touch: Establishing and Maintaining Boundaries in Service to People with Developmental Disabilities.* Eastman, Quebec: Diverse City Press.

Hingsburger, D. & Haar, S. (2000). *Finger Tips: Teaching Women with Disabilities about Masturbation through Understanding and Video.* Eastman, Quebec: Diverse City Press.

Kaeser, F. (1996). Developing a Philosophy of Masturbation Training for Persons with Severe or Profound Mental Retardation. *Sexuality and Disability 14* (4): 295-306.

Monat-Heller, R. (1992). *Understanding and Expressing Sexuality: Responsible Choices for Individuals with Developmental Disabilities.* Baltimore: Brookes Publishing.

Planned Parenthood Federation of America (March 2003). Masturbation: From Myth to Sexual Health. *Contemporary Sexuality 37* (3): i-viii.

Chapter 7

Social and Emotional Development in Adolescence

In addition to the adjustments that arise from physical growth and maturation, your child will experience psychological growth as well. Robert Havighurst, a developmental psychologist, first introduced the unique role changes that occur during adolescence. He labeled these changes as *developmental tasks of adolescence,* accurately implying that work is required as we prepare for the new roles we will be expected to take on in adulthood. You may hear these tasks referred to as "psychosocial" tasks because they involve changes in the way we think about ourselves (psychological) and how those mental shifts affect how we relate to others (social).

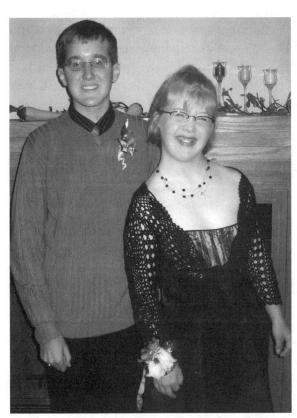

Your child's ability to move through the various psychosocial tasks of adolescence is strongly influenced and affected by life and social experiences, so the rate at which any person progresses through these tasks can vary considerably. At this time, there is little research about psychosocial development in people with developmental disabilities. However, as I speak with self-advocates, parents, and professionals, it is clear that much of the emotional maturation that all teens experience occurs at varying levels and rates for people with Down syndrome and other cognitive disabilities as well. For example, many teens with Down syndrome are quite excited and motivated to take on new responsibilities typical of adolescents; others need more prompting and encouragement. Some teens begin seeking increased independence during middle school, while others do not seem ready until later, sometimes beyond high school.

Remember, there is significant variability among all teens. Although there is really no need to "teach" your child about these tasks, understanding what to expect can help you identify stages your child may be in. This may help you more easily recognize and create opportunities for maximizing mental and social growth during adolescence and beyond.

Developmental Tasks of Adolescence

INDEPENDENCE: NEGOTIATING CHANGES IN RELATIONSHIPS

In the past, the typical adolescent drive for independence was seen as a separation from parents as the teen developed a desired need for self-sufficiency and autonomy. More recent literature views independence as a collaborative process between the parent and child as they work together to negotiate a change in their relationship that reflects an appropriate balance of autonomy and connectedness.

When an adolescent has a developmental disability, the process of achieving independence typically takes longer and is more complex. Drs. Brian Chicoine and Dennis McGuire, who run the Adult Down Syndrome Center in Chicago, have noted that many people with Down syndrome do not seem to experience the typical adolescent drive for independence until their early twenties or even later (McGuire & Chicoine, 2006). Even when the person expresses a desire to be independent, his ability to move away from his family and into an alternative living arrangement is often dependent on family and community resources and supports.

At a recent workshop I did for new parents of babies with Down syndrome, a parent asked, "How does a person become independent?" He was right to be thinking about independence while his child was so young. Because the ability to develop independence is strongly linked to life and social experiences, parents need to routinely examine their roles in promoting or inhibiting independence.

Usually, progress occurs naturally over time. Let's look at the example of dressing. In early childhood, we generally select appropriate clothing for our children and focus on helping them master zippers, buttoning, shoe tying, getting clothes on and off, etc. Later, we realize they should know how to make their own choices about clothing. We explain how to match colors and patterns or purchase coordinated clothing so decision making is fairly easy and error-proof. Perhaps you also did some teaching about how weather affects clothing choices. As an adolescent, your child may develop an interest in trendy styles or fashions and want to buy or select his own clothes. You take his lead and teach him how to purchase clothes that are appropriate for his body type (and as an adolescent, he often chooses to ignore your advice) and you help him find stores that appeal to him.

Parental Pause

1. Has my child expressed a strong desire to be independent in certain aspects of his life? What are they?
2. What obstacles have prevented progress for my child (obstacles for my child or that prevent me, the parent, from moving forward)?
3. What preparation does my child need to move closer to independence (skill development, information, support)?

Essentially, independence happens as you allow your child to begin making his own decisions—small ones at first, and then gradually, more difficult ones. Your job as a parent is to regularly evaluate and balance the level of challenge you are providing with your child's ability to handle those challenges. Even if your child never becomes fully independent, keep in mind that most individuals still experience the need for increasing power and control in their lives as they develop and mature.

A PROCESS FOR THINKING ABOUT AND ENCOURAGING INDEPENDENCE

One of the great dilemmas of parenting a child with a disability is wanting to create opportunities for developing his independence without jeopardizing his health and safety. Giving your child the opportunity to engage in experiences without knowing if he has the ability to succeed is downright scary and requires some ability to take risks. And when he is offered a chance and he fails, there is a natural desire to protect him from further failure by restricting his participation in experiences that may, in fact, be beneficial for learning and growth. Described below is a three-step process for thinking about your role in developing autonomy and independence in various areas of your child's life:

STEP #1—PREPARATION

It's unfair for anyone to be thrown into a new situation and be expected to perform a task or skill without proper preparation. The preparation phase is the "learning how" step that helps your child understand the basics for performing a task or developing a skill. Preparation most often occurs through a combination of watching and observing someone else perform the task. Individuals with Down syndrome, for example, may learn a skill by simply watching others do it repeatedly over time. Ordering from a menu, calling a friend on the phone, or emptying the dishwasher are examples of this. Complex tasks generally require more intense preparation and teaching time.

STEP #2—PRACTICE WITH SUPERVISION

Once your child has been prepared, practicing with supervision is the key to evaluating progress toward independence and fine tuning learning. Supervision means you are close by or within view in case you need to step in quickly. The length of this phase is highly variable and dependent on the complexity of the skill, your child's individual abilities, and other unique aspects of the experience (e.g., who your child is with, past experiences, etc.). Often it means literally increasing the distance between you and your child until he has mastered the task on his own.

When our daughter was first learning how to order at restaurant counters, we started sending her up to order the dessert. This order was easy and always the same: four chocolate chip cookies. During her first *practice with supervision* session, she came back to the table with a ham and cheese sub. She was frustrated and discouraged, and we were confused. After some inquiries, we realized she had not made eye contact or spoken clearly and when the person at the counter had guessed at her order, she had nodded her head in agreement even though the guess was wrong! We discussed the experience, wrapped up the sandwich, and left.

During the next visit, we reminded her about the importance of eye contact and diction and then had her order again. This time she got it right and her reward was a chocolate chip cookie (never underestimate the power of natural consequences as a learning tool). In *Protecting The Gift* by Gavin De Becker, one mom described the "practice with supervision" session she went through while teaching her eight-year-old son (without a disability) to buy a hot dog from a street vendor on his own:

> *"I started by buying them for him. Then I had him buy them with me standing there. Then I stood a little ways back when he went and asked for them. Then I parked the car in front of the vendor's cart and let him get out and buy a hot dog. Then I parked the car on the other side of the street, so he could cross the street, go up to the vendor, buy a hot dog, get the change, and return across the street."*

Unless you allow your child to try things without your assistance, it becomes difficult to identify new learning that must occur in order to make progress. The glitches that surface during this phase help reveal the obstacles that need to be addressed in order to move closer to independence.

Step #3—Coaching to Autonomy or Interdependence

With enough repetition, motivation, practice, and support, your child may be able to master a skill enough to manage on his own or with significantly less supervision and support. By this phase you'll have a clearer idea of specific aspects of the skill that may be too difficult for your child and will require assistance.

As you look for opportunities to develop independence, begin with lower risk situations. Experiencing episodes of success is more likely to boost your child's confidence and self-esteem as he prepares for more difficult challenges. Evaluating ways to reduce harm, rather than prohibit and ban participation in an experience, is often more effective.

IDENTITY: UNDERSTANDING ASPECTS OF SELF

Although identity formation, a sense of who you are, continues into adulthood, most researchers agree that key aspects of identity are "forged" during adolescence. The physical, emotional, and sexual growth your child experiences during this time, combined with added social demands and responsibilities, can lead to internal questioning about who he is and how he fits in with family and society. Your child may become more aware of differences at this time and begin comparing himself to others. Discussions about a variety of aspects of self frequently surface during adolescence.

AWARENESS OF DOWN SYNDROME OR OTHER DISABILITY

One aspect of identity development for individuals with Down syndrome or other cognitive disabilities involves understanding their disability. If you have not already talked with your son or daughter about his or her disability, adolescence is a time when discussions are usually necessary.

Individuals with obvious physical differences such as Down syndrome may struggle with identity issues earlier than other children. In a study of 77 families with teens ages 17 to 24 with Down syndrome, families reported that their children began noticing their own differences between the ages of 9 and 12. They also reported that when their children were at the developmental age of 6, most could recognize Down syndrome in others and had some ideas about what it meant.

Case Example: Going to the Movies with Friends Unchaperoned

Step 1—Preparation

At some point when my daughter was in middle school, I decided I wanted to be able to drop her off at the movie theater so she could see movies independently with friends. I had been accompanying her and her peers for quite some time. She seemed to know the routine, and I knew this activity would continue to be an important part of her social life as an adult. I talked with my daughter and her friends' parents to share my plan. My preparation began with teaching her aspects of the process I was doing for her. **Preparation** included teaching her how to:

- Locate the entertainment section of the newspaper that included movie listings;
- Identify the name of our movie theater so she could locate start times (we had been going for years but she didn't know the actual name);
- Money skills—determining actual cost of movie and refreshments;
- Movie planning—Previously I had called parents to coordinate outings, but I wanted my daughter to learn these skills. I made a list of things she needed to ask and tell when inviting a friend to the movies.

Step 2—Practicing with Supervision

When I felt I had adequately prepared my daughter, she agreed to a **practicing with supervision** phase. We both decided I would come along until she and I felt routines had been established and skills had been learned. I informed her that I wanted her to do as much as she could on her own and that I would not step in unless she asked me to.

During this practice with supervision phase, I realized how complex the skill actually was. When purchasing her ticket, for example, it took her forever to find the appropriate amount of money in her wallet while a line of impatient moviegoers formed behind her. Although I did not help her, during her next outing to the movies I encouraged her to prepare her money in advance or use a gift card. In the refreshment line, her friend wasn't paying attention to the movement of the line and stayed in one place as the people behind him moved forward. I intervened with some information about lines. After they had purchased refreshments, they headed into the wrong theater (an R-rated movie—perhaps this was intentional). I verbally redirected them and did some quick teaching on ceiling signs and how to locate a movie, all things I assumed they had known! The remainder of the day was uneventful, but the experience sticks with me.

Step 3—Coaching to Interdependence or Autonomy

At age seventeen my daughter is now able to find a movie (in the paper or online) that she and her friend jointly agree to, and can pretty much coordinate an outing with minimal help from me. Ongoing coaching related to this experience has been necessary, however. During the last trip to the movies, two theaters in the same movie house were playing the movie they chose to see. Unfortunately, they walked into the one that had started earlier and missed a good portion of the movie. The new learning involved being clear about their movie start time and matching it with the movie start time listed on the ceiling sign. The important point is there has been considerable progress over time.

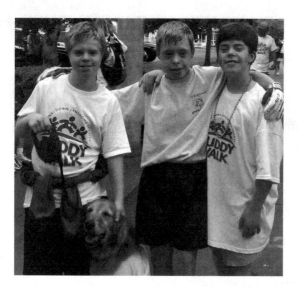

In the same study, 65 percent of parents stated that they spoke openly about Down syndrome within the family. Some families used a reactive approach; in other words, they waited until their child gave them some indication he had an awareness of his Down syndrome. Experiences that prompted these discussions included seeing another person with Down syndrome, the child with Down syndrome being aware of people staring, or the child noticing his own differences and beginning to compare his abilities with others. Other families in the study used a proactive approach, preferring to look for opportunities to raise awareness before it was necessary. These families wanted information about Down syndrome presented in a positive way rather than taking the chance that their child would learn in situations that were negative or distressing.

Observing your child come to grips with his or her disability is a poignant and powerful experience that's difficult to forget. My daughter's realization came quite unexpectedly during fall of fifth grade, her first year in middle school. Although she had been able to recognize other people with Down syndrome as a child and we had talked about Down syndrome fairly regularly, I'm certain she didn't truly understand what it meant for her until that year. For the first time since kindergarten, she had another student (new to the district) with Down syndrome in her homeroom. My daughter is a visual learner and I'm convinced that by observing her classmate with Down syndrome, she more clearly understood what it meant for her. I was unaware of these internal struggles with identity until one October evening when we were doing homework. She was having some difficulty with an assignment when she suddenly put her pencil down and asked, "Mom, do I have Down syndrome?" "Yes, you have Down syndrome," I responded. She sighed, shrugged with frustration, hung her head in her hands, and said, "I just want to be a regular kid."

It wasn't until then that she began to see with accuracy her differences. As much as I wanted to paint a rosy picture, I knew deep down we needed to discuss her limitations. She was noticing them on a daily basis and I needed to be honest. We talked about what it meant to have Down syndrome—how it took her a bit longer to learn new things, that sometimes people had a harder time understanding her—but I also reminded her that Down syndrome was only a small part of who she was as a person. We discussed ways she was like other fifth graders. We talked about her talents, her abilities, her interests, and other aspects of who she was. We talked about her future, about having a job, living on her own, and doing many of the same things her classmates would be doing as adults.

We began using the words "Down syndrome" when my child was quite young. During a shopping trip, our son noticed a little boy with Down syndrome and was convinced the boy was another little guy in his class with Down syndrome. It was then I realized he was noticing the physical features or "look" of Down syndrome.

Our son understands that he has Down syndrome and has been able to verbalize this since fifth grade. We have always talked to him and his siblings about what Down syndrome is and how it affects him, related to health issues, speech, and learning. In middle school, he became very aware of people in the community settings who have Down syndrome. In a group of typically developing peers, he wants to participate but doesn't always know how to engage others in conversation. He completely understands that his speech is sometimes difficult to interpret, which often makes him reluctant to join in.

We also realized that he learned very well to use, or shall I say abuse, his disability. He likes to play the "I am special so I don't have to" card, much to the chagrin of his siblings. We no longer use the phrase "special needs" in the disability arena, because I believe every child has special needs.

We have been chatting with our daughter about the fact that she has Down syndrome since she was in kindergarten. I introduced the concept by reading Where's Chimpy? *to her, pointing out some physical similarities between her and Misty, the girl in the story. Since then, we've often mentioned Down syndrome to her when there are "teachable moments"—for instance, if I notice someone in a store who has Down syndrome, I'll quietly ask her if she thinks that person has Down syndrome too. Or sometimes when she's struggling with math, I'll mention that Down syndrome makes it harder for her to learn certain things so it's not her fault if she doesn't get it right away.*

Now she is eleven and generally has positive feelings about having Down syndrome . . . but still has questions about being "different" that she has not connected with Down syndrome. For instance, in fourth grade when she had trouble with the regular class homework, she would hit her forehead with her hand and say, "I wish I had a better brain." Telling her that everyone is good at some things and not so good at other things helped a little, but to this day she rarely admits she can't do something, because she doesn't want to acknowledge she is different. She's still trying to figure out why she has challenges that other kids don't. The other day when we were ordering dinner at a fast food restaurant, I put some coins in a collection box for UCP (United Cerebral Palsy) and she asked me what CP was. I explained that it was something that caused brain damage at birth and that kids with CP usually have some trouble walking and sometimes learn more slowly. She said, "Is that what happened to me?"

Helping your child understand his disability and the unique impact it will have on him is an important role you'll have as your child enters adolescence. Avoid emphasizing his disability as the sole aspect of who he is as a person. Although Down syndrome may contribute to a few of your child's specific characteristics (e.g., speech difficulties, drier skin, or almond-shaped eyes), the disability itself should not define who he is. Remember (and try to help others remember) that he has a unique personality, skills, abilities, strengths, interests, and gifts that are more likely to reveal his true person than the disability itself. Included in that broader definition of identity is the fact that your child is a sexual person. Accepting and acknowledging this is more likely to support healthy sexual development.

TALKING WITH
YOUR CHILD
ABOUT DOWN
SYNDROME
OR OTHER
DISABILITY

If discussions about your child's disability have not surfaced, think about beginning to initiate discussions during adolescence. Here are some ways to get the conversation going:

- Purchase books written by or about people with Down syndrome or other disabilities so your child can hear firsthand how others like him have lived and grown up with their disability. Mitchell Levitz and Jason Kingsley's book *Count Us In* is a great book for teens to read or for parents to read and discuss with their child. If your child has Down syndrome, subscribe to the *UpBeat*, an NDSS newsletter written by and for people with Down syndrome that highlights individual lives and accomplishments and promotes self-advocacy. Encourage your child to submit an article about his own life. National Down Syndrome Congress creates *DS Headline News*, a special publication to promote stories about people with Down syndrome.
- If your teen likes to use the computer, help him access web sites that contain information about his disability. A few years ago, the National Down Syndrome Society created a site specifically for young adults with disabilities called Club NDSS (www.clubndss.org). The site contains good basic information about a variety of issues and includes quick games for making healthy choices about a range of topics.
- Encourage your child to spend time with teens who have Down syndrome or other types of disability and who share similar interests, experiences, and capabilities. Being and talking with others like himself is a healthy and comforting way to connect with others, share feelings, accomplishments, frustrations, and coping strategies. Check to see if there are local chapters of People First or other self-advocate groups. These groups offer support, but, more importantly, encourage self-determination, independence, and advocacy, regardless of disability. If there are few people with Down syndrome in your area, consider attending a national or local conference with a self-advocate track so your child can participate in workshops, learn new things, build skills, and learn to celebrate who they are.

Although most teens eventually move toward a realistic understanding and acceptance of their disability over time, some have more difficulty adjusting and react more negatively to having a disability. These individuals will need more help and support accepting their disability. Get professional counseling for your child if:

- You notice increases in negative self-talk ("I'm so stupid"; "I can't do anything").
- Your child denies he has Down syndrome or a cognitive disability and refuses to connect with others who are like him.
- You notice changes in personality—perhaps he was previously social and outgoing and now he is more withdrawn, quiet, or angry.
- You notice new and different behavior changes such as inability to eat, sleep, concentrate, lack of interest in previously enjoyed activities.

Many of these signs could indicate a range of other health issues, so check with your physician or a Down syndrome clinic if you have concerns. They can link you with local community or national resources that may be helpful.

FUNCTIONAL IDENTITY

A second dimension of identity development involves anticipating how we will contribute to our family, community, and society in adulthood. This aspect of identity is referred to as functional identity. During adolescence, most teens are experimenting with jobs, thinking about careers, and volunteering as they figure out how they want to become productive members of society. Even though your teen may not verbalize a desire to help out, he should be expected to perform tasks and participate in activities similar to other teens his age. By taking on increasingly difficult roles and responsibilities, your child's sense of competence and self-confidence will increase.

When our daughter turned ten, we introduced her to the concept of "responsibility." We explained that as people got older, they tended to learn and practice new skills so when they become adults, they will be able to do more things on their own. To illustrate this point, we tried to add on new responsibilities with each birthday, helping her to associate getting older with growing up with additional responsibilities. As she became a teenager, she began to anticipate new skills she would develop with each year. Initially, we decided the task we wanted her to learn, but now she gets to choose. This year she wants to get better at cooking.

When our daughter was twelve, she began showing us she was interested in taking on more responsibilities. One day, for example, she took a stack of letters off the table and dropped them in a mailbox a few blocks from our house, even though most of the letters had no stamps or return labels. We positively reinforced her helpfulness, emphasized the fact that she should tell someone when she is leaving, and now have her put the stamps and return labels on the envelopes. A few days later, my husband found our daughter giving herself an Albuterol inhaler treatment. This required a little talk about medicines, the consequences of overdosing, label reading, and why adult assistance is a good idea. We did begin having her keep track of the time between doses so she could remind us when she is due. Shortly after that she started calling me at work when she got home from school. The phone numbers had been there for a while, but for some reason, she started using them.

Being able to perform meaningful roles and responsibilities within the family and community helps your child see how he will contribute in adulthood.

Here are some other ways families have involved their child in new roles and responsibilities:
- Managing and organizing homework
- Coordinating, planning, and scheduling social activities
- Doing basic household chores
  - recycling papers or plastics and can-crushing;
  - filling bird feeders;
  - sorting, washing, folding, putting away laundry;
  - loading, starting, emptying dishwasher;

- dusting;
- vacuuming;
- taking out garbage;
- making their bed;
- setting the table;
- yard work;
- feeding pets
- Opportunities for "home alone" time
- Tracking family birthdays and mailing out cards
- Assistance with remodeling or other home projects
- Babysitting or supervised babysitting of nieces or nephews
- Caring for the family dog or pet
- Making out grocery lists and then finding the items
- Paper routes or other jobs that encourage skill development and responsibility
- Volunteering in the community

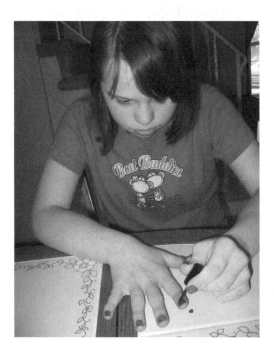

BODY IMAGE

Coming to grips with our physical appearance is another aspect of identity. In a society that glorifies beauty and thinness, it's easy for most of us to feel insecure about how we look. Considering that most of our children are comfortably acquainted with the media, they receive these same messages. Increasingly, I hear anecdotal stories from parents indicating that their children are aware of these messages and internalizing them.

My daughter asked me the other day if I thought she was fat. I have no idea where it came from.

*Recently my 13-year-old daughter saw a picture of someone with Down syndrome who was quite overweight. Since then she has asked me several times if I think **she** will be overweight when she grows up. She has also skipped lunch at school on the grounds that she doesn't want to get "fat."*

Strategies for helping your child feel good about himself and his body:

- *Model respect and acceptance of your own body* —Our nation's obsession with thinness and outward appearance is a tough message to battle. Begin at home by modeling a respect and acceptance of your own body. Avoid modeling negative self-talk ("I'm so fat," "I wish I was skinny"). If reasons for changes related to diet or exercise are justified, communicate motivations that emphasize an improvement in health and well-being ("I need to lower my cholesterol"; "eat more vegetables"; "feel more energetic"; "build up my muscles") rather than incentives that focus solely on looks and appearances ("I need to wear a size 8"; "get skinnier"; "lose weight").

- *Regularly communicate life affirming, positive messages.*
- *Encourage physical movement/activity*—Find a physical activity your child feels good about and encourage him to stick with it. Yoga, Tai Kwon Do, dance, walking, swimming, exercise videos, Special Olympics, or weight lifting may be good choices. Physical movement improves body awareness, and as skills are mastered, self-esteem.
- *Reveal the lies*—In an effort to illustrate self-acceptance, flaws and all, Jamie Lee Curtis appeared in a popular magazine in nothing but her bra and underwear. Her goal was to show the world that her body—untouched by cosmetic surgery—looked pretty much like everyone else's (and it really did, cellulite and all). On my fridge I have two pictures of Katie Couric side by side. The first is a real picture, the other an identical, digitally altered photo that makes her look twenty pounds thinner. It was a great way to remind my girls (and me) that the famous people they see in the media are usually airbrushed, photographed with special lenses, and in many cases surgically or digitally altered.
- *Make the most of what you have*—Help your child choose clothing that fits/compliments his body type. When out shopping and trying on clothes, identify styles that are appealing and flattering. Praise your child often when he takes the time to look nice and obviously takes pride in his appearance (see Chapter 8).

It bothers my daughter that people can tell by looking at her that she has Down syndrome and that they then jump to conclusions about her. For example, they assume she won't understand what they are saying and so they talk down to her. When I asked her if I could use her picture for a project, she said, "Yes, but do I have to look like I have Down syndrome in the picture? I just want to look like I'm a normal girl."

SEXUAL ORIENTATION

Another aspect of identity involves realizing what one's sexual orientation is or who we are sexually attracted to and have the potential for loving. Adolescence is a time when awareness of these attractions sharpens. Although there is very little literature on sexual orientation and individuals with developmental disabilities, it's important to be aware that diversity in sexual orientation exists among individuals with cognitive disabilities just as it does in the general population.

Determining sexual orientation in adults with cognitive disabilities is often more complicated since they experience restrictions in living arrangements, have limited access to partners, and generally have less privacy. For example, among people with developmental disabilities who live in homes that are segregated by gender, residents often choose same-sex encounters simply because they have limited options for choosing with whom they will form relationships (much like behavior that occurs in prisons). This phenomenon is called situational homosexuality because the behavior results from the situation itself rather than a true choice. When these same residents are allowed to choose partners, they often return to heterosexual behavior.

When a person is gay and also has a developmental disability, he faces the same and sometimes more intense ridicule and prejudice as any other gay person. A few years ago I was asked by a county case worker to provide safe-sex information to one of her clients, a young gay woman with a developmental disability. Although this woman was interested in the information, it became clear that her real need was for support and acceptance. Her efforts at seeking help from a non-supportive staff person had resulted in more rigid social restrictions (preventing her from seeing her partner), alienation from her family, and ridicule and isolation from roommates who lived in her group home.

Some things to remember regarding sexual orientation:

- One same-sex encounter, crush, or dream does not necessarily mean your child is gay or lesbian. Homosexual experiences are common among teens and not a good predictor of sexual orientation. Many males and females in the general population report homosexual emotions or experiences during their adolescent years; however, they still feel attraction to the opposite gender.
- Although many individuals who are homosexual remember feeling different from others early in life, acceptance of identity usually occurs in adulthood.
- Thoughts and fantasies are a better indicator of sexual orientation than behavior.

If you suspect your child may be gay, he or she will need information and support just like anyone else. Refer to the list of organizations in the Resources and be prepared to help your child locate materials that can help him feel good about who he is. Feeling okay about every aspect of who you are is an important foundation for healthy self-esteem and relationship building.

GENDER IDENTITY

Gender identity refers to our internal sense of whether we are male or female. This is different from who we are attracted to or have the capacity to fall in love with (sexual orientation). Most professionals agree that we all possess a blend of masculine and feminine characteristics and adhering to rigid stereotypes about what it means to be male or female is limiting or even damaging.

For some people, their inner sense of being male or female does not match their assigned biological gender. This can create confusion for the individual. We know now that this mismatch can often be traced to specific medical conditions that affect the sex chromosomes or development of the external genitalia or internal reproductive organs. For example, children born with ambiguous genitalia (requiring that their parents "assign" a gender at birth), Turner syndrome, Klinefelter syndrome, androgen insensitivity syndrome, or hypospadias may be more at risk for experiencing gender identity disorders.

The term "transgender" is an all-encompassing term used to describe people whose biological gender differs from their gender identity. If you suspect that your child is experiencing difficulties in this area, try to locate a professional or clinic specializing in transgender issues. If you're unsure about clinics in your area, call your local Planned Parenthood or an AASECT professional.

Learning to Think—Making Decisions and Solving Problems

It is common to become so used to thinking, problem-solving, or making decisions for your child that you forget how much this inhibits his ability to develop these skills on his own. Being able to solve problems and make decisions requires some level of abstract thinking. In typical teens, this skill usually improves on its own as physiological changes occur in the brain during adolescence. For teens with Down syndrome and other cognitive disabilities, abstract thinking is considerably more difficult. Reasons cited in the literature that contribute to this difficulty include:

- *Reduced perceptions of control*—If someone feels he has little control over what happens to him, he is less empowered or motivated to make his own choices. When people with cognitive disabilities try to participate in independent decision making, their efforts are often sabotaged by caregivers. For instance, others may encourage choice-making when there really is no choice, use persistent persuasion to try to get the individual to make a particular choice, or ignore the person's efforts to communicate choices. This eventually reduces the person's sense of control, self-efficacy, and motivation to make decisions.
- *Limited life and personal experiences* People need to have a variety of life experiences and opportunities to make meaningful decisions to become proficient at making decisions.
- *Decreased access to problem solving/decision making training*— Unlike individuals in the general population, students with cognitive disabilities usually require intentional instruction within a variety of situational contexts (on the job, in a relationship, etc).

Teaching problem solving is an important life skill. Researchers have documented many instances in which individuals with a wide range of cognitive limitations were successfully taught these skills, proving that with effective instruction and practice, your child can improve his problem-solving abilities. Common characteristics of effective learning include:

- Using real-life situations where the ability to problem solve is important;
- Providing information on the problem-solving process coupled with social skills training;
- Facilitator-guided instruction within a variety of simulated contexts (occupational, interpersonal, environmental);
- Ensuring that individuals have regular opportunities to make choices and experience problem solving and decision making in their daily lives so they can become more proficient at applying skills.

Teaching Activity: "Decision Clouds"

In middle school, our daughter's speech and language pathologist used *decision clouds* as a way to help students visually identify steps in the problem-solving process and apply it to everyday problems. Problems were identified by parents, the kids themselves, or staff based on skills needed for safety, autonomy, and independence. As situations arise that require your child to use problem solving-skills, use the template in Appendix B-1 to illustrate a way to work through a specific situation.

A Process for Teaching

1. What is the problem/decision? The first step is to clearly identify the problem or decision at hand. (Note that the Decision Cloud tool works best when applied to a situation your child is directly involved in rather than a hypothetical one.) For example, knowing how to handle sales-people or telemarketers on the phone or dealing with people who steal things are examples of problems you could write at the top of the cloud.

> *Example: I miss the bus after school.*

2. What are my choices? The second step involves generating a list of possible things your child can do to handle the situation. Your child may have a hard time coming up with a wide range of solutions or possibilities and tend to rely on strategies used in the past, even if they were unsuccessful. If the problem is one your child is familiar with or has actually experienced, he will have some ideas about options. If the scenario is new, it may be more difficult to come up with ideas. Encourage him to think about what could happen or share a few of your own experiences to help them get started. As you identify possible solutions, write possible ways to handle the situation on the lines (or use symbols or pictures of your child performing various options if your child is a nonreader).

> *Possible options: I could:* Go to the office and call home.
> Go to the office and call Mom on her cell phone.
> Walk home.
> Ask someone for a ride.

3. Which solution will work best? Figuring out which of the choices will work best is the next step. In classroom settings, this is typically done through modeling, watching others role play solutions incorporating realistic consequences, use of videos (where consequences are obvious), scripting, or pictures. Social Stories are another strategy for teaching outcomes and expectations related to problematic scenarios. Social Stories, originally created by Carol Gray for use with students with autism, are stories that are written for a particular person to communicate what behaviors are expected within a specific situation before the person encounters that situation. Based on the results discussed or illustrated above, allow your child to select the one that is the safest and makes the most sense.

> *Agreed upon best option: If I miss the bus, I should:*
> Go to the office and call Mom on her cell phone.

4. Practice. Ensuring that your child has opportunities to practice independently trying out the "best option" can improve success. Sometimes these practice sessions can be contrived or planned. Other times your child learns problem-solving abilities best by experiencing natural consequences and remembering consequences.

Intimacy: Connecting with Others

Although relationships with parents remain important in adolescence and into adulthood, friends, peer, and love relationships become more important for most teens during this time. It is during preadolescence or adolescence that your child may

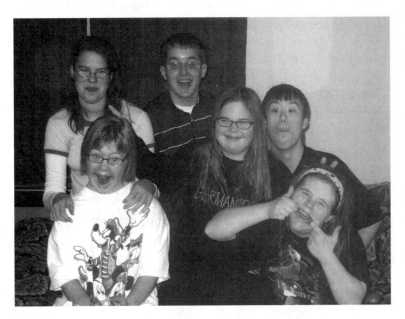

experience his first crush or become involved with his first romantic relationship. Having best friends and stable relationships with peers becomes more important and can act as a training ground for learning about and understanding more mature relationships.

Families that have a child with a disability often notice that peer relationships change after elementary school. Some parents find that shifting to a middle school (usually larger than the elementary school) offers more options for cultivating friendships and improvements in social life. Wider ranges of extracurricular activities can make it easier for your child to explore his interests and become part of a group. More often, however, families experience a decline in social activity levels in middle and high school years. Invitations to birthday parties subside, scout troops fold or disband due to lower interest levels, and friendships that worked well in elementary school now seem forced and unnatural. At a time when socialization becomes increasingly important, opportunities to socialize may become more limited for your child.

We experienced a gradual diminishment of social life during our daughter's first year in middle school. Although she was well liked by her peers (children with and without disabilities), there seemed to be few opportunities to interact with kids outside of school. Over time, we noticed her becoming less animated and more irritable, not typical for her. At the same time, she began spending more and more time in her room engaging in repetitive, nonproductive tasks or chatting with "pretend friends." We decided to more aggressively seek out opportunities for socialization.

Toward the end of her first year of middle school (fifth grade) we did some collaborative planning for her sixth grade year. After discussions with both her teacher and principal, our daughter expressed an interest in joining the sixth grade choir (which she loves) and a community service club at school. I did some research on activities that she could participate in outside of school. We enrolled her in Special Olympics (almost every sports season that first year). That summer we also sent her to a camp designed for kids with mild cognitive disabilities.

We began teaching her social planning skills so she could begin to understand what was required for planning social activities (the first step was getting Mom to put it on her calendar) so she could initiate activities with her preferred friends. I attempted to reconnect her with kids from her past to experi-

ment with compatibility (since she hadn't seen them in a while). Sometimes it worked and other times it didn't, but we kept trying. We did, however, notice improvements in her overall mood. Now as a high schooler, she continues to have an active social life.

Although my son seems to be well-liked and respected among his high school peers, these same kids are not calling him up on the weekends to do things. In our experience, being included at the high school has not created the kind of friendships or sense of community we had hoped for.

IMPROVING SOCIAL CONNECTIONS

If you notice negative downturns in your child's social life, you may need to make increased efforts to identify barriers and create a plan. Below are some common factors that often contribute to isolation:

Troubleshooting: Barriers for Connecting with Others

Inadequate social skills	■ Refer to Chapter 9 for ideas and resources for improving social skills
Minimal opportunities to be with others	■ Evaluate child's interests and gifts—explore appropriate opportunities in your community ■ Connect with local disability organization to identify social networks and activities
Problematic societal attitudes/alienation from typically developing peers	■ Consider increasing opportunities to connect with people with disabilities if not already doing so. Try Special Olympics, activities with your local Down syndrome support group, summer camps or programs for children or teens with disabilities. ■ Advocate for packaged programs that support relationship facilitation and development between disabled and non-disabled children (Best Buddies, PALS, Circle of Friends, etc.).

PEERS WITH DISABILITIES OR WITHOUT?

Although many families believe strongly that their child should be fully included in every aspect of community life, research suggests that having friendships in both groups (people with and without disabilities) is beneficial.

If your child is not developing fulfilling relationships with the "typical" classmates or coworkers he spends most of his day with, consider exploring ways for helping him connect with other people with disabilities. Finding friendships that are mutually beneficial takes considerable time and effort. All friendships evolve out of common experiences, mutual understanding, and shared interests, and the rewards are great. Active social lives for people with Down syndrome have been linked to improved mental and physical health (Chicoine, Fujiora).

Our daughter went through a time when she was younger (and fully includ-ed in a school with no other children with disabilities) when she didn't want to have anything to do with others who had disabilities. It was like she was embar-rassed by their actions. I noticed it most when we'd do activities (holiday party, etc.) with our local parent group. But as she got older, and was taking some classes in child development, she began to enjoy seeing babies and little ones with Down syndrome and they always seemed to like her too. When she was in high school, she had the opportunity to join a social group of teens with developmen-tal disabilities. The social group went against everything her dad and I believed in and had worked for. We didn't want her out in the community with a whole bunch of other kids with developmental disabilities; we wanted her included in the community like everyone else.

We decided to let our daughter be the main decision maker, even though I thought I knew what was best for her. Turns out she LOVED her outings with "the group." Thinking back, it was probably the first time that she could just be herself and not try 150 percent to keep up with everyone else. This is her life, not ours. She is more than capable of telling us what she likes and doesn't like. She has the right to make her own choices.

Resources that include information on facilitating relationships are listed at the back of the book.

References

Benson, B. (1995*)*. Psychosocial Interventions Update: Problem Solving Skills Training. *The Habilita-tive Mental Healthcare Newsletter 14* (1).

Buckley, S., Bird, G. & Sacks, B. (2002). *Social Development for Individuals with Down Syndrome.* Southsea, Hampshire, UK: Down Syndrome Educational Trust.

Couwenhoven, T. (2001). Sexuality Education: Building on the Foundation of Healthy Attitudes. *Dis-ability Solutions (4)* 6.

Cunningham, C. & Glenn, S. (2002). Parents Telling Their Offspring about Down's Syndrome and Disabil-ity. *Down Syndrome Association Malta Magazine* (http://www.dsa.org.mt/magazine_jan02_11.htm).

Fujiura, G. et al. (July/August 1997). Predictors of BMI among Adults with Down Syndrome: The Social Context of Health Promotion. *Research in Developmental Disabilities 18* (4): 261-74.

Haffner, D. (1995). *Facing Facts: Sexual Health for America's Adolescents.* New York: National Commis-sion on Adolescent Sexual Health, SIECUS.

Haffner, D. (2001). *Beyond the Big Talk: Every Parent's Guide to Raising Sexually Healthy Teens.* New York: NewMarket Press.

Kaufman, M. *Disability and Sexuality: Supporting Our Clients, Supporting Ourselves.* AASECT Confer-ence presentation, Chicago, IL, May 2004.

Levy-Warren, M. (2000). *The Adolescent Journey: Development, Identity Formation, and Psychotherapy.* New York: Jason Aronson.

McGuire, D. & Chicoine, B. (2006). *Mental Wellness in Adults with Down Syndrome: A Guide to Emo-tional and Behavioral Strengths and Challenges.* Bethesda, MD: Woodbine House.

Pueschel, S. (2001). *A Parent's Guide to Down Syndrome: Toward a Brighter Future.* Baltimore: Brookes Publishing.

Pueschel, S. (1997). *Adolescents with Down Syndrome: Toward a More Fulfilling Life.* Baltimore: Brookes Publishing.

Rubin, K. (2002). *The Friendship Factor: Helping Our Children Navigate Their Social World and Why it Matters for Their Success and Happiness.* New York: Skylight Press.

Shibley-Hyde, J. & DeLamater, J. (2003). *Understanding Human Sexuality* Boston: McGraw-Hill.

Simpson, A.R. (2001). *Raising Teens: A Synthesis of Research and a Foundation for Action.* Boston: Center for Health Communication, Harvard School of Public Health.

Thorin, E. et al. (1996). Dilemmas Faced by Families during Their Young Adults' Transitions to Adulthood: A Brief Report. *Mental Retardation 34* (2): 117-120.

Wehmeyer, M.L. et. al. (1998). *Teaching Self Determination to Students with Disabilities.* Baltimore: Brookes Publishing.

CHAPTER 8

Caring for the Body during Puberty

During a presentation at a national conference, I introduced examples of visual tools that could be used to help people with cognitive disabilities become more independent in caring for their own bodies. The father of an eleven-year-old son with Down syndrome mulled over my messages and eventually shared that I was contradicting every professional who had ever supported his son. He had been told over and over again that his son would never be independent with self-care, and consequently no attempts at teaching self-care had been initiated. This was disheartening, sad, and a very discouraging message—especially considering his son was only eleven!

Key Teaching Messages:

- Bodies require care.
- Taking care of my body helps me look my best.
- Now that I am older, I can learn to help take care of myself.

Preparing your child to take care of his or her body is one of the most important things you can do to help your child become an independent adult. Self-care skills typically revolve around proper hygiene, grooming, and dressing. Proper self-care skills influence societal attitudes and perceptions and greatly enhance social acceptance. When you have a child with Down syndrome or other cognitive disability, progress will often be painfully slow, but many individuals can make significant progress towards independence. Remember that every little bit of independence can be helpful in boosting your child's self- esteem and dignity, as well as reducing reliance on others to perform these tasks.

How quickly your child will learn self-care skills will depend on her own unique strengths and abilities. Many adults with Down syndrome learn to care for themselves with minimal assistance. Others require more assistance. Mastering these skills does take longer, however, and will require gentle persistence over time.

Commonly Taught Self-Care Skills

Hygiene
- ___ uses toilet and toilet paper
- ___ washes hands
- ___ washes face
- ___ takes showers or baths
- ___ washes hair
- ___ brushes teeth
- ___ manages menstrual hygiene
- ___ skin care

Grooming
- ___ combs/brushes hair
- ___ uses deodorant
- ___ shaves
- ___ applies make-up appropriately (optional)
- ___ nail care
- ___ uses tissues or handkerchief

Dress
- ___ dresses independently
- ___ chooses appropriate clothes for weather and occasion
- ___ wears clean, age-appropriate clothing
- ___ coordinates outfits

Whose Responsibility Is It?

Direct teaching about how to perform hygiene tasks falls squarely in the lap of parents. Caring for the body is private so learning experiences in which students are being taught to care for their body should be shrouded in a respect for privacy and modesty. Teaching these skills at home, in a bathroom that is private, is more likely to preserve and reinforce these concepts.

Although many school sexuality education programs designed for people with cognitive disabilities *do* include units on health and hygiene, most do not (and should not) involve instruction that requires your child to remove clothes and expose private body parts. Appropriate special education goals for programs that address hygiene and grooming within the classroom include:

- Defining good hygiene;
- Emphasizing personal responsibilities associated with caring for the body;
- Helping students recognize consequences of poor hygiene;
- Reinforcing proper hygiene technique using videos, slides, or pictures.

What Do I Teach?

Before you create a plan, it's important to do some assessment of where your child is related to self-care. There may be skills your child is in the middle of learning how to do, tasks that require considerable help from you, or other skills she does well

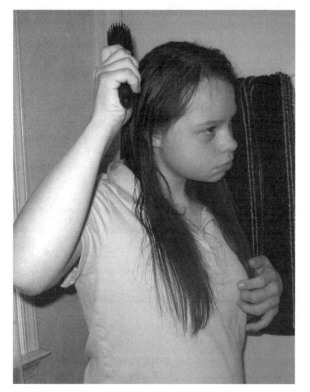

on her own. For example, your child may know how to turn on the shower and adjust the water temperature, but relies on you to do most of her body washing and shampooing. Maybe your child can brush her teeth and get dressed in the morning, but has difficulty choosing appropriate clothing. Perhaps your child has the skills to perform morning hygiene tasks independently but needs reminders from you to move from one task to the next. Here are things to consider as you make decisions about where to begin:

- Which tasks seem most urgent? For example, if my child learned how to _____ it would:
  - make the daily routine much easier,
  - make school inclusion more likely,
  - enable my child to have more privacy with something that really should be private.
- What tasks does your child show an interest in learning?
- Which tasks would be easiest to learn and could create early success?
- What skills do you (the teacher) feel most confident teaching?

How Do I Teach?

It's easy to forget how complicated self-care tasks can be. After all, we've been doing them for so long, they've become automatic, requiring very little thought or effort. Individuals with cognitive disabilities often learn more effectively when self-care tasks are broken into smaller, more manageable steps and appropriate instruction is provided.

STEP 1: TASK ANALYSIS

Any skill you are trying to teach your child can first be broken down into tinier steps and then taught one step at a time. A good way to conduct a task analysis is for you to perform the task you want to teach your child. Move through the task slowly, writing down all of the steps that are a part of doing the task. For example, if you wanted to teach your child how to wash her hands, you would wash your own hands, paying attention to each step. When you're done your list might look like this:

1. Turn on water.
2. Adjust water temperature.
3. Get hands wet.
4. Pump soap dispenser to get soap on hands.
5. Rub hands together.

6. Rinse soap off under faucet.
7. Turn off water.
8. Dry hands with towel.

Once you have some idea of the steps involved, use your list to teach the skill to your child. Breaking the skill into smaller tasks can be helpful as you monitor progress and evaluate learning. For example, you may find in the process of moving through the steps that your child has difficulty manipulating faucet handles and therefore can't perform steps one, two, and seven. This new information will help you know where to provide support or come up new ideas for facilitating independence.

STEP 2: DIRECT INSTRUCTION

Once you've listed the individual steps that are a part of the skill, some type of direct instruction should be provided. Teaching each of the steps of a task usually involves one or more of the following:

VERBAL EXPLANATION

Many people simply need auditory instruction or someone "telling" them how to perform a particular skill in order to learn. When using verbal explanations, pay close attention to words that you are using. Brief explanations with simple words that you know your child understands will work best. Move through the explanation one step at a time and make sure your child is paying attention.

DEMONSTRATION

Demonstration involves modeling or showing your child how to perform individual steps—the "seeing" part of instruction. Most of us are aware of how much more effective learning is when we can watch someone perform a task at the same time verbal instructions are provided. This is especially true for individuals with Down syndrome and other cognitive disabilities.

PHYSICAL ASSISTANCE

For many individuals, a combination of verbal and visual instruction will be sufficient. Others may also need physical guidance or "doing with help" as a part of the teaching process. At first, physical assistance may mean you are actually doing the task for your child but over time, as she learns the skills, you can fade your assistance. (See the box on prompt hierarchy.)

COMBINING TEACHING METHODS

Most people learn best with a combination of teaching methods. For example, a demonstration with verbal instructions or physical assistance with verbal clarification usually works better than one method alone.

- When you are teaching personal hygiene skills, you may need to invade your child's space and privacy as part of the teaching process. Begin with the least invasive teaching strategy and increase only if your child has difficulty learning. For example, if your child is unable to learn to wash her hair with verbal instructions alone, move to demonstration or some physical assistance.
- When using physical guidance, use the least restrictive prompt that is necessary to learn the skill.

Hierarchy of Prompts

Prompt hierarchies identify the levels of assistance that can be offered if your child needs help learning a new skill. As you introduce a skill through verbal instruction and demonstration, observe her performing the task you are trying to teach. If a physical prompt is necessary, begin with one that is most appropriate for your child and provides the least "hands on" contact. Determine how many times the physical prompt will be provided before fading out. For example, if you are teaching shampooing and your son or daughter has difficulty with scrubbing the head, a full physical assist may be appropriate for the first three times. After the third time, move to a partial assist, etc. Varying levels of support from most to least are listed below.

- **Full Physical Assist** means you are essentially performing the task but involving your child as you provide assistance. For example, putting your hand on your daughter's hand as you teach her to shampoo her hair would be a full physical assist.

- **Partial Physical Assist** means less physical assistance is provided. Rather than use complete hand-over-hand assistance to teach shampooing, you might steer your child's hand from her wrist, forearm, or elbow to encourage a scrubbing motion.

- **Modeling** means demonstrating for your child what you want her to do. If your child is a good imitator, physical touching may not be needed. Instead use task analysis to break down steps into smaller steps that make sense for your child. Demonstrate smaller steps, one at a time, and then have her model the smaller steps until the larger task is learned.

- **Gestures** are nonverbal ways of cueing your child to perform a task. Pointing, miming an action, mouthing words, or using facial expressions helps her know what to do.

- **Direct Verbal** refers to the use of spoken directions to prompt your child to do the steps involved in performing a task or prompting. "Now, it's time to wash your hair." You can start here if your child is able to follow directions.

- **Indirect Verbal** alerts your child that something comes next, but doesn't tell her exactly what it is you want her to do. "Good, you have the shampoo on your hand, now what do you do? Or, "You've got your hair nice and wet—what's next?"

- Break down larger skills into smaller, more doable steps. Taking a shower, for example is a skill, but can easily be broken into many smaller skills (see below).
- Remember to fade assistance over time. Continually performing the steps for your child without reducing assistance leads to dependency, not competence. For example, help her two to four times, then let her try.

EXAMPLE: DIRECT INSTRUCTION FOR SHOWERING

Before your child begins to learn to shower on her own, do a spot check of your bathroom to help you anticipate and prevent problems. For example, rubber mats placed on the floor of the bathtub can help prevent falls. Soap and water in the eyes during showering can be annoying, so figure out a way your child can reach a towel quickly if

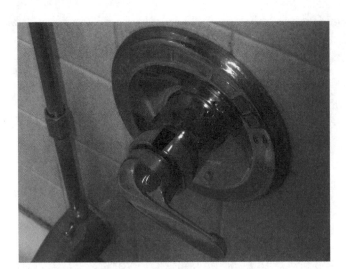 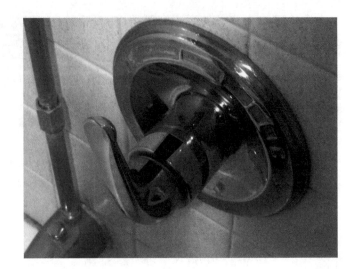

necessary. It can help to hang towels on racks placed on the opposite end of the shower or just outside of the shower curtain. If you have sliding shower doors, throw the towel over the top of the door. Purchase a shower caddy or make sure there is a flat surface to place soap and shampoo to prevent items from falling and injuring toes. If your child has difficulty getting in and out of the bathtub, a bar to hold onto can help.

Think about aspects of showering that your child may have difficulty with and consider how a visual tool may help. For example, markings on the faucet can prevent "too hot" and "too cold" accidents (in the photo above, note the position of the black tape on the faucet before (left) and after (right) the water is turned on for a shower). Consider adjusting the temperature setting on the water heater to prevent accidental scalds.

TASK ANALYSIS—TAKING A SHOWER

1. Bring items needed to the bathroom.

If your child has her own bathroom or shares a bathroom with siblings, the supplies she needs will likely already be there. If she does not have permanent space for shower items, encourage her to bring soap, shampoo, and a clean bathrobe and towel with her to the shower. A hygiene bucket or container that holds these items can help her stay organized.

2. Turn shower on and adjust water temperature.

There is no correlation between water temperature and hygiene. In other words, showering with warmer water does not get you cleaner than showering with cooler water. Your child should decide what water temperature feels most comfortable for her. Adjusting the faucet to ideal water temperatures each time can be tricky. When our daughter struggled with this, we created a "visual marker" so she knew how far to turn the handle. Brightly colored electrical tape (it's waterproof) worked like a charm. Generally, warmer, tepid temperatures are better for dry skin than hot temperatures.

3. Get wet.

Encourage your child to wet her entire body, including hair. If the shower nozzle is far above your child's head, sometimes getting wet enough is a challenge. Handheld shower heads can help your child put water exactly where it's needed.

4. WASH HANDS.

It's fine to use the hands to clean the body, but hands should be clean. Begin by washing hands. Loofahs, washcloths, or other items are not really necessary and may prove to be more cumbersome.

5. SHAMPOO HAIR.

Explain to your child that a general rule for showering is to begin at the top of her body and move down. If she is first learning how to shower, you may want to teach shampooing as a separate skill, after shc has mastered other aspects of showering.

    a. **Place shampoo in hand.** Once the hair is wet, ask your child to place a small amount of shampoo, about the size of a quarter, in the palm of her hand. This task sounds easy, but for many children, manipulating caps on shampoo bottles or knowing how much squeeze pressure will produce the correct amount of shampoo takes practice. Consider using small bottles that are easy to manipulate or pump dispensers. If your child has long hair, extra shampoo is not necessary. In fact, too much shampoo makes rinsing more difficult and can irritate the scalp, resulting in dandruff-like conditions. As long as the scalp is lathered, the lower parts of the hair will be cleaned during the rinsing phase.

    b. **Lather head.** Once she has shampoo on her hand, have her rub her hands together so shampoo is distributed on each hand. Place both hands on the head and gently massage the scalp in the front, back, and sides. Your child will need to massage firmly enough to create a lather. When she is first learning this skill, you can model the appropriate amount of pressure or use a shower mirror to help her know if she has done this sufficiently.

    c. **Rinse shampoo.** Place head directly under the water stream and rinse thoroughly. Again, if your child is shorter, the shower stream may not be powerful enough to rinse thoroughly. A handheld showerhead may work as an alternative. Give your child concrete ways to know when she has rinsed sufficiently. For example, if your hair no longer feels slippery, or if you can squeak the hair between your fingers, the shampoo is gone. Having your child count to a certain number (one that you know will allow time for sufficient rinsing) while under the showerhead is another idea.

6. WASH BODY.

Physicians who work with people who have Down syndrome typically recommend soaps like Dove that include moisturizing lotions. Used in small amounts, these soaps are less irritating and drying, and prevent exacerbation of dry skin conditions common in people with Down syndrome. Many of these brands come in pump dispensers for easier use.

There are a number of ways to teach steps to body washing. One approach is the **head-to-toe strategy.** Using this approach, your child begins at the top of her body and moves down. The steps in this process would look like this:

    a. Wash face (including ears and behind ears)

    b. Upper Body
      shoulders
      arms (elbows)
      underarms
      chest
    c. Lower Body
      stomach
      genitals
      buttocks
      feet

Another approach is to focus on **key body parts** that, when washed inadequately, produce the most odor. This is an abbreviated way to wash the body when your child is not excessively dirty or sweaty but is due for a shower. Washing these parts of the body should be nonnegotiable.

    a. face
    b. underarms
    c. private body parts (genitals & buttocks)
    d. feet and toes

7. Rinse body.

Thoroughly rinsing soap can prevent skin irritation. Encourage your child to turn in a circle under the shower stream two or three times. This helps rinse soap from all areas of the body.

8. Turn off water.

9. Dry body.

Your child should remain in the shower stall or tub after the water is turned off and use her towel to dry her hair until it is damp and no longer dripping wet. Next, dry the remaining parts of the body.

10. Apply moisturizer (optional).

If your child has Down syndrome and has problems with dry skin, encouraging her to apply a good moisturizer immediately after a shower or bath when the skin is still damp will provide the most benefit. You may want to introduce this as a responsibility that comes with caring for the body at certain times of the year. Focus on the skin areas that tend to be most problematic for your child. Moisturizers such as Lubriderm, Eucerin cream, and Aquaphor are more effective for people with dry skin conditions.

11. Put on robe.

Encourage the use of a robe while your child is moving from the bathroom area to her own room to dress. This is an opportunity to reinforce modesty and remind your child that her body is private and should be covered in public areas of the house.

You probably noticed that some steps are more complicated than others and could be broken down into even smaller steps. Monitoring your child's progress will help you to know if more detailed instruction is needed.

Incorporating Modesty into Teaching Self-Care

Because many self-care tasks involve modesty and privacy issues, thinking about messages your child may be getting can determine how difficult it may be for her to understand modesty.

- *Use your child's chronological age as a guide.* Considering typical sexual development can help guide your decisions about when to begin teaching self-care skills and help you decide which teaching strategies may be most appropriate. For example, knowing that most children tend to become more modest about their bodies sometime during late elementary school can help you know when to begin teaching your child self-care skills. Similarly, if your daughter has a good sense of modesty, jumping in the shower with her to teach proper showering techniques is disrespectful and probably not an appropriate teaching strategy. If your child needs physical prompts, brainstorm ways you can provide assistance in minimally invasive ways. For example, if your child has difficulty with shampooing, reach around the shower curtain to perform the task requiring assistance, then leave. Or help your

Empowering Individuals Who Need Help with Intimate Care

David Hingsburger, in his book **I Openers: Parents Ask Questions about Sexuality with Children with Developmental Disabilities,** describes key elements of modeling that can help your child begin to understand the difference between necessary intimate care (hygiene assistance, diaper changing, or health care) and exploitative touch:

The first step involves getting permission. Remember the body rights described in Chapter 3? Teach your child that her body is her own and no one has the right to touch her body without her permission. Before you provide assistance with any hygiene, grooming, or dressing routine, always ask **permission using a private voice,** then wait for a response. If your child does not use words, wait for some kind of response, eye contact, a head nod, or other cue that indicates readiness.

Second, with a soft nonthreatening voice, **describe** what you are doing throughout the process. Talking as you are performing intimate care invites questions and creates an atmosphere of openness.

Third, encourage your child to **participate** in the process as much as possible. Use hand-over-hand techniques to guide her through the self-care tasks if she is unable to perform them on her own. Involve her to the greatest extent possible.

And finally, **talk with her** about the experience and observe how she responds. For example, comment, "You smell so good" or, "Now you're clean and ready for school." After you've assisted her, ask her how she feels now that she is clean. Talk openly about what just happened and learn to read her responses and moods following intimate care.

If your child receives assistance with intimate care at school, ask the school care providers to follow these same guidelines.

child practice specific parts of shampooing over a sink until she has mastered the skills and can perform them in the shower.

■ *Evaluate spaces where intimate care is provided.* It's easy to become desensitized when helping with bathing and toileting routines, but observing from your child's perspective can help you identify areas where improvements can be made. Are doors closed? Are there ways to minimize body exposure? Are others moving in and out of the room when your child needs privacy? What else can be done to maximize privacy and encourage dignity, modesty, and a general respect for the body?

■ If your son or daughter has significant care needs, *help her distinguish between necessary touch and exploitative touch.* If your child is used to receiving assistance with intimate care, she may be more confused about the purpose of the touch and the caregiver's intent, making it harder for her to differentiate between appropriate affection and exploitative touch. See box on page 141.

Teaching Frequency—How Often Is Enough?

How often your child showers will depend on your individual standards for cleanliness, culture, geographic location, and your child's age and lifestyle. People who live in warmer climates and are more active in sports and activities, for example, will require more frequent bathing. During puberty, when oil and sweat glands are active, or when your daughter is menstruating, daily showers may be necessary.

When children are young, parents decide how often bathing needs to occur. Eventually, if you want to promote autonomy, your child should know how to make those decisions on her own. Here are some suggestions for facilitating independence:

1. *Establish consistent routines and expectations for hygiene.* All children benefit from structure and consistent expectations. Some families find that integrating bathing into the daily schedule helps their child adapt more quickly. Using a picture schedule or marking shower days on a calendar can help your child plan in advance and become less reliant on you for reminders.

2. *Help her tune in to bodily signs.* One way to help your child make decisions about when showers are necessary is to increase her awareness of her own unique body signs that help her know it's time to shower or bathe. In the throes of puberty, signs typically become more obvious. Hair gets greasier faster or body odors surface more quickly. Helping your child recognize these signs can encourage independent decision making about hygiene and cleanliness.

3. *Link hygiene routines with events and activities.* If your child is physically active, it makes sense to link bathing routines with sports nights or other physical activities. For example, if she plays basketball on Tuesdays, identify Tuesday night as bathing night.

Teaching Activity: "Puberty Products"

Once the need for more frequent bathing is necessary, a trip to the store with your son or daughter to purchase hygiene products that will be needed during puberty can be a fun way to review body changes, new responsibilities associated with caring for the body, and participate in consumer decision making. Create a handout with three column headers similar to the ones below. Under the first column, review with your child, or have her list, body changes she remembers that are specific to her gender. In the second column, list responsibilities she will need to learn. Then ask your child to come up with products or hygiene items that will be needed as she takes more responsibility for caring for her own body. List these items under the third column and use them as your child's shopping list. A sample list for girls might look like this:

Body changes	My responsibilities	Things I will need
Sweat/body odor	shower more often use deodorant	soap deodorant
Oilier skin & hair	shower more often wash hair more often	shampoo
Zits/acne	shower more often wash face AM & PM	zit cream face soap
Grow hair	shave	shaver/razor
breasts	wear a bra	bra
get period	use menstrual pads	pads

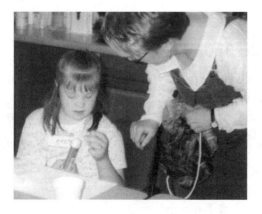

Let your child select items based on what appeals to her (smell, packaging, etc.). The more involved she is in the process, the more likely she will be motivated to actually use the products. At home, have your child identify the items you purchased and explain why they were (will be) needed. For example, if deodorant is grabbed from the bag, your child might tell you it is needed to prevent body odor, or because the sweat glands become more active during puberty. One-word answers like "B.O." or "stink" will do as well.

Common Obstacles to Independence with Self-Care

HEALTH ISSUES

Most of us experience times when illness or disability affects our motivation or ability to care for ourselves. Individuals with cognitive disabilities, however, often have a harder time communicating symptoms that accompany health and medical problems, so they may go undetected for extended periods of time. Speak with your child's healthcare provider if:

- you notice changes in motivation levels (your child previously took pride in her appearance and now seems apathetic);
- you notice changes in her ability to learn new tasks; or
- she experiences skill regression (she once had self-care skills mastered and now requires help).

INCONSISTENT EXPECTATIONS

If independence with hygiene issues is a goal you have for your child, communicate those goals with family members or others who help with intimate care routines. Often one person ends up performing tasks for the child because it's faster and easier while another is trying to help her develop these skills on her own. When expectations are inconsistent, learning is slowed and teaching less effective.

INSISTENCE ON PERFECTION

Achieving independence with self-care will take time. Try to acknowledge and praise any and all of your child's efforts, remembering that your goal is independence, not perfection. If she is trying to be more independent, but repeatedly fails to meet your high expectations, she will easily become discouraged. If you jump in and do things for her, she will begin to see herself as less capable and eventually will stop trying.

Accept every step in the right direction. For example, as long as your child smells clean and looks presentable after a shower, praise her for becoming responsible about caring for her body. If obvious problems surface, reevaluate your teaching strategies.

Our daughter was tactually defensive for so long and her motor development was so delayed that she is just now gaining independence in personal

Teaching Activity: "Caring for My Body Kit"

Having all hygiene and grooming items in one place can make self-care easier and more efficient. Think about purchasing or having your child select a bucket, travel bag, or other cool container to keep frequently used items together in one place. Besides the items that may become necessary during puberty, kits could also include:

- soap
- wide tooth comb or vent brush
- toothpaste
- nail clipper
- perfume or aftershave (optional)
- body lotion
- shampoo
- toothbrush
- dental floss
- nailbrush
- electric shavers or razors
- lip balm

grooming. We have had to choose between having her hair look fluffy, gleaming, and clean and letting it look slightly oily because she scrubs her scalp by herself using feather-light touches and isn't able to get all the shampoo out by herself.

Dressing

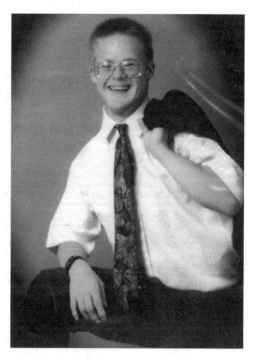

Whether we like it or not, clothes play an important role in helping your child blend in with her social environment, especially in middle and high school. If you want your child's clothing to be an asset and not a liability to her, you need to pay attention to, and teach your child about, clothing selection, fit, and style choices.

FINDING CLOTHES THAT FIT

As children with Down syndrome enter adolescence and their bodies take on new dimensions, many parents notice it becomes more difficult to find clothes that fit. Shorter and stockier body shapes, shorter arm lengths, and limited fine motor skills can limit clothing options for people with Down syndrome, making clothes shopping a trying experience. Here's a list of ideas parents have shared with me that have made my life easier and have allowed their children to dress stylishly and age-appropriately.

PAY ATTENTION TO STYLES AND FASHION TRENDS

Paying attention to current styles and fashion trends among your child's peers can help you and your child make clothing choices that are age-appropriate and stylish. Here are some ideas:

- Frequent shops where your child's peers shop to evaluate current trends that may be flattering.
- Page through teen fashion magazines with your child to get ideas of styles that would work for your son or daughter.
- Pay attention to current styles and fashion trends.
- If your child is a teen or adult, watch style shows such as "What Not to Wear" to enhance understanding about clothing styles that work for certain body types.

Some clothing styles can actually make life easier for people with Down syndrome. For example, ¾ length sleeves and capris may prevent the need for time-consuming alterations in arm or pant lengths. Collars can help sloping shoulders appear squarer. When you see a clothing style that seems to work and meets your expectations, take advantage of it.

MAKE MINOR ADJUSTMENTS

Difficulties with manipulating snaps and buttons often limits clothing choices. Sometimes small adjustments can make a huge difference in clothing choices and independence. For instance, one mother told me she used a razor blade to make buttonhole openings on jeans a bit larger. The slightly larger opening helped her daughter become independent with buttoning, allowing her to wear button/zip jeans for the first time in her life (she had resorted to elastic waist pants). Velcro or slip-on shoes might be easier and more practical if your child continually struggles with keeping shoestrings tied or she ties shoes too loosely and they continually come undone.

ALTER AS NEEDED

The need for clothing alterations at some point is inevitable. If you already have the ability to alter clothes, you're in good shape. If you don't sew, find someone who can. Altering clothes can help your child look more polished and presentable. Some companies such as Land's End or L.L. Bean will hem pants for no extra charge.

SPECIALTY CLOTHING FOR PEOPLE WITH DOWN SYNDROME

Understanding that finding appropriate, good-fitting clothes for an older child with Down syndrome can be hard, companies that specialize in clothing for people with Down syndrome have been created. Various options are listed in the back.

Tips for Girls

Try the Boys' Section. I had great difficulty finding pants for my daughter in the girls' department. When she was younger, pants were too long and didn't seem to fit right. When she became a teen, the pants were much longer and seemed to be designed for girls with long, slender legs, which again made finding a good fit difficult. When my daughter began wearing a Boston brace for her scoliosis, we were forced to buy all new clothes (the brace instantly increased her waist by two sizes). Another mother whose daughter was also in a brace suggested I purchase boys' pants. The waists were larger and pant legs shorter, requiring little or no alterations. I took her advice, and, even after my daughter was out of her brace, continued to find gender-neutral jeans in the boys' department.

If your daughter wears orthotics or has wide feet, boys' shoes often carry wider widths. Since sports shoes are generally not gender distinguishable, shopping in the boys' section may result in a more comfortable fit.

Petite Departments. Nicer department stores often have petite departments where clothing is designed for shorter women. If your child has moved beyond the Juniors department, a petite section may offer more age appropriate options.

Tips for Boys

Finding pants that fit boys with Down syndrome may be easier than finding pants for girls, since there are usually more choices of waist sizes and inseams available for males. If your local stores do not offer pants with short enough inseams, however, bigger cities sometimes house specialty stores designed for shorter men where more flattering clothing choices are offered.

Sometimes when their son has trouble fastening buttons and snaps, parents may fall into the habit of letting him wear sweatpants as an alternative to jeans or dressier pants. Although sweatpants may be acceptable in some situations, in others, they are not. Some parents find that a good alternative is to buy canvas "climber" pants, which often have adjustable cinch waists and are available from stores such as Land's End.

MATCHING CLOTHES

There is nothing that makes your child stand out more than mismatched, improperly assembled outfits. One way to alleviate stress and confusion associated with dressing is to make clothing choices error-proof. Purchase simple, basic, comfortable clothing items that require no matching or coordination. A few pairs of well-fit, stylish black or denim jeans, for example, can be worn with just about any colored or patterned top or T-shirt. A good, classic black skirt or dressier black pants can be matched up with most any top or jacket. Try to choose clothes that are appealing, but also interchangeable and versatile.

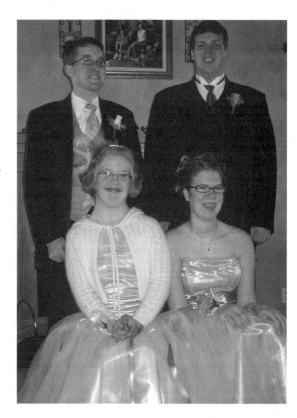

Another possible solution is to organize clothing by "outfits." Purchase hangers that allow tops and bottoms to be hung together so minimal decision making is required and "outfit" choice is foolproof. One mom told me that by organizing her son's wardrobe this way, he eventually memorized what things went together. Although there were some elements of rigidity to their method (he refused to mix and match), it did help him choose appropriately coordinated outfits independently.

WEARING CLOTHES THAT ARE CLEAN AND IN GOOD REPAIR

As soon as your child understands the difference between "clean" and "dirty," help her apply these concepts to clothing. Explain that clothes are "dirty" and need to be washed if:

- they smell, or
- they have spots or stains.

If your child spills a drink on herself, rather than taking off the shirt without an explanation, explain that her shirt is now "dirty" or "stained" and that she needs to put on a "clean" one. Teach your child where to put clothes that are ready for the wash when she takes them off at night.

Once your child is done growing, sometimes clothes are kept for longer than they should be. You will probably need to coach her so she knows what to do with clothing that's not suitable to wear in public. Communicate your own expectations with your child. Usually clothing that's permanently stained, faded, or looks worn (excessive pilling or stretched out of shape) should be tossed. If a piece of clothing is simply ripped, missing a button, or needs some simple mending, start a repair pile and ask your son or daughter to throw clothes that are in need of repair on the pile. If your child seems interested in knowing how to do repairs, teach her.

Having disposable income for replacing well-worn clothing is frequently an issue for adults with developmental disabilities. As your child reaches adulthood, encourage sibs or other family members to monitor her clothing needs or offer new clothes as gifts when finances are tight.

BALANCING APPROPRIATENESS WITH EASE OF DRESSING

Sometimes people with cognitive disabilities wear clothing that's inappropriately matched for age or social occasion. For example, they may be much smaller or more petite than their peers, making clothing choices more limited. Or they might want to wear favorite clothes in situations that aren't appropriate. For instance, I have a friend whose daughter, following her high school prom, wanted to wear her prom

Troubleshooting—Clothing Inappropriateness

Potential problem	Possible Strategies
Clothing inappropriate for age	■ If child is unusually petite, opt for plain clothes. Sometimes lettering, pictures, logos, or other distinguishing features are clues to where clothing was purchased. ■ Remind gift givers that even though your child can still wear a child's size, she wants to wear clothes like the other teens or young adults ■ Consider taking a sibling or same-aged peer clothes shopping so he or she can tell your child what clothes are and are not "cool"
Clothing inappropriate for occasion	■ Offer suggestions for appropriate types of clothing for different areas in person's life. ■ Organize clothing by function (school, work, special occasions, etc.) to facilitate decision-making. ■ Make clothing for special occasions less accessible (put on a higher shelf or store out of sight) so fewer errors are made
Clothing inappropriate for season	■ Involve your child in seasonal closet cleaning (making shift noticeable) to make transitions clearer ■ Have your child be temperature reporter ■ Make visual thermometer with clues for what to wear based on temperature ■ Make out-of-season clothing less accessible
Clothing unclean, worn, or in need of repair	■ Identify clear standards for clothing that can be worn in public ■ Encourage family and friends to purchase presentable clothing for gifts if finances are tight

dress to almost every "special" occasion that came up. This included a self-advocacy conference, a more casual high school dance, and a funeral! Some individuals have difficulty making the transition from clothes for warmer weather to colder weather clothes. If you've experienced any of these scenarios, see the suggestions in the box on page 148.

> *My two daughters are only about a year apart. One day when they were both preteens, my younger daughter went through her sister's drawers and closets with her and helped her weed out the "uncool" clothes. My daughter with Down syndrome wasn't terribly pleased with some of her sister's judgments, but after that day I noticed that she stopped wearing colored knee socks with shorts (which looked out of fashion)—this was something I had been unable to convince her to do.*

Teaching Activity: "Mirrors, Mirrors Everywhere"

Taking care of the body can be an abstract concept. Brushing and shampooing hair, showering, shaving, putting on makeup, or evaluating clothing choices are difficult to do unless you can see what you're doing *while* you're doing it. Evaluate mirror availability in the areas where your child showers, dresses, and performs (or will be performing) grooming activities. Although mirrors on dressers are helpful, have at least one full-length mirror so your child can view her entire body close-up before leaving the house. Purchase magnetic mirrors for your child's locker at school so she can do spot checks or freshen up throughout the school day.

Chapter 8—Framework for Teaching about the Body

Concepts	Key Messages	Goal Behaviors
Names for private body parts	<ul><li>All body parts have a name, including private body parts</li><li>Girls have a vulva, clitoris, breasts, buttocks (outside of body)</li><li>Boys have penis, testicles, scrotum, buttocks</li></ul>	<ul><li>Uses correct names for genitals</li><li>Identifies self as male or female</li></ul>
Functions of private body parts	<ul><li>All body parts have a job to do</li><li>Private body parts (male & female) needed to make babies (reproduction)</li><li>Private body parts feel good when touched (pleasure)</li><li>Private body parts are used for elimination</li></ul>	
Societal rules for private parts	<ul><li>Private body parts stay covered in public places</li><li>If I want to touch my own private parts, I should be in private</li></ul>	<ul><li>Keeps private parts covered in public places</li><li>Moves to private space when touching genitals</li></ul>
Body rights	<ul><li>My body belongs to me</li><li>No one should touch my private parts without my permission</li><li>No one can make me touch their private parts if I don't want to</li><li>If someone forces me to share my body in ways I don't like, I should tell ___</li></ul>	<ul><li>Reports illegal or unwanted touch</li><li>Respects boundaries of others</li></ul>
PUBERTY		
Bodies change during puberty	<ul><li>Bodies grow and change during puberty</li><li>Bodies change on the outside and inside</li><li>Some changes are the same for boys and girls; some are different</li></ul>	
Functions of private body parts	<ul><li>Girls begin to ovulate and menstruate during puberty</li><li>Boys begin making sperm and ejaculating</li><li>People are physically able to have babies after they have reached puberty</li><li>Genitals feel good when touched</li></ul>	

Concepts	Key Messages	Goal Behaviors
CARING FOR THE BODY Hygiene and grooming/self-care	■ Like other body parts, private parts need to be cleaned and taken care of ■ Taking care of my body is one of my responsibilities as I get older ■ If I need help, I can ask _____	■ Practices good hygiene
Reproductive healthcare	■ Private parts need healthcare just like the rest of my body ■ Breast self-exam /gynecological exam ■ Testicular self-exam	■ Practices preventative healthcare

CHAPTER 9

Social Skills for Healthy Relationships

Social skills involve knowing the rules for how interactions occur in different situations. When your child learns and understands these rules, he'll more easily connect with others and interact in appropriate ways. Most children learn social skills with little or no instruction. They watch adults or peers and figure out the unwritten norms of social behavior. They understand when they've made mistakes based on cues or feedback from others and then learn not to make the same error again.

Individuals with cognitive disabilities have more difficulty learning social skills incidentally and almost always require concrete instruction and coaching over longer periods of time. A few factors contribute to their difference in learning. First, they have more difficulty reading and interpreting verbal and nonverbal cues from others. For example, your child may not notice or may misinterpret what is happening when someone moves away from him because he or she is uncomfortable with the physical closeness of the interaction, or your child may miss a look of embarrassment when he mentions something private. Second, individuals with cognitive disabilities generally have fewer opportunities to socialize and practice these skills in social situations. Having opportunities to generalize skills to real life settings is a critical component of social skills training. Understanding how to apply learned skills in a variety of settings contributes to social acceptance.

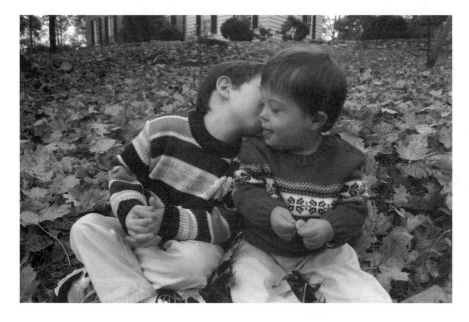

Social Skills for Connecting with Others

SOCIAL ETIQUETTE

____ greets others appropriately
____ maintains appropriate social distance
____ says please and thank you
____ offers to help another person when assistance is needed
____ gives compliments
____ receives compliments
____ introduces self to others
____ introduces new person to group

CONVERSATIONAL SKILLS

____ adjusts voice volume to social situation
____ knows how to start a conversation
____ joins a conversation
____ keeps the conversation going (question-asking)
____ identifies appropriate topics to discuss
____ faces person who is speaking
____ make eye contact
____ stays on topic
____ listens actively while others are speaking
____ takes turn talking
____ can change subjects
____ can end a conversation

FRIENDSHIP SKILLS

____ can call a friend on the phone
____ can answer the telephone
____ finds common interests
____ makes apologies
____ compromises
____ recognizes feelings in self
____ expresses own feelings in appropriate ways
____ identifies emotions in others
____ responds to feelings in others in appropriate ways
____ recognizes peer pressure
____ responds assertively to peer pressure
____ gives and takes in relationship (shares power)

DATING SKILLS

____ asks someone out on a date
____ handles rejection
____ assertively identifies limits
____ respects limits of others (hears and responds to "no")
____ recognizes partner pressure
____ responds assertively to pressure from partner (can say no)
____ expresses unpleasant feelings
____ expresses positive feelings
____ gives and takes in relationship (shares power)
____ asks partner to use a condom

What Skills Should Be Taught?

There are literally hundreds of ways to categorize social skills that are helpful in life but I've chosen to focus on skills that will likely be needed to improve your child's ability to connect with others and enhance relationships. Use the table below to identify areas where your child may need assistance.

Social Skills that Enhance Relationships

UNDERSTANDING EMOTIONS

Within the context of sexuality education, being able to identify, communicate, and manage feelings is a basic interpersonal social skill. Sharing feelings and responding to others' emotions enhances closeness and intimacy. And, feelings are often at the crux of discussions surrounding relationships, body changes, touching, and sexual expression, so being able to identify and express them is critical.

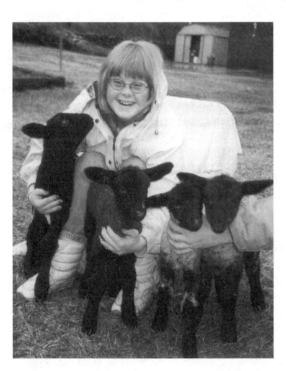

Although there is some research demonstrating that individuals with Down syndrome have difficulty labeling emotions shown in pictures of facial expressions, other experts have found that people with Down syndrome demonstrate clear abilities for recognizing and responding to emotions in others in real life. (Buckley; Chicoine). Individuals I work with seem to have more trouble with labeling their own feelings and expressing them in appropriate ways than with recognizing others' emotions.

Recently I was asked to provide some individualized instruction for a young adult on how to say no assertively. She shared with me her difficulty with this skill, especially in dating situations. During one session, I worked on helping her understand the nonverbal component of refusal skills, specifically how to use her body (in addition to words) to help her convey a serious message. Reviewing digital photos of her face proved to be insightful. She saw that when she was under stress, she smiled. She then readily understood how smiling could confuse people in serious situations. After I spent some time helping her match her facial expression with what she was feeling in her body, she became more successful at getting others to respond to her attempts at being assertive.

TEACHING ABOUT FEELINGS

My daughter was still quite young when I grew weary of people telling me how lucky I should feel because individuals with Down syndrome are always such "happy" children. It seemed to me that my child experienced the same range of emotions as her sister. She has good days and bad days, just like all of us.

Key Teaching Messages:

- Everyone has feelings.
- Four common feelings are happy, sad, angry, and afraid.

Feelings are essentially our way of responding to the things that happen around us. Helping your child become aware of these responses is the first step in feelings education. A good place to begin is by introducing your child to basic feelings.

If your child seems pretty familiar with the four basic emotions, introduce other feelings vocabulary. For example, feeling embarrassed, disgusted, disappointed, worried, frustrated, etc.

Teaching Activity: "Books That Teach about Feelings"

Happy
- *What Makes Me Happy?* by Catherine Anholt (Walker Books, 2006).
- *When You're Happy and You Know It,* by Elizabeth Crary (Parenting Press, 1996).

Mad/Angry
- *Andrew's Angry Words,* by Dorothy Lachner (North-South Books, 1995).
- *I Was So Mad,* by Mercer Mayer (Random House Books, 2000).
- *I'm Mad,* by Elizabeth Crary (Parenting Press, 1992).
- *Mean Soup,* by Betsy Everitt (Harcourt Brace Big Book, 1995).
- *Now Everybody Really Hates Me,* by Jane Read Martin (HarperCollins, 1993).
- *When I Feel Angry,* by Cornelia Maude Spelman (Albert Whitman & Co., 2000).
- *When I'm Angry,* by Jane Aaron (Golden Books, 1998).
- *When Sophie Gets Angry—Really, Really, Angry,* by Molly Garret Bang (Blue Sky Press, 1999).
- *When You're Mad and You Know It,* by Elizabeth Crary (Parenting Press, 1996).

Sadness
- *Fishing,* by Diana Engel (MacMillan Publishing Company, 1975).
- *Franklin's Bad Day,* by Paulette Bourgeois (Scholastic, 1997).
- *Sylvester and the Magic Pebble,* by William Steig (Aladdin Paperbacks, 1986).

Fear
- *All Alone After School,* by Muriel Stanek (Albert Whitman & Co., 1985).
- *The Bravest Babysitter,* by Barbara Greenberg (Puffin Press, 1986).
- *Goggles!,* by Ezra Jack Keats (Simon & Schuster, 1998).
- *Harriet's Recital,* by Nancy Carlson (CarolRhoda Books, 2006).
- *Ira Sleeps Over,* by Bernard Waber (Houghton Mifflin, 1975).
- *There's a Monster under My Bed,* by James Howe (First Aladdin Paperbacks, 1986).

Ranges of Feelings
- *Feelings,* by Aliki (Harper Trophy, 1986).
- *The Feelings Book,* by Todd Parr (Little Brown Young Readers, 2005).
- *The Feelings Box,* by Randy M. Gold (Aegina, 1998).
- *Glad Monster, Sad Monster: A Book about Feelings,* by Anne Miranda (Little Brown Co., 1997).
- *The Grouchy Ladybug,* by Eric Carle (Harper Trophy, 1996).
- *How Do You Feel?* by Norma Simon (Albert Whitman & Co., 1977).
- *My Many Colored Days,* by Dr. Seuss (Knopf Books, 1996).
- *Today I Feel Silly,* by Jamie Lee Curtis (Harper Collins Publishers, 1998).
- *The Way I Feel,* by Janan Cain (Parenting Press, 2000).

Possible discussion questions:
1. Tell me about a time you felt _____ (scared, happy, sad, mad)?
2. Can you show me how your face looks when you feel _____ (scared, happy, sad, mad)?
3. What are things you like to do when you feel _____ (scared, happy, sad, mad)?

IDENTIFYING
FEELINGS
IN SELF

Key Teaching Messages:

■ You're the expert on how you feel.

Teaching Activity: "My Personal Feelings Book"

Use photos of your child and the sample captions below to create a personalized book about your child's feelings. Laminate the pages, punch holes, and place them on a connector ring or in a binder. The assembled pictures are a concrete way to review feelings vocabulary and help your child understand the unique ways he experiences and manages his own emotions. If your child is younger, start with the top two captions. As he gets older, create additional pages using the more complex concepts (events that trigger specific emotions, physical sensations associated with different feelings, healthy ways to handle feelings particularly negative ones). Use the template below to create pages that address each of the four basic emotions (happy, sad, mad, scared) and others if you can.

I am mad!
(include a picture of your child's mad face)

I feel mad when …
(things, events, or experiences your child associates with the emotion)

When I am mad my body …
(identify gestures, voice characteristics, posture, or other nonverbal cues your child exhibits while expressing a particular emotion)

When I feel mad I can …
(identify healthy ways to handle negative emotions. See the section on "Expressing Negative Feelings in Healthy Ways" for ideas).

Teaching Activity: "I Would Feel…"

Read off the list of situations one at a time and ask your child to tell or show you what feelings he might have related to the event. If your child is less verbal, use the pictures from his own personal feelings book above, and have him point to the picture of the face that most accurately reflects his feelings. Or, have him demonstrate how he would feel using facial expressions.

■ It was your birthday.
■ You were being teased by kids at school.
■ You were invited to a friend's party.
■ You lost your wallet (purse).
■ You got yelled at by your teacher.

■ You won an award.
■ Your pet died.
■ Your team won the tournament.
■ A close friend was very sick.
■ Someone took your favorite sweatshirt.

<table>
<tr><td>

DISSING
FEELINGS

</td><td>

According to research, how someone learns to view and handle his own feelings is greatly influenced by his parents' or other caregivers' attitudes. When those around us minimize feelings, we learn to ignore, suppress, or deny our feelings rather than figure out ways to adjust to and manage them. For example, telling your child "it's not that bad; get over it" suggests that experiencing the emotion is not okay. Using distractions or avoiding discussions about feelings provides a similar message. When your child is struggling with events that create stress and anxiety, try to help him label the emotion, validate the feeling, and assist him in handling his feelings in healthy ways.

</td></tr>
</table>

IDENTIFYING FEELINGS IN OTHERS

Key Teaching Messages:

- People express feelings in different ways.
- People express feelings with words, their bodies, and sometimes both.
- Paying attention to how others are feeling helps us know what to do.

My daughter seems to be gifted with a remarkable emotional intelligence. She has this ability to really pick up on the emotions in others and respond. If I am angry, she senses it. If I am sad, she seems sad as well. I've noticed that she tends to mirror the emotions of those around her but has difficulty knowing what to do. Noticing this helped me realize how important it was to talk with her about what I was feeling and why. I want her to understand why I feel the way I do and know that it's okay to experience all feelings, not just happy ones.

Teaching Activity: "Feelings Charades"

The goal of this activity is to introduce ways we use our bodies to express feelings. Write the feeling words below on strips of paper. Then take turns picking slips of paper out of the hat. Without talking, use exaggerated facial expressions and body language to see if your child can guess how you're feeling. If your child is a nonreader, decide on a feeling, act it out, and have your child guess the feeling. If he guesses correctly, ask him to show you what parts of the body helped him guess. Then let your child have a try. Watching your child will help you know his unique body language for expressing feelings and emotions. Here are examples of feelings that can be acted out:

Happy	Sad
Disgusted	Mad
Scared	Surprised
Embarrassed	Worried
Frustrated	Proud
Tired	

Remind him that although we can sometimes guess how another person might be feeling, we're not always right. Asking is the only way to know for sure how another person is feeling.

Teaching Activity: "Feelings Game"

Take *facial* photos (or encourage your child to take photos, if he's old enough) of family members or other people he knows expressing different emotions. Create and cut out feeling labels in large print, making a set of four for each person photographed. Have your child match the face photos with the appropriate word labeling the emotion. (Mad face with mad label.) Ask him to point out specific facial or body details that helped him determine the emotion. When he notices something specific, help him connect that part of the facial expression with the emotion. For example, "Yes, he is smiling. Most people do smile when they are happy" or, "Yes, grandpa's forehead wrinkles when he is angry."

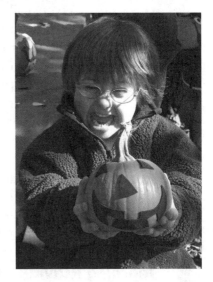

After your child is able to match the faces with the correct labels, include new photos of the same family members experiencing a variety of *situations that triggered different emotions*. Try to make the situation obvious—for example, a picture of a sibling winning or losing a game, a death in the family, a new baby, the expression of a family member after a family pet created a mess, etc. Using the same labels, ask your child to match the event with the emotion it triggered. Remind your child that people can feel differently about the same event. For example, performing in a school play can make one person feel excited, while another person may be nervous or afraid.

It may be difficult to pinpoint the feelings being exhibited in some of the pictures. This is an opportunity to explain that we're not always right when we try to guess what another person is feeling and illustrates why talking about feelings is important. Remind your child to ask if he's not sure. Things he can say if he is trying to respond to emotions in others can include: "Are you okay?"; "What happened?"; "Can I help?" ; "What's the matter?" or "I'm happy for you!"

Teaching Activity: "Feelings of the Rich and Famous"

Facial expressions and emotions exhibited by actors on televisions or in movies are often more dramatic, animated, and exaggerated. Use your child's favorite video or DVD to observe facial expressions, body language, or to talk about experiences that lead to certain emotions. During the show, ask your child questions about events that trigger a particular emotion. For example, "Lizzie looks sad. What happened that made her sad?" Point out specific body changes (sagging shoulders, tears, smiles, etc.). If your child has trouble being specific, it can help to turn off the sound to remove contextual clues and force attention on faces and bodies.

EXPRESSING
NEGATIVE
EMOTIONS IN
HEALTHY WAYS

Key Teaching Messages:

■ Learning to express feelings in healthy ways is part of growing up.

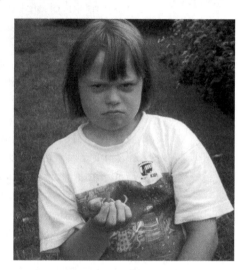

As your child gets older and his communication skills improve, encourage him to label, then talk about his own feelings. Your own modeling can go a long way in helping him understand that all people have feelings and that talking about them is healthy. Use phrases like "I felt so happy when…" or "I got mad when…" during everyday conversations with your child. Although expressive language skills may be delayed in children with developmental disabilities, they often notice nonverbal cues that may indicate you are feeling a certain way.

Teaching Activity: "Managing My Feelings"

Help your child generate his own unique list of things he can do when dealing with feelings of sadness, anger, fear, or frustration. Remind him it is okay to feel all kinds of emotions, but learning how to manage them in healthy ways is a part of growing up. Use the list below to help him evaluate actions and behaviors that would be helpful. Common examples of ways people manage their feelings in healthy ways include:

- talking with someone about what happened and what feelings you're experiencing;
- writing about feelings (journaling);
- exercising or participating in sports or other physical activities;
- relaxing with slow, deep breathing;
- engaging in a favorite hobby or interest (let him pick);
- listening to music;
- doing something fun (laughter is a great stress reliever!);
- watching a funny movie;
- reading or looking at a favorite book.

Not so healthy ways might include:

- hitting another person;
- hurting yourself;
- yelling at someone;
- saying mean things;
- doing things that hurt the feelings of others;
- destroying things;
- eating a whole package of cookies;
- talking about the incident over and over (perseverating).

Teaching Activity: "Coping List"

With your child, generate a list of things he can do when experiencing feelings that create uncertainty, anxiety, or undue stress (fear, sadness, frustration, etc.). Your child's lists may look different for each emotion. Write at the top of the list, "When I feel _____ I can…" Then suggest choosing from the healthy list above to create a menu of actions your child would prefer to use. Keep the list in a convenient place where your child can find it.

If your child benefits from visual cues, take pictures of him doing his preferred activities and use them to create a visual list of ways to manage his emotions. During times when he needs help coping with emotions, remind him of the list and have him choose an activity he believes will help him feel better.

Teaching Other Social Skills

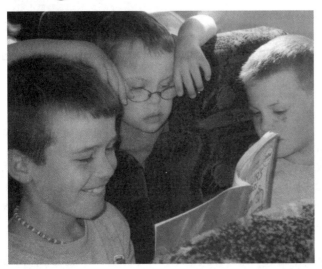

There are a variety of approaches for teaching social skills. Most models for teaching are grounded in social learning theory, which means skills are learned through a combination of watching others perform the skill, practicing, and then experiencing feedback from the natural consequences that result (positive and negative).

Individuals with Down syndrome or other cognitive disabilities benefit from formal social skill instruction that is repeated and reinforced over time. In the early years, you will be your child's social skills instructor. Below is a step-by-step process for teaching social skills.

STEP 1: DECIDE ON A SKILL YOU WOULD LIKE TO TEACH YOUR CHILD

If you're not confident you know where to start, you can gather considerable information by observing your child in everyday social situations at home, school, or in the community. Over a period of time, patterns become obvious and provide clues for where you can jump in. If your child attends school, teachers or professionals working closely with him can offer feedback on specific skill areas that need work. Talking with them can help you come up with ideas on how to teach and reinforce these same skills at home and other environments.

STEP 2: EXPLAIN WHY THE SKILL IS IMPORTANT

Your child may be more motivated to learn a new skill if you explain to him why it matters. Learning ways to start conversations, for example, can help him meet new people more easily or feel more comfortable in new social situations. When he understands how to be assertive, others will be less likely to take advantage of him, and you can then allow him more freedom and independence. Offering a brief explanation for why the skill is important also helps put the skill in a social context that makes sense for him.

STEP 3: BREAK IT DOWN

Most social skills can be broken down into smaller steps, making teaching more concrete and understandable for your child. For example, the social skill for helping your child introduce himself to others might include the following steps:

1. Look the person in the eye.
2. Say "hello, my name is _____."
3. Ask the person his or her name.

For social skills that seem more complex, consider creating cheat sheets that break down the skill in a visual way for your child. These tools can be created with words (like the one above) or pictures.

STEP 4: DEMONSTRATE THE SKILL

Students with developmental disabilities learn best when they can observe what it is you are trying to teach them. Model for your child each step of the skill so he can see how it's done. Or involve siblings in the demonstration while your child watches.

STEP 5: PRACTICE THE SKILL IN A SAFE SETTING

After you've demonstrated the steps, give your child a chance to practice and imitate the skill. Use everyday opportunities at home, with siblings, or relatives to practice skills. For some individuals, setting up a contextual scenario can help make the practice session more relevant. For example, "Okay, let's pretend I'm a kid in the park and you want to introduce yourself. Why don't you act out the steps?"

STEP 6: PROVIDE CORRECTIVE AND POSITIVE FEEDBACK

Immediately after your child demonstrates the skill, offer corrective feedback. Always begin with positive feedback in order to build confidence and motivate your child to try again. "Not bad for a first try" or "You spoke very clearly." If there are ways to improve the skill, offer specific suggestions. For example, "It was hard for me to hear you because you were looking down. Let's try it again, but this time I want you to look me in the eyes so I can hear you better."

STEP 7: PRACTICE SKILL IN A REAL LIFE SETTING

Once you feel confident that your child has learned the skill, look for opportunities for him to use his skills in natural settings. Generalization of social skills from individual teaching situations to a variety of real life settings will be a critical component of successful learning.

Other Strategies for Teaching Social Skills

- *Play and Recreational Time*—Play time is an excellent way to begin assessing the social skills your child may need and to start social skills teaching. Teaching manners, taking turns, or sharing are good foundations to build from.

- *Social Stories*—Social Stories, created by Carol Gray, are stories or narratives used to teach social expectations and appropriate responses in specific social situations. These stories can be created in narrative form or by using pictures. Typically these stories include a descriptive sentence about the environment, a directive or appropriate response that helps the child understand expected behavior, and typical responses by others to inappropriate behaviors. This strategy has been found to work particularly well with individuals who have autism, but many families whose children have Down syndrome or other cognitive disabilities have also had success using Social Stories to teach social skills. There are collections of Social Stories commercially available, or you can write and illustrate your own with photographs or clip art.

- *Role Models*—Ensure your child has opportunities to be around peers who can model appropriate social skills. At home, help siblings understand the role they play in teaching and modeling appropriate social skills for their sibling. Sometimes brothers and sisters allow their sibling to get away with inappropriate behavior because "he's so cute" or because they tire of the work involved in negotiation or conflict.

- *Videotaping*—With increased access to technology, it is easier than ever to create tools your child can view and learn from. Record yourself or your child performing skills you are trying to teach using strategies from this chapter, then have your child view them.

Video Self-Modeling: An Effective Approach for Teaching

Video Self-Modeling is a teaching technique used to help motivate individuals with intellectual disabilities to learn new skills or accept new situations more comfortably. The process involves the production of a 2- to 3-minute video clip of the student performing a skill or activity successfully. Typically, many videotaped sessions of the person attempting the skill are recorded and then painstakingly edited so that in the end the student can watch himself successfully performing the skill (all unsuccessful attempts are edited out). This process is often used to teach appropriate social interaction, communication skills, and even daily living skills. Professionals who have studied this technique believe it works so well because it improves self-efficacy (individuals see themselves being successful and therefore believe they can perform the task) and also acts as a powerful visual tool for sharing detailed instructions.

Social Skills Instruction in Adolescence and Adulthood

Although your child will continue to need to learn, practice, and reinforce social skills into adolescence and adulthood, it is completely normal and developmentally appropriate for him to tire of you as his instructor. When this happens, you'll need to explore other ways that social skills coaching and instruction can continue to happen. Some common resources for social skills instruction include:

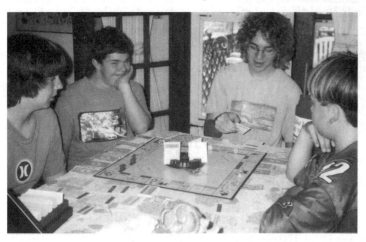

■ *School*—If your child struggles in his interactions with others or behaves in ways that make it hard to connect with others, advocate for social skills instruction. Since many individuals (with and without disabilities) have difficulty understanding social etiquette, there may already be opportunities for learning and practicing social skills in your district. Some schools may already have social skill groups for kids who need extra help understanding how to get along with others. Speech and language pathologists may be able to assist in teaching the pragmatics of learning conversational skills or facilitate social skills groups as a component of speech services. Guidance departments usually play an active role in teaching aspects of the curriculum involving social skills and friendship development. At the high school level, peer mentor programs or community service classes (courses that require so many hours of school or community service) might be an opportunity for your child to be matched with, or mentored by, a peer. Although this doesn't usually involve formal teaching, the peer feedback, modeling, and coaching that occurs as a part of these programs is often beneficial in reinforcing social appropriateness in natural settings.

■ *Community Agencies*—Professional counseling agencies sometimes offer classes designed to help kids or teens who struggle with social skills. Disability agencies that recognize the benefit of social skills instruction might be able to offer classes or at least structured opportunities to get together so social skills can be practiced and reinforced.

References

Benson, B. (1995). Psychosocial Interventions Update: Resources for Emotions Training. *The Habilitative Mental Healthcare Newsletter 14* (3).

Buckley, S., Bird, G. & Sacks, B. (2002). *Social Development for Individuals with Down Syndrome: An Overview.* Hampshire, Southsea, UK: Down Syndrome Educational Trust.

Couwenhoven, T. (May/June, 2001). Sexuality Education: Building on the Foundation of Healthy Attitudes. *Disability Solutions 4, 5:* 8-9.

De Freitas, C. (1998). *Keys to Your Child's Healthy Sexuality.* Hauppauge, NY: Barron's.

Foxx, R. M. & McMorrow, M. (1983). *Stacking the Deck: A Social Skills Game for Adults with Developmental Disabilities.* Champaign, IL: Research Press.

Ludwig, S. (1989). *Sexuality: A Curriculum for Individuals Who Have Difficulty with Traditional Learning Methods.* Newmarket, Ontario: The Regional Municipality of York Public Health.

MacDonald, J. (August, 2003). *Observations on Conversations with Young Adults with Down syndrome.* National Down Syndrome Congress Conference presentation.

Madison, L. (2002). *The Feelings Book: The Care and Keeping of Your Emotions.* Middletown, WI: Pleasant Company Publications.

Maksym, D. (1990). *Shared Feelings: A Parent's Guide to Sexuality Education for Children, Adolescents, and Adults Who have a Mental Handicap.* North York, Ontario: G. Allan Roeher Institute.

Moreno, K. (1998). Surviving in Society: The Importance of Teaching Social and Problem Solving Skills. *Down Syndrome News, 22* (8): 103.

Sexuality Information and Education Council of the United States. (1991). *Guidelines for Comprehensive Sexuality Education K-12.* New York, NY: Author.

Siperstein, G. & Rickards, E. (2004). *Promoting Social Success: A Curriculum for Children with Special Needs.* Baltimore: Brookes Publishing.

Valenti-Hein, D. & Mueser, K. (1990). *The Dating Skills Program: Teaching Social-Sexual Skills to Adults with Mental Retardation.* St. Joseph, MI: International Diagnostic Systems.

Chapter 9—Framework for Teaching Social Skills That Enhance Relationships

Concepts	Key Messages	Goal Behaviors
Identify basic feelings	■ Everyone has feelings ■ Four common feelings are happy, sad, angry, and scared	
Label feelings in self	■ You are the expert on how you feel ■ Learning to express feelings in healthy ways is part of growing up	■ Identifies emotions in self ■ Expresses own emotions in healthy ways
Recognize feelings in others	■ People express feeling in different ways ■ Feelings can be expressed with words, bodies, and sometimes both ■ Paying attention to how others are feeling helps us know what to do	■ Recognizes emotions in others ■ Responds appropriately to feelings in others
What is a social skill?	■ Social skills are rules for how to act around others ■ Learning these rules can help you act appropriately with others	■ Interacts with others in socially acceptable ways

CHAPTER 10

Friendships and Dating

A few years ago, I drove my daughter to a camp for individuals with cognitive disabilities. When we entered her cabin, one of her cabin mates (someone whom she had never met) immediately approached her, took her hand, and informed her they were going to be best friends. This is a scene I had witnessed many times before. People with developmental disabilities want, often in a very desperate way, to connect with others and experience friendships, yet they often overlook or are unaware of the important roles that time and choice play in forming relationships. I'll never forget the day a teenaged boy on my daughter's track team called her his "girlfriend." There was a new energy in her step and a gleam in her eye for the entire week. (The following week, I observed him win over a few of her female teammates in a similar manner, but I didn't have the heart to tell her!)

Being able to develop friendships and spend time with people your child appreciates and who appreciate her is a need she will have throughout her life. The early part of this chapter will focus on connecting with peers and general aspects of socialization. The good news is, sometimes relationships do happen with little or no intervention at all. In other situations, varying levels of support, facilitation, or assistance are necessary in order for relationships to grow.

There are now large bodies of literature that have been developed and practiced by people far more experienced than I. Amidst the information are some fairly consistent themes for how parents and/or professionals can increase the number and quality of an individual's relationships. Some basic premises that support relationship development at any age include:

- *Having a goal or vision* for what you want for your child. As your child matures, let her develop and create her own vision.
- Recognizing *key interests, skills, assets, or gifts* in your child that can provide a basis for connecting with others.
- Becoming familiar with *formal and informal groups* in your community where assets can be shared, valued, and appreciated.

■ Ensuring there are opportunities for your child to connect with the *same people over a period of time.*

■ Assisting or teaching your child to *give and contribute* within relationships (rather than just take and receive).

Categorizing Relationships

A good way to begin teaching about relationships is to introduce your child to some basic categories of relationships that you can use as a context for teaching other concepts. A teaching sheet with examples of common relationship categories is presented in Appendix B-3. This tool is designed to help you explain relationship concepts and prepare for discussions that typically surface. You can elaborate or simplify relationship categories and teaching messages based on your child's individual experiences and capacities.

Key Teaching Messages:

■ I have many different people in my life.

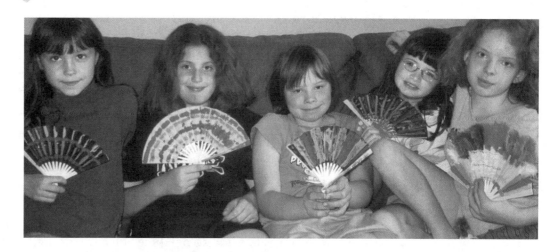

Teaching Activity: "People in My Life"

Use the worksheet in Appendix B-3 to help your child categorize different people in her life. This can help her see how relationships are similar or different and improve her ability to understand teaching concepts presented in the chapter. Use the *Guide to Teaching about Relationships* in Appendix B-6 to help explain different relationship categories and give examples.

List people's names or gather photos of people who might fit into categories on the diagram (digital cameras will work well for this). Ask permission before you take photos. Let people know you are working on a "relationships" project. After giving your child some basic definitions for each category, have her place photos of the people in her life into the correct relationship category. Remove and add new people as relationships change, grow, or are discontinued.

Connecting with Others: Friendships

The following story, which appeared in a National Association for Down Syndrome newsletter, was written by a Chicago-area parent who developed her own strategy for ensuring that her teenaged son had an active social life:

The group emerged a little over a year ago when I invited a few of my son's friends over for pizza and a movie to mark the end of the summer and the return to school. As the kids were heading out the door at the end of the evening, one of them turned to me and said, "This is the most fun I ever had." Suddenly it dawned on me—these kids are no different than their average counterparts. They love to hang out, have fun, share conversation and laughter just like every other teenage I know. The only difference is, these kids need a little help in getting it all to come about. That's where the parents come in.

In the age of e-mail, this is a fairly easy activity to organize. I contacted about six or seven families with students roughly my son's age from the same high school. All of them were kids he knew through school, special recreation, or even our NADS baby playgroup! I told the parents what I wanted to do—get the kids together on a fairly regular basis for pizza and a movie. I gathered e-mail addresses, sat down and looked at the high school calendar in order to avoid conflicts with school events, and came up with a list of dates. All of the families signed up for a convenient date to host and voila—the "Pizza and a Movie Group" was born.

I now set up a calendar for three or four months at a time. The gatherings are always held on a Saturday night about twice a month and we have settled on a regular drop off and pick up time. I e-mail everyone a reminder a few days before each party night. Some of the hosts have added their own touches to the gathering. The group has also played bingo for small prizes and engaged in hilarious rounds of charades. In the summer, some activities have taken place in the backyard. The size of the group has grown to 12 now, and the enthusiasm they all have for the get-togethers is amazing!

My son starts talking about the pizza parties a few days ahead of time, and he usually asks me about five times during the day, "Mom, what time is the party?" For the first time in his life, he has a social life—and he knows it. To say he loves being part of the Pizza Party group is an understatement.

(Reprinted with permission from **NADS News**, January 2004)

Teaching Activity: "Getting Together with Friends"

Helping your child learn how to plan and coordinate time together with friends is a skill worth teaching. Use the worksheet in Appendix B-7 to clarify decisions that need to be made when planning social activities with friends. The finished planning sheet can act as an invitation. (See "A Process for Thinking about and Encouraging Independence" in Chapter 7 for more information on teaching this kind of planning.)

Boundaries in Relationships: Context Is Everything

TOUCH AND
AFFECTION IN
RELATIONSHIPS

Key Teaching Messages:

■ The type of relationship I have with a person helps me know what kind of touch is okay (appropriate).

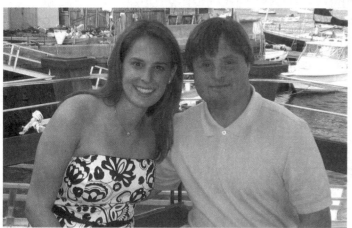

The type of relationship we have with another person helps us determine physical closeness or distance. Within marriage, family, and certain friendships, for example, there are ranges of physical and emotional closeness. In contrast, we usually keep some physical and emotional distance from acquaintances and strangers. Although we as parents inherently understand this concept and have the ability to adapt our levels of touch and affection based on the relationship we have with the person, children with developmental disabilities usually need considerable help with this. Labeling relationships for your child and then helping her understand greetings or types of affection within these relationships can help her become more socially appropriate.

Connecting with Others: Romantic Relationships

Keep in mind that as your child moves into adolescence, it is normal for her to want to experience what it feels like to be loved and cared about by people outside of her family. Remember, there are powerful messages on television and in the media that having a boyfriend or girlfriend is normal, if not inevitable. Even if your child mostly watches programming geared toward younger kids, she will see a great deal of idealized dating and flirting behavior on the screen. When she is in middle school, she will see real-life couples and hear conversations centered on boyfriends or girlfriends. By high school, expect that your child will routinely witness couples expressing physical affection in the hallways, dances, and other school functions.

At around age 13, my daughter discovered teen magazines such as Tiger Beat *and* M. *She reads them from cover to cover and is very up on which heart-throb actors already have girlfriends and which ones are still looking. She beams when there's a kissing scene on TV or the movies, and tells her younger sister (who is still disgusted by kissing) that she is soooo immature.*

SEXUAL
ATTRACTION
AND CRUSHES

This whole idea of acknowledging that a person is cute and how to let that person know what you think has been an ongoing topic of conversation in our house and I imagine it will continue for some time, especially as our son begins to date. We have used role playing as a strategy to help him practice in this area.

Teaching Activity: "OK Touch with People in My Life"

Explain to your child that when we have known people for a long time, we can get physically closer to them and sometimes touch them, if that is OK with them. For example, if Grandma is having a bad day or is upset about something, it would be okay to give her a hug, but if a stranger on the bus seems upset, hugging would not be okay.

Use the *Guide to Teaching about Relationships* in Appendix B-6 to help you identify suggested rules for appropriate touching in various relationship categories. Visual examples of different forms of affection are available to use in Appendix B-5. Identify pictures that represent your standards for appropriate affection. Organize them on the "Okay Touch" diagram from Appendix B-4. When finished, tape the "People in My Life" (B-3) and "Okay Touch" (B-4) pages together so your child has a visual display of acceptable ways to express affection (or not express affection) within the different relationship categories. Use this tool to positively reinforce appropriate touch and behavior, and review touch in the context of relationships if she does any inappropriate touching. Remind your child that the most intimate touching (sexual) occurs only in the context of romantic relationships.

A list of possible ways to interact—from least intimate (least body contact) to most intimate:

- Nod of the head
- Say "hi"
- Smile
- Wave
- Handshake
- High five
- Touch on the arm
- Touch on the shoulder
- Pat on the back
- Arm around shoulder
- Quick, brief hug
- Front body hug
- Arm around waist
- Brief kiss on cheek
- Brief kiss on mouth
- Touching private parts with clothes on—(sexual)
- Looking at private parts—(sexual)
- Touch private parts with clothes off—(sexual)
- All forms of sexual intercourse—(sexual)

He has become more discreet, able to keep his thoughts in his head when he sees a cute girl in passing. Now he often turns to me or his father and says more quietly, "She's hot!!"

Our daughter has crushes on boys in her class who are about her same age. They do not seem overwhelming but fairly normal. We have told her that all boys and girls have strong feelings and want to be close to people they like. We have told her it is important to make sure the other person feels the same way and that learning to be a good friend is good too. We expect that she will want a close physical relationship with a boy at some point. I try to keep the lines of communication open. She is not a strong communicator, but we still try.

Key Teaching Messages:

- Sexual feelings become stronger during puberty.
- When you have sexual feelings for another person it's called having a "crush."
- Crushes are normal and happen to everyone.
- Crushes can be mutual (both people have feelings for each other) or one-sided.

Last year in fifth grade, our daughter seemed to learn from her friends that it was important to have at least one boy you "like." She would say things like "I kind of like this boy named David." If I asked why, she'd just say that he was nice or something equally vague. So, I was reasonably sure she didn't give him any thought when she wasn't with her friends. But this year, I think she has a real crush on a boy. She has told me there is a boy in her class who has blond hair, brown eyes, and is "c-u-t-e." She is clearly spending some time observing him, because she will come home from school and tell me things she learned about him— for instance, that he has a twin brother, he got a hair cut, or his mother says he was born sucking his thumb.

Maybe your child has talked to you about a particular person she has strong feelings for or you've noticed shyness, giggling, blushing, or flirty behavior around certain people. Perhaps your child has a poster of some famous person she likes to stare at or talk about. When I bring up the concept of "sexual feelings" in my workshops, I ask participants to describe what happens in their bodies when they get close to or think about a person they like. They say things like: "I get butterflies," "I get nervous," "My hands sweat," "I blush," "I feel sexy," "Heart beats fast," or, my favorite, "My tummy vibrates." Descriptions like these are a concrete way for your child to talk about sexual feelings and associate those feelings with sexual interest or attraction. Label these sensations as "sexual feelings" and explain that when a person has these feelings, it usually means they are "attracted to," or have a "crush" on that person. Perhaps talk about sensations you had when you were your child's age. Make sure she knows these feelings are normal and happen to most kids her age.

Crushes can be hard when feelings of attraction are not reciprocated or the object of the crush is unattainable. Although these are painful experiences, they are common and happen to most kids during adolescence.

When our daughter was in 4th grade she had a crush on the cutest and most popular boy in her class. At one of her IEP meetings I found out she had been writing him "love" notes for about a year. We were so lucky that this kid "got it." He always took the notes and read them, put them in his pocket, and went on. Even with friends, he wouldn't make fun of her or say anything mean to her. He never encouraged her—just went along with it—and I thank this kid to this day.

My daughter made the assumption that because she had strong feelings for a boy, he automatically felt the same way about her. I had to tell her that wasn't always the case. I could tell this hurt her a bit, but I reminded her that she was a beautiful person and at some point in her life, she would be attracted to someone who would have similar feelings for her. This seemed to please her.

Our son has had major crushes! They seem to be on the most popular girls, cheerleaders, and his brother's female friends, as well as on popular movie and musical stars. We have tried to handle crushes the same way as for everyone else. Some people are just not available to us. Crushes can hurt, but they are also part of life.

Sometimes crushes can become obsessive and uncomfortable for the person who happens to be the object of your child's affections. If your child makes phone calls, writes notes, emails, or makes frequent verbal announcements about her feelings and they go unreciprocated your child may need some help with limit setting and boundaries. Use these situations to talk with her about how crushes can be one-sided and that in order for relationships to start, *both* people need to be attracted to each other. If the person your child is attracted to is giving her obvious signals that he or she isn't interested (teachers or other caregivers may be able to help you with this), talk to your child and help her learn to respect the feelings of others. Consider sharing your own experiences with unreciprocated crushes to help her understand this is a common experience. Remind her of the aspects of her personality that are unique and positive and that finding someone who has similar feelings for her will take time.

Our daughter's first obvious crush occurred in middle school and continues today with the same boy (without a disability). He's a popular student and very cute. When I noticed his name written on a steamy bathroom mirror (about 6th grade) I decided it was time to talk. We talked about her feelings, and that they were normal. I told her that when people had strong sexual feelings like she was feeling, it was called "having a crush." We talked about reasons she liked the boy. She told me he was nice to her, was funny and cute. Without my knowledge, she became more open about her feelings at school until one day I got a call from her teacher. On a field trip she had been very vocal about her feelings for this boy with her entire class. When she got home I had to tell her crushes were personal feelings that were private. I told her she could talk about her feelings with me. I suspect other girls her age are indeed talking about boys, but in more subtle ways, with girlfriends probably.

ROMANTIC RELATIONSHIPS AND DATING

When your son or daughter experiences a relationship where there is mutual interest and attraction, dating issues will likely surface. There is great variation in attitudes, desires, and readiness for dating among individuals with developmental disabilities, much like there is for others. Some young people are very vocal about wanting a boyfriend or girlfriend, but have difficulty finding a compatible partner. Others

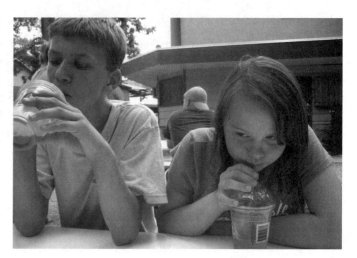

have no desire to date until later when a love interest is discovered in adulthood. Still others may be uninterested in forming romantic partnerships. The remainder of this chapter will be most relevant for families who have a son or daughter who has expressed an interest in dating or is currently involved in a romantic relationship.

Parental Pause—Relationships and Dating

1. What thoughts, concerns, or feelings surface when I think about my child dating?
2. What informal learning messages has my child received about dating and relationships? (from media, siblings, etc.)
3. What formal learning has he or she received?
4. What skills and information would I like my child to have before she dates?
5. What values do I want to share with my child about dating and relationships?

DEVELOPMENTAL PATTERNS OF DATING

One goal of dating is to get to know a person better, but how that happens can vary depending on the age and maturity level of the individual. In the general population, there tend to be developmental patterns in how people learn to date. In the early stages, crushes and sexual feelings move from being somewhat private to more public. Girls and boys begin talking with friends about who they "like," in hopes that these divulgences make it to the ears of the intended recipient and that feelings will be mutual. Much of this occurs through flirting, passing notes, phone calling, or, nowadays, instant messaging. This process is often called *"pairing off"* and even though actual face-to-face time is quite limited, the exchanges can be viewed as early dating experiences.

As teens mature, *group dating* becomes more popular. A group date is essentially a group of males and females who plan to participate in a social experience together. The motivation for getting together is almost always driven by some level of interest and sexual attraction between all or some members of the group. Group dates are a less threatening way to build comfort and social skills, and can act as practice sessions for understanding how relationships work and develop. I observed one of these "practice sessions" recently while waiting at a concession stand during a high school football game. Four young-looking teen couples huddled in a circle, each appearing to have a designated partner, were all watching each other closely for cues for what to do next. Finally, one bold male placed his arm around the waist of the girl standing next to him. By the time I had purchased my hot chocolate and headed back to the stands, the other three couples had followed suit. Watching the circle reminded me of ways typical kids ease into romantic relationships and learn how to express affection in gradual, safe ways.

It's a little harder when your oldest child has Down syndrome. I was dreading how I would handle the whole Homecoming scene during my daughter's first year in high school. I assumed she would need a date and that I would have to figure out logistics of getting them to a place to eat, etc. Then a neighbor who had three kids in high school told me that most students go with friends as a group rather than as dates. She told me she was planning a meal at her house so the kids would have someplace to go before the dance. Her plan inspired me to make my own plan and I went from there.

In high school, college, or for some, adulthood, *one-to-one* dating becomes more popular and represents the most mature form of dating requiring the most skills. If your child has had little experience with dating and is now an adult, consider group or couples dating as a way to develop social skills. Here are other factors to consider:

ASSESSING DATING READINESS

Each family has their own views on when dating should begin. For many families the standards applied to siblings will be the same as for the child with Down syndrome. If your child is obviously too young but already likes the idea of dating, get her perspective on what dating is, explore her motivation for dating, and then share your own views. For example, if she wants to date but is chronologically too young, you could say, "At your age, it's common to develop crushes and have strong feelings like you do, but kids your age don't usually date. When you're older, and you find someone you really like and they like you too, I can help you learn more about dating and what it involves." Or, "Most people don't begin dating until ___. By that time you will have more practice getting along with others in relationships."

If your child has expressed an interest in dating and is at a developmentally appropriate age (his or her peers *are* dating) but has little information or experience, ideas for topics and skills that can enhance the dating experience are listed below. This list is by no means comprehensive but does address much of the misinformation and skill deficit areas I frequently encounter in my work with individuals with cognitive disabilities. While it is not necessary for your child to know or have all of these skills prior to dating, the list can help you identify teaching goals and evaluate progress over time. The remainder of this chapter offers ideas for teaching these skills and information.

Our son will be allowed to date when he turns sixteen, six short months away. He already knows who he wants to ask out. She is a young woman who also has Down syndrome, attends his high school, is the same age, but a year ahead of him in school. He has known her for over nine years. He is comfortable with her. By watching them you would think they are an old married couple when they discuss things.

DATING SKILL ASSESSMENT CHECKLIST
- ❏ Does your child understand what a date is and why people date?
- ❏ Can she identify a person who is appropriate to date?
- ❏ Could she ask someone out on a date?
- ❏ Can she plan a date?
- ❏ Can she evaluate whether a relationship is healthy or unhealthy?

Teaching Dating Skills

WHAT IS A DATE?

If your child has expressed an interest in dating, begin by getting her perspective on what she thinks "going on a date," "going with," or "going steady" means. Often children with cognitive disabilities use words they have heard others use but are unclear about what they mean. It's hard to stay current with changing terminology and criteria kids use to describe courting behaviors. When my youngest daughter (without a disability) was about twelve, she asked my permission to "go out" with a boy from school. When I asked her what "going out" actually meant, she told me it meant talking to the guy at school and sending notes back and forth. Her definition of "going out" had been much different than mine. Making sure you both have a common understanding can make discussions clearer.

Key Teaching Messages:

Dating is:
- a planned activity;
- a way to spend time together with someone you like;
- a way to learn more about each other;
- a way to decide if you are a good match for each other.

It will be important for you to emphasize the reciprocal nature of dating. Remind your child that dating requires some level of interest from *both* people, not just one. It is also helpful to remind your child that dating is a planned activity that two people agree to and prepare for in advance.

FINDING SOMEONE TO DATE

When people have limited access to a pool of dating partners, they tend to reach out to people closest to them even if they're inappropriate. Identifying some specific criteria for distinguishing "inappropriate" from "appropriate" dating partners can be helpful. For example, you can explain that an appropriate person to date is someone who:

- is close in age;
- is unrelated (dating relatives is inappropriate);
- is available to be in a relationship (not already dating someone else, in a serious relationship, or married);
- is interested in getting to know your son or daughter;
- has similar interests and abilities.

Many parents feel uncomfortable when their teen or adult expresses a desire to date someone without a disability. Healthy relationships are about shared power and reciprocity. When one person has a cognitive disability and the other does not, the risk

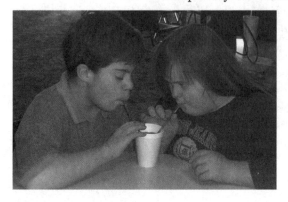

for exploitation increases dramatically. As younger generations of children grow up in inclusive settings, it will become more common for people with disabilities to want to date the non-disabled peers they interact with. Remember that people with developmental disabilities see the same role models we do in the media and in life. The milder the cognitive disability, the more aware your child will be of the prejudices, negative stereotypes, and pejorative attitudes toward people with disabilities in our society. As a result, your child may come to see dating a "normal" person as a more appealing and acceptable option.

When I talk with teens and adults about their experiences with dating nondisabled partners, it always leads to an animated discussion involving their personal thoughts and experiences. I have yet to hear of a successful romantic relationship between a person with Down syndrome (or other cognitive disability) and a typically developing peer. Unfortunately, many young people with disabilities have shared their feelings of frustration, rejection, or unhealthy consequences related to these dating experiences. Over time, with experience and sometimes counseling, many of these individuals learned to recognize the value in dating another person with a disability.

In a recent session I conducted, self-advocates talked about how they felt when they dated another person with a disability:

"For the first time I am with someone who understands about my seizures and is not afraid of me."

"I know what his disability is and he knows about mine."

"We belong to the same group…it feels comfortable."

It can be very difficult to address your child's frustrations if she wants to date, but is unable to find a compatible partner. The interest, skill level, and desire to connect with someone may be there, but the well is dry. It's easy to dismiss this problem as something all people experience, but people with disabilities clearly face more obstacles than the general population. The use of power and control by parents and providers, fewer opportunities for socialization, transportation issues, lack of privacy, and pejorative attitudes and societal stereotypes about people with disabilities and sexuality make finding a partner, getting together, and developing and maintaining a relationship much more complicated.

My son was always wanting to date girls who were clearly out of his league. One day I finally sat down with him and just said, "You know, your best chance for a long term-relationship will be with someone who understands what it's like to have a disability, probably another girl who has a disability just like you do." It seemed like once I gave him permission, he became more interested in girls with disabilities.

Some time ago during a clinic visit, a mother approached us regarding her nineteen-year-old son with Down syndrome. The mother was concerned about a mutually developing relationship between her son and a girl in his special education class at high school. The mother came to us seeking some ideas on how she could "nip-it-in-the-bud" (the relationship) before it developed into something serious! It's important to remember that in the area of relationships, your son or daughter has the same need to love and be loved as anyone else. It's helpful to view early dating experiences as "practice sessions" for understanding the work involved in learning how to make a relationship successful. Most of us learned these skills over time in the context of various relationships through adolescence and adulthood. Your child will require similar opportunities to experience a variety of relationships before finding a compatible partner and understanding what it means to be in a committed, exclusive relationship(s).

There are no magic solutions for resolving this issue, but if your child is interested in developing a romantic relationship and is unable to find a person to date here are some ideas:

■ *Work at helping your child develop an active social life*. The self-advocates I meet who have succeeded in finding compatible partners are actively involved in organizations that support people with cognitive disabilities. They belong to friendship groups, People First, Special Olympics, job training programs, or attend ARC sponsored social events, and are well connected to agencies in their community that exist to support and improve the lives of individuals with developmental disabilities. If your son or daughter has few connections outside of the family, think about ways to improve opportunities to meet other people. Contact local organizations, get on mailing lists, and ask about socialization opportunities that already exist in your community. Or, have your child contact local agencies and ask about events and activities designed for self-advocates. Find a reason to host a party. Birthdays, graduations, or holiday-themed parties can be a good excuse to get together with friends or meet new people. If you live in a rural area, consider attending a national conference or exploring the possibility of connecting with others via written correspondence or email.

> *We have a hotel party every year for my daughter's birthday. It started out small with just a few girls. Over the years we have added new people, and the party part is now coed (the sleepover is still girls only). The teens who are invited really look forward to it now.*

■ *Support and encourage ongoing self-improvement*. Take every opportunity to help your child continue to work on improving herself. Expect her to use good manners and continue to develop social skills that will help her make a good impression on others. Help her look her best by encouraging good hygiene and grooming. (Not surprisingly, when I ask self-advocates to identify appealing traits in a romantic partner, looking and smelling good are right at the top of the list!) Encourage your child to identify self-improvement goals. Support her in finding and developing new interests, hobbies, and skills. Expose her to the world of self-advocacy so she can learn new skills and work to improve the lives of others.

■ *Encourage persistence*. Finding a partner will require persistent effort over time. If a relationship does not work out, encourage your child to try again. Help her learn from each relationship so she can continue to grow and develop as a result of these experiences.

Teaching Activity: "Safe and Unsafe Ways to Meet People"

Write each of the items below on separate slips of paper (if you have other ideas, add them to the list). Explain to your child that the slips of paper identify different ideas for finding people to date. Let her know that some of these places are safer than others. Ask her to sort the items into what she believes are red light (unsafe) and green light (safer) piles. For items in the red light pile, explain why it is unsafe, using comments below.

Red light (Unsafe)	**Green Light (Safer)**
At work (sexual harassment laws)	Special Olympics
At the mall (sexual predators)	School
On the street (sexual predators)	Self-advocacy groups
Internet sites (sexual predators)	Other social clubs or groups
Bars	Friends of friends

Remind your child that even meeting people in safer places requires good judgment. For definitions of sexual predators, see Chapter 12. Use chaperoning or practice with supervision strategies (identified earlier in the chapter) if your son or daughter is in a new relationship and feels uncertain or unsafe in the early dating stages.

ASKING SOMEONE FOR A DATE

If all goes well and the person your son or daughter asked accepts the invitation to get together, celebrate with your child! Encourage her to move to the next step and make a more detailed plan for what they will do together.

Key Teaching Messages:

- Both you and the person you ask have to want to date each other.
- If the person is not interested, he or she can say no.
- If you are not interested, you can say no.

Teaching Activity: "Planning a Date"

Use the worksheet on planning a date in Appendix B-8 to identify a list of things your son or daughter should decide before the date. If this is your child's first date, go through the list together. As she becomes more experienced, she can use the sheet to plan dates with a partner.

CHAPERONES AND DATING— PRACTICING WITH SUPERVISION

Once you've shared basic information about dating with your son or daughter, moving forward with practice sessions is a logical next step. How much supervision is needed will, of course, vary. Supervision through the use of a chaperone is advisable if your child:

- has minimal information about the dating partner;
- has little experience with dating;
- has little information and few of the social skills identified earlier in the chapter;
- will likely need assistance with handling money, communication, etc.

Chaperoning—Practicing Dating with Supervision

Types of Assistance That May be Needed	Role of Chaperone—Most Supervision	Role of Chaperone—Less Supervision
Communication (your child or the partner is difficult to understand or is nonverbal)	■ Work with your child to plan the date (use planning sheet). ■ Gather information about partner from others who know him/her best. ■ Communicate plans and expectations for the date with dating partner's parents. ■ Accompany couple on date in order to act as interpreter until used forms of communication are more familiar and mutually understood by dating partners.	■ Intervene to clarify communication with others (ticket seller, restaurant staff) only as needed. ■ Provide written or verbal instructions beforehand if specific teaching is needed (e.g., how to find your seats at a play or stadium).
Money	■ Handle money issues as chaperone.	■ Use gift cards. ■ Prearrange payment prior to date (e.g., get menu from restaurant ahead of time so choice can be made). ■ Have child overestimate costs and use larger bills.
Transportation	■ Act as driver. ■ Use radio to tune out conversation.	■ Have peers or sibling drive couple to destination. ■ Have couple use public transportation.
Privacy	■ Accompany couple. ■ Assess and teach skills (see above). ■ Encourage dating in public locations initially. ■ Sit closer to couple.	■ Increase physical distance from couple over time (sit in separate part of theater, separate table at restaurant). ■ Increase alone time as skills are taught and demonstrated.

Parents often do the chaperoning at first, especially with less experienced couples who need effective teachers and coaches. Later on, siblings, peers, or anyone else who is willing and responsible can fill this role.

Planning an initial date at home or in public places such as the mall, movies, or restaurants can be a good way for a couple to get to know each other and establish comfort and trust in a safe environment. Your goal is to help them practice the art of dating and become increasingly independent. As your child learns to handle herself, it's appropriate to reduce supervision over time.

So far the affection and sexual behavior in our son's current relationship has been appropriate in public settings—hand holding, arms around each other, and an occasional kiss. There are times when I am transporting them home that I feel awkward and avoid looking in the back seat. I just keep telling myself, I am just the driver, I am just the driver….

Parental Pause—Dating and Supervision

1. What types of affection do I feel okay with my child demonstrating in my home?
2. What types of affection are okay in public?
3. Are there ways I can allow privacy for my child at home? What are they?

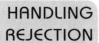
HANDLING REJECTION

Not all invitations to go on a date are accepted. Prepare your child for possible verbal and nonverbal responses she might see or hear if the person she asks is not interested in dating. Remind your child that these are usually signs the person is not interested in dating or spending time with you and that the person she is asking has the right to make a decision about whether or not to go out with her. Discuss how rejection is a fairly common experience and she should expect it to occur now and then. (This might be a good time to share one of your own personal rejection stories.) Talk to your child about the

Teaching Activity: "Recognizing Rejection—Saying No"

Introduce your child to both verbal or nonverbal examples of ways people tell or show you they are not interested in going on a date. Remind your child that in order for a relationship to work, both people have to want to date each other. If the person asked is not interested, your child needs to hear the no, stop, and respect the person's choice. Your child can use these same verbal and nonverbal responses if she is not interested in dating someone who asks her out.

Things the person might say…	**Things the person might do…**
"No thanks"	Not answer
"I'm not interested"	Look away
"I have other plans"	Walk away
"I'm busy"	Avoid you (turn away when they see you coming)
	Ignore you (e.g., start talking to someone else)
	Not return phone calls

feelings that go along with being rejected but encourage her not to give up just because one person is not interested. Try to be positive; remind her there will be other chances to meet new people. Persistence and tenacity are important qualities in the dating world.

EVALUATING RELATIONSHIPS

When two people have a chance to spend time together, they begin to learn more about what they like or dislike in each other. How long it takes to really get to know another person varies. Some individuals will know after one or two dates whether they

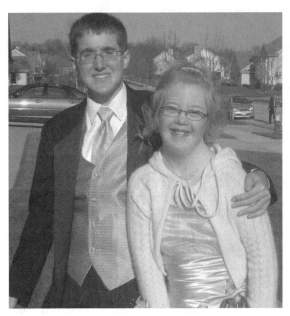

want to continue to work on the relationship. I have known many teens or adults who date a person once and have no interest in a second date with the same person. For others, evaluating whether a relationship is working out requires considerably more time. If your son or daughter is involved in a relationship, encourage him or her to openly discuss aspects of the relationship that are going well and not so well. If things don't appear to be going well, remind your child that not all relationships work out and that it takes a while to find someone who is a good match. Inexperienced couples, disabled or not, sometimes need help with this.

Key Teaching Messages:

- After I get to know a person better, I may feel differently about that person.
- I get to choose which relationships I want to continue and which to stop.

RESPECTING BOUNDARIES

When we talk about "respecting boundaries," we are really talking about demonstrating a respect for each other's boundaries related to physical affection within a relationship. Most individuals I work with don't understand the term "consent" but are familiar with the term "permission." Teaching your child to ask permission before moving into someone's personal space is a good way to illustrate respecting boundaries in dating relationships.

Remind your child that in healthy relationships, the person you are dating will care about how you feel and won't want you to feel pressured or uncomfortable. You may want to talk about some common forms of affection acceptable within early dating experiences (e.g., hand holding, hugging, kissing, etc.). Then identify ways to ask permission before touching ("How about a kiss?"; "Is it all right if I give you a hug?"; "Would you feel okay if I kissed you?").

Also let her know that not all dating situations will be ideal and remind her that two people can have different ideas about what boundaries are okay. Even if boundaries are different, remind your son or daughter that her body is her own and no one has the right to make her do things with her body that she doesn't want to do. Encourage your child to talk to you or another person she trusts if she feels pressured or limits are not being respected.

Key Teaching Messages:

- My body belongs to me.
- I decide what touch feels comfortable for me.
- I can say no to touch or sexual behavior that makes me feel uncomfortable.
- Talking with my partner about my boundaries is important.

Teaching Activity: "Ingredients of Healthy Relationships"

Once your child starts dating or becomes interested in dating, the "Ingredients of a Healthy Relationship" worksheet in Appendix B-9 can be used to identify and discuss key elements of healthy relationships or evaluating whether the relationship is working. Some ideas for explaining and discussing each of the concepts are listed below:

■ *You are both interested in each other (Mutual Interest)*—In healthy relationships there is usually something that draws us in and makes us want to spend time with each other. We might think the other person is interesting in some way, or like the way a person looks. Over time, as we get to know the person better, we may learn things about who they are as a person (they are funny, always have nice things to say, make us feel good, use good manners, are caring or treat us with respect, etc). Discussion questions:
  - *What do you like about _____? (person your child is dating, if involved in a relationship)?*
  - *What things about a person make you want to date them? (if not dating now)*
  - *What happens if you like someone more than they like you? Do you think the relationship would work? Can you make someone like you?*

In order for a relationship to work, *both* people have to *want* to be a part of the relationship and keep it going. Relationships take work and when one person has no interest or loses interest, the relationship doesn't usually continue.

■ *You both have things in common (Common Interests)*— If two people have things in common, it's easier to find things to do that you both will enjoy. Discussion questions:
  - *What things do you both like to do together?*
  - *If you were going to date someone, what would be a fun thing to do on a date (if not dating now)?*

■ *You get to know each other slowly over time (Time)*— Healthy relationships develop slowly over time and are not rushed. It takes time to get to know a person for who he or she really is and decide if he or she can be trusted. How the person treats us helps us to know whether or not we can trust them. Sometimes it takes time for people to show us their true selves. Discussion questions:
  - *How long do you think it takes to get to know a person? (weeks, months, years?)*
  - *What things would make you not want to trust a person? (The person breaks promises, makes me feel nervous or anxious, takes things from me, lies, is mean to me, is bossy and decides everything, hurts my feelings, etc.)*
  - *What things would help you decide a person could be trusted? (He or she tells the truth, keeps promises, makes me feel safe, respects my limits, cares about how I feel, etc.)*

■ *Boundaries Are Respected*—Dating couples express affection in many different ways, but in healthy relationships, limits and boundaries are respected. A person who cares about you will not want to hurt you or touch you in ways that feel unsafe or uncomfortable. Remind your child that her body is her own and she can say no to touches or affection that make her feel uncomfortable. A partner who respects her will listen and stop if she says no. (See Teaching Activities below on saying no.)
  - *What forms of affection do you enjoy?*
  - *What could you do if your date (partner) was touching you in ways you didn't like? (Emphasize saying no, getting away, telling someone, yelling so chaperone hears, etc.)*

■ *Shared Power*—In healthy relationships there is sharing and turn-taking; one person should not always be in charge. You take turns paying, deciding how to spend time together, talking and listening.
  - *Do you feel like you get to make decisions in your relationship?*
  - *Do you feel like you have power? How about _____ (the partner)? Does he/she get to make decisions?*

Teaching Activity: "Recognizing Pressure to Change Boundaries"

Introducing pressure lines that are commonly used to get people to move beyond their boundaries can help your child recognize and be better prepared to respond. Here are common pressure lines identified by self-advocates who have dated, along with their ideas for possible responses:

Pressure Line—"I'll break up with you if you don't have sex."
Response—"Go ahead."

Pressure Line—"If you loved me, you'd have sex."
Response—"If you loved me, you'd respect my limits."

Pressure Line—"If you really cared about me, you would do this."
Response—"If you really cared about me, you would respect my limits."

Pressure Line—"Everyone else is doing it, why can't we?"
Response—"Everybody is not doing it."

Being assertive in high pressure situations like these is not easy and requires considerable skill. Most of us need help learning to be assertive in situations where stakes are reduced before we can function in situations like these. Look for opportunities in which your child can practice assertiveness in her everyday life.

Teaching Activity: "Responding to Pressure to Change Boundaries"

Let your child know that if she feels uncomfortable or pressured by her partner to do something she doesn't want to do, she should say "No." Explain that saying "no" is one important way to help others know your boundaries. When teaching this skill, remind your child that most of us say no two ways: with *words* and with our *bodies*. Here are some basics for improving your child's ability to communicate an effective "no":

Saying "No" with words
- firm, strong voice
- clear message
- "No" scripts:
  - ❏ "I don't want to do that"
  - ❏ "I want to stop"
  - ❏ "I won't go any further"
  - ❏ "I don't feel comfortable doing that"
  - ❏ "I'm at my limit, we should stop"
  - ❏ "No, stop!"

Saying "No" with the body
- serious face (no smiling)
- look the person in the eyes
- sit up or stand up straight
- push person away
- turn and move away from person

Review with your child the verbal and physical elements of an assertive "no" and then demonstrate using exaggerated examples. It may be helpful to contrast an ineffective demonstration with an effective one. For example, smiling while saying no or saying no very softly can be contrasted with a serious face and loud, firm no. The obvious differences can help your child make distinctions between an ineffective and effective response. After you think she understands the difference, take on the role of the pressurer, using the pressure lines above. Practice until your child seems comfortable with an assertive response.

Being able to say no and refuse sexual advances is an incredibly complex and difficult skill, particularly for people who are usually rewarded for doing as they're told. Human sexuality curricula geared towards teens without disabilities include a variety of techniques for responding to unwanted sexual pressure that may be transferable to individuals with cognitive disabilities. Some may be too complex, but you can decide if they might be usable with your own child. The literature suggests that individuals who have a wider repertoire of skills may be more effective at responding to pressured sexual encounters.

Verbal Ways to Respond to Pressure Situations

Technique	Example	How it works
Say "No"	"No thanks"	Assertive verbal and body language sends "I'm serious" message
Repetitive "No"	"No, I don't want to" "No, I don't want to" "I said 'No!'"	Helps pressurer know you're not going to budge
Give a reason	"No, I'm not ready, I want to wait" "No, I don't know you well enough" "No, I am not protected" "No, because this is as far as I go"	Offer reason for refusal
Reverse the Pressure	"You say that if I loved you I would have sex. But if you loved me you'd respect my limits"	Pressurer is forced to respond
Suggest doing something else	"I don't want to go to your apartment. Let's get some coffee instead"	■ Helps cool down situation ■ Buys time to think about what to say if it happens again ■ Distracts other person ■ Allows for continuation of friendship if desired

Physical Ways to Respond to Pressure Situations

Technique	Example	How it works
Walk away or leave		Helps pressurer know your friendship is in jeopardy
Avoidance	Don't go with the person again	Prevents pressure situation from occurring

Teaching Activity: "Hearing No"

When a partner says "stop" or "no," or seems uncomfortable, the sexual behavior should stop. Let your son or daughter know that stopping when a partner says "no" or "stop" is a way to show respect for your partner. If you care about how your partner feels, an assertive "no" should be all that is needed. Tell your child that when force, bribes, or tricks are used to force people into unwanted sexual behaviors or touching, it's called sexual exploitation. Forcing people to go past their limits is against the law (see Chapter 12) and a clear sign the relationship is unhealthy.

Teaching Activity: "Red Light/Green Light"

Having information about specific characteristics that make relationships healthy and unhealthy can help your child improve decisions related to when to continue or end a dating relationship. Review the symbolism associated with the red and green stoplight symbols. For example, "When we're in a car and we get to a red light what do we do? Right—we have to stop."

Introduce this activity by saying, "Now that you are starting to date and spending time with different people, I want to give you some information that can help you know if a relationship is a red light relationship—one you should stop because it is not healthy—or a green light relationship—one that should be continued because it is healthy." Go through the list of characteristics listed on the green light sheet in Appendix B-10 with your child and clarify, using concrete examples if necessary, to make sure she understands the characteristics. For example, for the first characteristic, "you both like to do the same kinds of things," ask your son or daughter, "Tell me some things you and Anna both like to do.... That's neat that you both enjoy basketball and going to the movies." Provide concrete examples for each characteristic.

Next, show your child the red light list (Appendix B-11). Explain that not all relationships will be perfect, but you want her to recognize warning signs that could signal the relationship is not a healthy one and should be stopped. For example, talk about what it would feel like if one person in the relationship was always in charge and got to make all the choices about where to go and what to do. If your son or daughter has had experiences in relationships like this (friends or romantic relationships) use them to illustrate examples. For example: "Remember Daryl from school? Remember how you didn't like to hang out with him because he was bossy and always told you what to do? You stopped spending time with him because you decided you liked to make your own choices. In healthy relationships, people take turns making decisions; one person doesn't get to always be in charge." Discuss the list and provide clarification using words or experiences your child can relate to.

To review comprehension, make copies of the lists and cut them up, making sure there is one characteristic on each strip. Mix them up and ask your child to separate healthy characteristics from the unhealthy ones. In workshops, I use two boxes, a red one (stop) for collecting unhealthy characteristics and a green box (go) for gathering healthy traits. At home, you can cut out the stoplight symbols on each page, color one red and one green, and use them to produce two separate piles. It may be helpful to review these lists each time your son or daughter enters a new relationship or to reassess and evaluate current ones as they develop and evolve.

RESPECTING MY PARTNER'S BOUNDARIES
- My partner's boundaries may be different than mine.
- My partner has the right to say no to touch or sexual behavior that feels uncomfortable.
- I need to respect my partner's boundaries.

WHAT IS A "YELLOW LIGHT" RELATIONSHIP?

It's normal for all couples (new and experienced) to encounter problems, conflicts, or difficulties in relationships. During workshops with teens and young adults, we identify common difficulties and how to work through them. In my workshops, a yellow light relationship is one with a problem or conflict that might be fixable with action. Usually the "action" involves bringing up an issue and sharing feelings, concerns, and possible solutions with the partner so he or she knows that something needs to change in order for the relationship to continue. Yellow light relationships, then, are relationships that require some "action" (work). If actions don't result in changes or improvements (the partner doesn't listen, the problems continue, or things remain the same), the relationship moves to "red light" and a breakup is a logical next step.

BREAKING UP

When a relationship is unhealthy or your child comes to the realization that things just aren't working, you may be called upon to help her either initiate or recover from the "breakup." Breakups are never easy, but here are some things to remember as you educate and support your child:

- *Help her identify ways the relationship is not healthy.* Review the red light list to determine what characteristics make the relationship unhealthy in order to help her verbalize why she is wants to break up.
- *Encourage her to make a definite decision.* Some individuals are just so enthralled with having a romantic partner, they would rather cling to the thought of being in a relationship, even if it is unhealthy, than participate in an actual breakup. (We all know people like this, with and without disabilities.) Give your son or daughter permission to let go, and be encouraging about the future ("just because this relationship didn't work out doesn't mean there won't be others").
- *Discuss details of how to break up.* Discuss possible locations if she is doing the breaking up in person and create some scripts and rehearse them. I recommend that breakups occur in public places where others are around if it's in person or on the phone. Encourage your child to be direct and to the point.
- *Expect uncomfortable feelings.* Even if your child initiates the breakup, he or she is likely to feel lonely and unhappy, and a sense of loss. Your child may question her decision and focus only on the positive aspects of the relationships rather than on what went wrong. You may have to remind your child why her decision to end the relationship was a good one and reassure her that her feelings are a normal part of the breakup process. If your child is the one being left behind, try to be supportive and empathetic. Remind her that both people have to want to be in a relationship in order for it to work.

Sexual Expression in Romantic Relationships

Few topics generate more anxiety and debate among parents of children with disabilities than a discussion about their child becoming sexually active. Nevertheless, becoming a sexually healthy adult means understanding the responsibilities that go along with being in a sexual relationship.

Before talking with your child about sexual behavior, take time to clarify your own thoughts and values about the issue. What sexual behaviors would be acceptable? Which ones are not? Obviously, there's a wide continuum of attitudes among all parents. Some common parental perspectives regarding sexual activity in relationships are listed at right. See which one most closely fits your own beliefs.

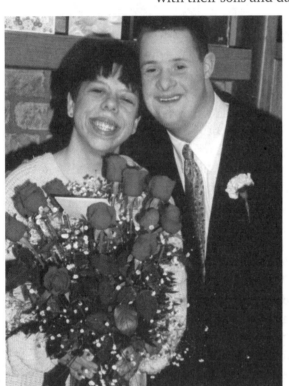

> **GETTING HELP WITH TEACHING ADVANCED TOPICS**

Most professionals agree that parents play a critical role as primary sexuality educators. However, there is disagreement over who should actually teach about more in-depth and complicated issues such as protection from pregnancy, prevention of AIDS and sexually transmitted diseases, and pleasure. Educators argue that most parents have inadequate levels of knowledge, skills, or comfort to address these issues with their sons and daughters. Others feel that adults with disabilities have rights to privacy about their sexual lives much like the rest of the adult population and that placing parents in the role of teacher violates those rights. Still others think that the intimate bond between a parent and child makes it too difficult to provide sexuality education in a factual, unbiased manner.

There are wide ranges of comfort levels among parents regarding sexuality topics. Many parents do want their children to experience lives that include healthy sexual relationships but feel unprepared to assist them and would rather rely on trained professionals. If you fall into this category it's completely understandable and acceptable to use outside experts. Ideas for where to go for assistance with education are listed below.

LOCAL DISABILITY ORGANIZATIONS

Most agencies supporting individuals with developmental disabilities (ARC, UCP, People First) by now recognize their needs and rights related to sexuality. Often these agencies have lists of resources, classes, counseling services, organizations, or staff experts who may be able to address your child's needs.

PLANNED PARENTHOOD CLINICS/FAMILY PLANNING AGENCIES

Family Planning agencies specialize in providing reproductive healthcare services to individuals who may otherwise not have access to services. Not all of these agencies have staff trained or experienced in working with individuals who have cognitive disabilities, but more often than not they have a good level of comfort and training regarding pregnancy and sexually transmitted disease (STD) prevention, pleasure, and consent.

Common Perspectives Regarding Sexual Activity

Common Beliefs	Refining Your Stance:
Denial /Elimination of Sexuality You don't believe your child has the same drives or needs as the general population or the capacity to form a relationship with another person. You believe it's best to avoid or eliminate the possibility of romantic relationships.	■ What are acceptable ways for my child to express his/her sexuality? ■ How do I feel about masturbation as a possible form of sexual expression? ■ Even if I believe my child will not be sexual in a relationship, is there information that would be helpful to her?
Delaying Sexual Involvement You recognize your child may in fact be sexually involved at some point but believe important criteria or conditions should be present if and when sexual activity occurs. These conditions may include waiting until a certain age, or until specific rites of passage have been achieved (being able to live in his or her own place, having a job, being able to support self, etc.).	■ What criteria or conditions do I feel indicate readiness for sexual involvement in my son or daughter? ■ What if my child is not able to meet my criteria? Can the criteria change? ■ Is there information I want my child to understand prior to becoming sexually active?
Safe & Responsible Sexual Involvement You believe people who are sexually intimate should act responsibly. Although you don't condone sexual activity for people your child's age and/or with your child's disability, you recognize your son or daughter may choose to become sexually active against your wishes. If sexual activity does occur, you want your child to be safe, and act responsibly.	■ What does responsible sexual activity look like? As a parent, how would I be able to determine if my child was acting responsibly? ■ Am I willing to help my child if she or he wants to be responsible? ■ If I can't help, who can?
Abstinence Until Marriage You value your child's right to form relationships but believe intercourse and more intimate forms of sexual expression are unacceptable outside of a marriage relationship.	■ How do I define abstinence? ■ Are there shared sexual behaviors that are acceptable to me before marriage? What are they? ■ What information do I want my child to understand even if he or she is not sexually active? ■ If my child found a partner and was involved in a healthy, mutually respectful relationship would I support their right to marry? ■ What if my child is unable to find a compatible partner and marriage never happens? Will I feel differently?

If you call to make an appointment, ask them about their training and experience working with individuals with cognitive disabilities. Talk with them about your son's or daughter's needs and assess their interest and motivation in helping you meet your goal. If you sense they have little experience, give them some concrete suggestions for ways your child learns best. For example, "I don't have the resources to explain how to use a condom. How do you help to make these concepts concrete?" or, "My daughter understands better when pictures or models are used. Do you have pictures or models available in your clinic?" Often these clinics are used to working with teens who also benefit from concrete teaching methods.

FAMILY PHYSICIAN/HEALTHCARE PROVIDER

If your son or daughter has a good relationship with your family physician, talk with the doctor about the possibility of scheduling individualized education sessions on the responsibilities of pregnancy and disease prevention. He or she may also be familiar with resources, classes, counseling services, organizations, or other experts able to address the needs of individuals with cognitive disabilities.

AASECT EDUCATORS, COUNSELORS, AND THERAPISTS

AASECT (American Association of Sex Educators, Counselors, and Therapists) is the only organization devoted to training and certification of professionals in order to promote sexual health. AASECT certified educators, counselors, and therapists have extensive training in all aspects of sexuality and are available in most states. Not all of them have experience working with individuals with developmental disabilities. If you are fortunate enough to have one of these resources in your community, one of the agencies listed above probably knows who they are and how to contact them. A partial listing of certified professionals in the United States is available at www.aasect.org.

SEXUALITY RESOURCE CENTERS

Sexuality resource centers are increasingly being recognized as legitimate partners in sexuality education. Often the public views these establishments as "adult toy stores," but a handful of them are much more than that. Sexuality Resource Centers employ well-trained staff, sell quality products, books, and often offer individualized

What Should I Ask the Professional to Teach?

Adults with intellectual disabilities often receive very little information about rights and responsibilities associated with sexual expression in romantic relationships. If your child with Down syndrome is involved in a serious relationship, help him or her find information and resources that will help with informed and healthy decision-making. Suggested topics a professional can help with include:

- Importance of consent related to sexual expression
- Privacy and sexual expression
- Male and female sexual response cycle
- Risky sexual behaviors (related to pregnancy sexually transmitted infections/HIV)
- Protection from pregnancy/sexually transmitted infections/HIV
- Correct condom use

sexuality education sessions in a professional setting. Sometimes community classes on various sexuality topics are offered as well. For a listing of sexuality resource centers in the U.S., refer to the list in the back of the book.

References

Ames, T. and Samowitz, P. (1995). Inclusionary Standard for Determining Consent for Individuals with Developmental Disabilities. *Mental Retardation* (August): 264-67.

Cohen, W. et al. (2002). *Down Syndrome: Visions for the 21st Century.* New York: Wiley-Liss.

Couwenhoven, T. (2001). Sexuality Education: Building on the Foundation of Healthy Attitudes. *Disability Solutions 4* (6).

Engel, B. (1997). *Beyond the Birds and the Bees: Fostering Your Child's Healthy Sexual Development in Today's World.* New York: Pocket Books.

Griffin, L. (1996). *Informed Consent, Sexuality, and People with Developmental Disabilities: Strategies for Professional Decision Making.* Milwaukee, WI: ARC.

Haffner, D. (2000). *From Diapers to Dating: A Parent's Guide to Raising Sexually Healthy Children.* New York: New Market Press.

Hatcher, R. et al. (1998). *Contraceptive Technology.* New York: Ardent Media.

Hingsburger, D. (1993). *I Openers: Parents Ask Questions about Sexuality and Children with Developmental Disabilities.* Vancouver, British Columbia: Family Support Institute Press.

Hingsburger, D. (1998). *The Ethics of Touch: Establishing and Maintaining Appropriate Boundaries in Service to People with Developmental Disabilities.* Eastman, Quebec: Diverse City Press.

Hingsburger, D. and Tough, S. Healthy Sexuality: Attitudes, Systems, and Policies. *Research and Practice for Persons with Severe Disabilities 27*(1): 12-13.

Hingsburger, D. and Pendler, B. (1990). Sexuality: Dealing with Parents. *The Habilitative Mental Healthcare Newsletter 9* (4): pp. 29-34.

Hubbard, B. (1997). *Choosing Health—High School: Sexuality & Relationships.* Santa Cruz, CA: ETR Associates.

Kaser, F. (1992). Can People with Severe Mental Retardation Consent to Mutual Sex? *Sexuality and Disability 10* (1).

Katherine, A. (1991). *Boundaries: Where You End and I Begin.* New York: Simon & Schuster.

McCarthy, M. (1999). *Sexuality and Women with Learning Disabilities.* London: Jessica Kingsley Publishers.

Miron, A. and Miron, C. (2002). *How to Talk with Teens about Love, Relationships, and S-E-X: A Guide for Parents.* Minneapolis, MN: Free Spirit Publishing.

Montfort, S. and Brick, P. (1999). *Unequal Partners: Teaching about Power and Consent in Adult-Teen Relationships.* Planned Parenthood of Greater Northern New Jersey.

Rubin, K. (2002). *The Friendship Factor: Helping Our Children Navigate Their Social World—and Why It Matters for Their Success and Happiness.* New York: Penguin Books.

Sexuality Information and Education Council of the United States. (2004). Guidelines for Comprehensive Sexuality Education K-12. National Guidelines Task Force. 3rd Ed. New York: New York: SIECUS.

Stangle, J. (1991). *Special Education: Secondary Family Life and Sexual Health: A Curriculum for Grades 7-12.* Seattle, WA: Seattle-King County Department of Public Health.

Stein, N. and Sjostrom, L. (1994). *Flirting or Hurting: A Teacher's Guide on Student-to-Student Sexual Harassment in Schools.* Washington, DC: NEA Association.

Stengle, L. (1996). *Laying Community Foundations for Your Child with a Disability: How to Establish Relationships That Will Support Your Child After You're Gone.* Bethesda, MD: Woodbine House.

Strauss, S. (1992). *Sexual Harassment and Teens: A Program for Positive Change.* Minneapolis, MN: Free Spirit Publishing.

Valenti-Hein, D. and Mueser, K. (1990). *The Dating Skills Program: Teaching Social-Sexual Skills to Adults with Mental Retardation.* Orland Park, IL: International Diagnoses Systems.

Chapter 10—Framework for Teaching about Relationships

Concepts	Key Messages	Goal Behaviors
Types of relationships	▪ I have many different people in my life	▪ Experiences rich and diverse social connections
Boundaries in relationships	▪ The relationship I have with different people helps me know what kind of touch is okay ▪ An arm's length away is okay in most social situations	▪ Interacts with others in socially acceptable ways
Sexual attraction & crushes	▪ Sexual feelings become stronger during puberty ▪ When I have sexual feelings for another person it's called having a "crush" ▪ Crushes are normal and happen to everyone ▪ Crushes can be mutual (both people are interested) or one-sided	▪ Recognizes sexual feelings as healthy and normal ▪ Handles own sexual feelings in socially appropriate ways
Romantic relationships	▪ Romantic relationship is when 2 people have sexual feelings for each other (reciprocal) ▪ Sometimes we are attracted to people we know; other times we are attracted to people we don't know well ▪ There are people I cannot be romantically involved with (illegal relationships—boss, family, minors)	
Dating	▪ Dating is a planned activity that can help you decide if you are a good match for each other ▪ Both people have to want to date each other. If the person I like is not interested, he/she can say no. If I am not interested , I can say no. ▪ There are different ways to date (group, double, couple) ▪ I should speak with my family when I feel ready to date (family can discuss values, criteria, natural progressions)	▪ Plans a date ▪ Interacts with dating partner in socially acceptable ways
Evaluating relationships	▪ After I spend time getting to know a person, I may feel differently about that person ▪ I get to choose which relationships I want to continue and which to stop ▪ Healthy relationships improve my life ▪ Unhealthy relationships are destructive	▪ Sustains healthy relationships ▪ Avoids exploitive relationships

Concepts	Key Messages	Goal Behaviors
RESPONSIBILITIES OF SEXUAL EXPRESSION IN ROMANTIC RELATIONSHIPS		
Permission	■ I decide what forms of affection feel comfortable for me ■ Talking with my partner about my sexual limits is important ■ I can refuse sexual behaviors that feel uncomfortable ■ I need to respect my partner's limits	■ Communicates own boundaries related to physical affection ■ Respects boundaries of partner ■ Reports exploitative touch
Privacy	■ Affection that involves exposing body parts is private	■ Expresses affection in socially acceptable ways
Protection	■ Couples in sexual relationships show each other they care in many different ways ■ Some sexual behaviors can cause pregnancy, HIV, or STDs ■ Sexual behaviors that can cause pregnancy or spread STD/HIV(risky behaviors) require protection	■ Protects self/partner from unwanted pregnancy and STDs
Pleasure	■ There are many ways to give and receive pleasure ■ Sexual expression should feel good for both partners ■ Male and female bodies respond differently to sexual activity ■ Talking with your partner about what feels good can enhance pleasure	■ With partner, experiences mutual pleasure from sexual expression
Marriage/Committed Partnerships	■ Couples marry (commit to each other) when they love each other and want to share their lives together ■ There are roles and responsibilities in committed partnerships/marriage ■ It is helpful for couples to talk about these responsibilities so they can decide how they will handle them	

CHAPTER 11

Committed Partnerships, Marriage, and Parenthood

Twenty or thirty years ago, marriages involving individuals with developmental disabilities were still quite rare. During the years I was writing this book, I was surprised by the number of wedding or engagement announcements I heard about involving couples with Down syndrome or other cognitive disabilities. I do believe we are just now understanding how access to quality education and opportunities for full participation in the community has benefited individuals with cognitive disabilities. As they have become more deeply integrated into all aspects of society, it makes sense that some adults will want to experience the fulfillment that comes from being in a committed, intimate relationship.

Parents who have children involved in serious relationships have many questions about marriage as a possibility for their son or daughter. They ask me: Do I know any people who have been married? How are they doing? What steps did the families take to prepare them for this commitment? This chapter is a compilation of what I have learned from research, speaking with couples with intellectual disabilities, or parents whose sons and daughters have married or are in long-term, serious relationships.

Exploring Legal Options for a Committed Relationship

We often think that marriage is the only option for a committed relationship. Unfortunately, there are still many logistical obstacles for marriage between adults with cognitive disabilities. They include:

- *State Marriage Laws*—Before the 1970s, most states had laws that prevented individuals with mental retardation from marrying. These laws originated out of fears concerning adults with developmental disabilities procreating, their capacities to rear children, the economic impact these children placed on society, and/or the possibility of coercion and manipulation when only one of the partners within the marriage had a disability. In many states, antiquated laws prohibiting marriage between people with mental retardation have been repealed. Other states continue to retain discriminatory statutes that reflect little of what we know about people with developmental disabilities. In states that still retain these statutes, however, they are often not enforced.

■ *Financial implications*—If couples with Down syndrome receive Social Security benefits, there may be financial disincentives to marry. In some states, for example, two single people receive more benefits and income than a married couple. In other states money provided for support may also be jeopardized. Individuals with intellectual disabilities already exist on meager incomes, so further reductions in benefits can create a financial burden. Some families seek alternative living arrangements (e.g., commitment ceremonies, living together) in order to preserve benefits. Others have chosen to accept reductions in benefits and use alternative supplements when needed.

■ *Guardianship*—State guardianship laws vary from state to state. Most laws, however, clearly spell out the rights of the guardian in making decisions related to marriage. In some states, rights of couples with intellectual disabilities can be preserved even if the individual has a guardian. Normally, parents seeking guardianship for their sons and daughters are counseled and educated about their rights and responsibilities. Check with your local disability agency or an attorney who specializes in guardianship issues for information specific to your state.

If your son or daughter is seriously considering a legal partnership, you'll need to explore your state's laws and the specific impact those laws would have on your son or daughter's situation. Your local or state disability agencies should be able to direct you to individuals who have expertise addressing these issues.

SKILLS FOR A
COMMITTED
RELATIONSHIP

My 26-year-old son with Down syndrome has been living with his girlfriend for the last 6 months. They have been dating for a year and a half. It actually started quite slowly. Because we live outside the city and she lives in her own apartment, he would stay overnight at her home if they were going somewhere special. It was more convenient. Then he began to stay an extra day since her apartment was closer to his work. One day he said to me, "I really love her and want to live with her." I was actually quite astounded. It was a moment I had dreamed of happening but never really believed would. Both of our families agree that although they are not actually married, they have made a serious commitment to each other

Key Teaching Messages:

■ When two people have been dating awhile and feel they are in love, they may decide to make a long-term commitment to each other.

■ There are different ways to make this happen.

and we most certainly did not want to push them into marriage until they were really sure of what a long-standing relationship means. They have both matured enormously and are both learning how to take care of each other.

In Western society, parents of typically developing children usually don't give much thought to preparing their son or daughter for marriage or committed partnerships. They might teach them cooking or housekeeping skills, or make sure they know about birth control, but most of the time teens and young adults without disabilities learn the skills needed for a successful marriage on their own. If your child has Down syndrome or another cognitive disability, it is important to look carefully at the individual skills he might need in order to make a relationship work. Ultimately, it is your responsibility to assist your child in learning as many of these skills as possible before he or she moves out of your house, with or without a partner.

The chart below lists the basic skills an adult needs (with or without support) in order to have a chance at a successful long-term relationship with a partner.

Preparation for Marriage—Common Topics and Issues

Sexuality Issues	■ responsibilities of sexual expression ■ human sexual response cycle ■ pregnancy prevention ■ STD prevention ■ genetic counseling & testing ■ parenthood
Relationship Skills	■ handling conflict ■ communication skills ■ identifying and expressing emotions ■ delineating roles (if any) of partners' parents ■ roles & responsibilities of partners in the relationship
Managing Finances	■ budget planning ■ bill paying
Managing Home	■ food preparation ■ cleaning ■ home maintenance/repairs ■ laundry
Accessing Community Resources	■ transportation ■ health care ■ social services support ■ legal services ■ social/recreation/leisure

It is beyond the scope of this book to tell you how to teach your child all of the above skills. Instead I've focused on select issues that specifically relate to sexuality and relationships that build on information provided throughout the book. You may find it useful, however, to discuss the range of skills that would be helpful if you find yourself in conversations with your child about marriage or another type of committed relationship.

Learning from Others: The Couples

In writing this chapter, I talked to these couples and/or their parents.

Nate Greenbaum and Lydia Orso: Nate and Lydia have known each other since childhood. As children, they often accompanied their parents to activities they both enjoyed. When I interviewed the couple, they had been seriously dating for many years and were exploring the possibility of marriage.

Jeremy Martinsen and Simone Nelson: Jeremy and Simone were married in August of 2004. Jeremy and Simone met in March of 2000 while they were both on a trip with their families. They became acquainted while staying at the same resort. Because there seemed to be mutual interest and attraction, the families helped the couple continue the relationship over a distance. For three years, the couple traveled long distances to meet, sometimes Simone going to Jeremy's city and other times Jeremy traveling to Simone's part of the state. They married after three years of dating.

Andy Detienne and Beth Euclid: Andy and Beth met at their senior prom. After three years of dating they (and their families) understood their relationship was serious. They became engaged after dating for five years. They will soon be celebrating their tenth wedding anniversary.

MANAGING HOME AND FINANCES

Managing finances, developing skills to manage a home or apartment, and knowing how and when to use community resources are basic skills that any individual (with or without a partner) needs to master independent living. Although an adult with Down syndrome or other cognitive disability may never be completely independent in all of these areas, he or she still may want to marry.

The families I interviewed felt strongly that opportunities to live outside the home helped their son or daughter develop these skills and were important precursors to entering into a committed partnership or marriage.

"As in any marriage, the more solid you are as an individual, the happier you are in careers, the happier you're going to be in marriage."

—Rick Detienne (Andy's dad)

The Detiennes felt strongly that their son, Andy, needed to experience life independent from them before entering a marriage. Andy therefore lived independently with a roommate for two years before marrying Beth. During those two years, Andy learned basic household chores such as cleaning, laundry, and some cooking, and was able to improve his money and checkbook skills. Andy's parents felt these were critical learning years and contributed significantly in preparing him for marriage. For her part, Beth spent three years living independently with support in her own apartment before marrying Andy.

Increasingly, postsecondary programs being developed across the country for young adults with developmental disabilities are often designed to teach skills for living independently. Although expensive, some are appropriate for individuals with Down syndrome and other cognitive disabilities.

SEXUALITY ISSUES

When two individuals with intellectual disabilities share a committed relationship, they often need extra attention, training, and support related to sexuality issues. I recommend that the couple be offered the opportunity to spend time together with a trained professional who can answer their questions and address concerns in various areas of sexuality. Teaching about the human sexual response cycle may be especially valuable (see below). This type of information sharing may occur in the context of premarital counseling, if the professional is trained and comfortable working with individuals with Down syndrome or intellectual disabilities, or separately by a sex therapist or counselor.

HUMAN SEXUAL RESPONSE CYCLE

Understanding how a couple becomes pregnant is different from knowing how the body works and experiences sexual pleasure. The body of knowledge we have on the human sexual response cycle resulted from William Masters and Virginia Johnson's work back in the 1960s. Education in this area involves helping couples understand differences between the male and female body, understanding physiological signs of sexual arousal, and maximizing opportunities for experiencing sexual pleasure in a variety of ways.

Some would argue that this is not typically a component of education for other couples, but my experience is that couples with cognitive disabilities need considerable help with these issues and often get very little information. I recommend that adults with Down syndrome learn about these issues from professionals who are trained and experienced in addressing sexuality issues (see Chapter 10 for ideas). If the counselor has little experience with people who have cognitive disabilities, he or she will probably not use the pictures or videos that are often beneficial in teaching concrete learners.

One couple I interviewed, Beth and Andy, spoke frankly about the shortcomings of the sexual education they received before marriage. For example, Beth did not recall ever learning about sexual intercourse before marriage. Andy remembered getting information about the male and female body, sexual intercourse, and sexually transmitted diseases in high school but wasn't convinced he had the information he needed. Before the wedding he asked a friend to help him pick up some videos that might be instructional. He bought three educational-type videos (and he'll give you the exact titles if you ask him) and later Beth and Andy watched them together.

In contrast, another couple, Nate and Lydia, felt they had received sufficient information about sexuality during their counseling sessions. Their counselor spoke with them about the specifics of sexual intercourse and did address their concerns.

The families of Jeremy and Simone took a more informal approach to premarital instruction. Jeremy and Simone received help and support from Jeremy's sister who lives nearby. Before Jeremy and Simone married, she shared basic information about sexuality with the two of them.

PREMARITAL COUNSELING

Considering that individuals with intellectual disabilities often have fewer formal and informal opportunities to learn about sexuality and relationships, parents of the couples profiled in this chapter felt that premarital counseling was an important way for them to gain information and develop skills that would be beneficial in marriage. A variety of strategies, both traditional and not so traditional, were used to help acquire premarital counseling. It was clear that parents of the couples needed to play a more active role in seeking out and advocating for appropriate counseling services.

Since Lydia and Nate had been vocal and persistent about their desire to marry, Nate's mom began exploring resources for premarital counseling. In her search, she

Key Teaching Messages:

■ There are roles and responsibilities in committed relationships (marriage).
■ It is helpful for couples to learn and talk about these responsibilities so they will know how to handle them.

learned of a graduate student who was doing an internship at a local Jewish agency. She discussed her needs with staff, and the graduate student decided that modifying and then implementing the agency's pre-engagement counseling curricula with Nate and Lydia would be a worthy internship project. The curricula was intensive and com-

prehensive. The graduate student met with the couple once a week over an eight-month period. They discussed information about sexual intercourse, contraception, important aspects of marriage (honesty, communication, trust), handling conflicts in marriage, as well as decision making about children and the responsibilities associated with caring for them. Both Lydia and Nate felt the information was helpful.

Although Beth and Andy didn't participate in a formal premarital counseling program, they did view a series of videos about marriage provided by Beth's priest. They were also encouraged to attend a pre-marriage weekend retreat with other nondisabled couples who were considering marriage. The retreat was sponsored by a small, private, Catholic university near their community and involved spending time and speaking with other couples. Beth and Andy felt this experience was helpful, although Beth admitted she would have been more interested in speaking with married couples who had developmental disabilities.

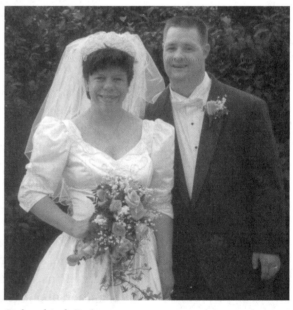

Beth and Andy Detienne

EXPLORING PARENTHOOD

There are several unique aspects to exploring parenthood for couples with cognitive disabilities that adults without disabilities do not generally need to consider. First, people with Down syndrome need to understand implications of having Down syndrome on fertility (is pregnancy even a possibility?) Second, if pregnancy is possible, what are the chances of having a baby with Down syndrome or other disability? And third, people with Down syndrome will likely need extra help understanding, in practical and concrete terms, exactly what having a baby would mean for them over the long term.

Teaching Activity: "What's It Like?"

At a recent sexuality conference, I was thrilled to see married couples with intellectual disabilities sharing their stories with other self-advocates. If you are aware of a couple(s) in your area with intellectual disabilities who are married or involved in a serious relationship, encourage your child and his or her partner to schedule some time together to ask questions. Help them prepare questions they would like to ask that address the unique aspects of being together when both partners have intellectual disabilities. Some ideas for questions:

- How did you meet?
- How long have you known each other?
- How long were you dating before you decided to get married (or commit to each other)?
- Is being married like you thought it would be?
- What kind of help have you needed? Who has helped you the most?
- What advice do you have for a couple with intellectual disabilities who are thinking about marriage?
- Has your relationship changed at all?

FERTILITY ISSUES IN MALES WITH DOWN SYNDROME

Studies have confirmed that males with Down syndrome have reduced rates of fertility, compared to males in the general population. In 1989, the first documented case of a male with non-mosaic Down syndrome fathering a child was described in the *Journal of Medical Genetics* (Sheridan, 1989). The male offspring was identified to be genetically normal. A second confirmed case of a man with trisomy-21 fathering a child was described in 1994 (Zuhlke). More recently, a third case of a genetically normal male child being born to a male with Down syndrome was reported in India (Pradham, 2006).

Although men with Down syndrome are often assumed to be infertile, the above cases illustrate that this is not a safe assumption to make. This means that men with Down syndrome or their partners should use contraceptives when they are interested in participating in sexual relationships but parenthood is undesirable.

Documented Outcomes of Pregnancy in Males with Down Syndrome

Male parents with Trisomy 21	Outcome
Pradham (2006)	Genetically normal male
Zuhlke (1994)	Not reported
Sheridan (1989)	Genetically normal male

Male Fertility Testing. Infertility in males with Down syndrome has most often been attributed to abnormalities in the sperm-making process (*spermatogenesis*) in the testicles. If your adult son or his partner have concerns about infertility, schedule an evaluation with a urologist or family physician. The initial work-up for male infertility generally includes a physical exam (to rule out structural problems that could contribute to infertility) and a semen analysis. For the semen analysis, your son will be asked to provide a sample of semen (obtained through masturbating in a private room, then ejaculating into a specimen container). The semen is then analyzed for presence of sperm, sperm count, motility abilities (how the sperm move), and morphology (form and structure of sperm).

When Andy and Beth expressed a desire to have children, Andy's parents were well aware of the higher incidence of infertility, so helped them explore their options. Andy's primary care physician suggested fertility testing in order to determine whether parenthood was even a real possibility. After testing, the doctor was able to verify that Andy would not be able to father a child. Andy's memory of hearing the news from his father continues to be a sad and poignant moment for him:

"I found out about my test results. I thought it was good news that I could father a baby. I was wrong! I found out from my dad in the car when he was driving. Found out I can't father a baby. We both cried so hard. I told Beth and she was bawling, I was bawling. I cried in front of my dad. It wasn't fun for either one of us. It was hard but we hung in there together and we decided together not to have kids."

FERTILITY ISSUES IN FEMALES WITH DOWN SYNDROME

There is some evidence that females with Down syndrome also have reduced fertility. In one study, half of the women had anovulatory cycles (cycles in which ovulation did not occur), which is one indicator of reduced fertility. Nevertheless, there have been numerous reports of pregnancies in women with Down syndrome. Based on the information currently available, it appears that mothers with Down syndrome have about a 50 percent chance of having babies with Down syndrome. An increased risk of miscarriages and delivering a baby prematurely also appears to be more common. Outcomes of all pregnancies in females with Down syndrome documented to date are listed below. Information about the women's partners and whether or not they had a disability is not available.

Documented Outcomes of Pregnancy in Females with Down Syndrome

Female Parents with Down Syndrome	Outcome
26 women (28 pregnancies)	10 normal
	10 Down syndrome
	1 set premature, nonviable normal twins 3 malformed
	1 slight microcephaly
	1 stillborn 2 aborted, no other information known

Fertility Testing in Females. Determining fertility in females is much more complicated and costly. The process typically begins with a pelvic exam in order to check for structural abnormalities of the reproductive organs. The woman may be asked to track and chart specific information about her menstrual cycles (e.g., basal body temperatures or cervical mucous) so the physician can look for patterns that indicate ovulation is occurring. Sometimes this is done using ovulation prediction kits. Samples of blood may also be taken to evaluate hormone levels that play a key role in ovulation and reproduction. If the above findings seem normal, additional testing designed to examine internal structures of the reproductive anatomy may be suggested. Many of these tests are costly, uncomfortable, and painful, so it may be advisable to test the male partner first and only proceed with infertility testing for the woman if her partner has been determined to be fertile.

GENETIC COUNSELING

If a couple is planning to have children and at least one of the partners has a genetic condition, they should be offered genetic counseling. This counseling should address the unique aspects of the disability and how it may or may not affect offspring. In the past it was assumed that the offspring of individuals with developmental disabilities would automatically have mental retardation. In fact, this myth actually spurred the development of institutions and mass sterilizations of residents. We now know that not all children of parents with developmental disabilities are affected and that some function within the "normal" range of intelligence.

Preparing your son or daughter in advance for a session with a genetics counselor is important. Here are some strategies:

- *Awareness of disability*—By adulthood, your child should have a good understanding of his disability, how it uniquely affects him physically and developmentally, as well as individual adaptations and strategies that have worked to support and maximize his independence. If your adult child or his or her partner is unaware of their disability refer to Chapter 7 for some ideas on increasing self-awareness.

- *Exposure to babies, children, teens, and adults who have a similar disability*—If your child has experiences being with or caring for others who have a similar disability, it will help him understand the range of abilities possible in any children he might have. One mother I know whose teenaged daughter is excited about the possibility of being a parent arranged for her daughter to spend time with babies with Down syndrome. She attends her local support group events regularly so her daughter is exposed to individuals of all ages with Down syndrome. The mother—who is a nurse—has also set up supervised babysitting times in her home so her daughter can more easily learn about common health issues and responsibilities faced by parents of children with Down syndrome.

Be sure to select a genetic counselor who is able to share information in understandable and sensitive ways and whose attitudes can support informed decision making. For example, it takes remarkable skill and sensitivity to explain the importance of finding out whether the couple's child might have Down syndrome without making the couple feel as if Down syndrome is a terrible thing. In addition, it is essential that the professional be able to share information in concrete ways that will enhance understanding and comprehension.

MAKING THE DECISION TO HAVE CHILDREN

Key Teaching Messages:

- Becoming a parent is a decision.
- Some people decide they want to be parents and have children; others decide they don't want the responsibilities that come with being a parent.

If, after genetic and fertility testing, parenthood is in fact a real and desirable option, counseling regarding the couple's motivations, feelings, and responsibilities of parenthood should be explored. In most cases, the reasons will be no different than anybody else's. Listed below are common motivations for wanting children that surface during counseling and education sessions.

MEDIA IMAGES OF PARENTHOOD

When we consider the important role media plays in our children's lives, it's easy to understand how becoming a parent may seem appealing. My younger daughter is quite fond of the old *I Love Lucy* episodes and we watch them often. During the later episodes we noticed how much little Ricky sleeps—morning naps, afternoon naps, and then off to bed before big Ricky gets home. I asked my daughter to compare Little Ricky to her real-life cousin. My youngest nephew rarely sleeps and seems to experience power surges throughout most of the day. In the TV world, the smaller details and logistics of parenting a child are routinely left out. Babies seen on television sleep a lot, are well nourished, hardly ever get sick, rarely cry, and require minimal effort. Frequently these are the images people latch onto (not just individuals with developmental disabilities) and come to see as reality.

My daughter loves to watch old videos of herself and her sister as babies and comment on how cute they both were. I think it's where she gets a lot of her ideas about wanting to be a parent.

There is a popular comic strip called "Baby Blues" that my daughter loves. In this strip, things that would be dreadful to deal with in real life are often depicted as hilarious and handled with a quick quip from the mom or dad.

PERVASIVE SOCIETAL EXPECTATIONS

Although attitudes have changed, many individuals still assume that part of becoming an adult means being a parent. In some families, moving away, getting a job, getting married, and having children is such an ingrained social script that it becomes difficult to believe that parenthood is a choice.

During the mid-1980s, I led what we called "Baby, Yes, No, Maybe?" workshops designed for couples who were struggling to decide whether or not they wanted to be parents. Many of the participants were undecided, but others pretty much knew they did not want children. They often expressed frustration with the pervasive cultural expectation of becoming a parent and had registered for the workshop in hopes of getting help responding to the pressure they felt on a daily basis. When people encounter married couples without children (or even those with one child), they are often aggressive about seeking an explanation.

My point is, when you are a parent, you don't always notice how pervasive the expectation is, but your child may be very aware of its presence. If societal expectations seem to be an important motivational factor for your child, be sure you (and/or the counselor) are presenting marriage and parenthood as two separate decisions rather than a package deal. Parenthood is a *choice* rather than an obligation within marriage.

Clearly, it's completely normal and acceptable to choose not to be a parent today. If you have immediate family members who have chosen this lifestyle, have them talk with your child about why they chose not to have children (if it was a choice). Your son or daughter should know it is perfectly okay and normal to be a grown adult and not have children.

DESIRE TO BE A GROWNUP

In some instances, the desire to be a parent stems from simple curiosity or a desire to be viewed by others as more adult-like. Often these desires are closely connected to a desire to truly participate in the adult experience. Decision-making is improved when couples (disabled or not) have opportunities to explore their own thoughts and feelings within the context of concrete experiences that capture the realities of what's it's like to be a parent.

Here are some ideas for exploring the realities of parenthood:

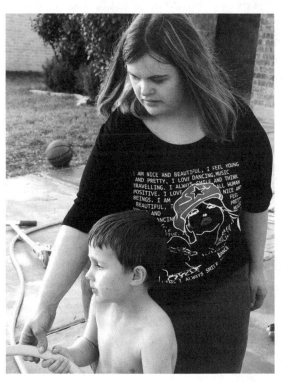

- *School and Community Coursework*—Most schools spend some time addressing the basics of a childcare and parenting. In middle school, for example, classes on babysitting and childcare are typically introduced. Although assigned time is limited, it's a starting point. Child development courses at the high school level are another possibility. Local YMCA's, recreation programs, hospital education departments, scouting groups, or community agencies such as the Red Cross may offer childcare certification courses. Usually these courses require spending some time caring for children.

- *Supervised Childcare*—If there are younger nieces and nephews in your family, let your son or daughter help you baby sit them, if possible. Supervised childcare means you're around and can step in quickly if help is needed. Make sure your child is truly participating in the experience and doing the work that would be required of a parent. Teach him how to change diapers, coordinate play activities, plan snacks, and put children down for naps, then allow him to practice his skills. Start with short timeframes and work up to longer increments of time. If your child tries to withdraw from the experience, be firm and remind him of his responsibilities and that parenting is a full-time job. If you have a daughter with Down syndrome who has expressed an interest in having children, there is a very real possibility her baby could have Down syndrome, so arranging for her to help provide care for a child with a disability should also be a part of the experience. Following these opportunities, discuss aspects of the experience that she liked and didn't like.

- *Career Exploration, Job Training, Volunteer Experiences*—One of the goals of school-to-work transition programs is to explore a variety of jobs in different professions. If parenting or taking care of children interests your child, advocate that he spend time in local daycare facilities, elementary school programs, church nurseries, or other experiences that involve caring for children. At a conference I attended a while back, a young woman with Down syndrome talked about the variety of jobs she had held, including one at a child care center. During her speech, she shared her feelings about this position: "I didn't like this job; taking care of kids was sooo hard."

- *Mentoring Experiences*—After Andy and Beth discovered they would not be able to have children, Beth was devastated and continued to feel a need to "mother." At some point, Beth's mom was contacted by a family whose young daughter also had William syndrome (like Beth). The contact proved to be useful for everyone involved. Beth was able to play with and care for the younger girl from time to time, helping her fulfilling her desire to mother. The girl's family appreciated Beth's role as a mentor and inspiring role model for their daughter.

SIMULATED CHILDCARE EXPERIENCES—ARE THEY EFFECTIVE?

In order to provide concrete ways to help students begin to understand the responsibilities associated with caring for a "baby," many schools require participation in simulated childcare experiences. Typically the "babies" are sacks of flour, eggs, or dolls that are programmed with computer chips to cry intermittently. Although these activities may be helpful in initiating early conversations about concrete responsibilities of being a parent, they shouldn't be the only experience. Individuals with (and without) intellectual disabilities who are interested in becoming a parent need real-life, repetitive opportunities to experience child-rearing responsibilities at different ages and stages.

In school, my daughter used that computerized doll "Baby Think It Over" at two different times. She hated the experience both times. The first time she used the baby, she had to start by filling out a form with information on how many

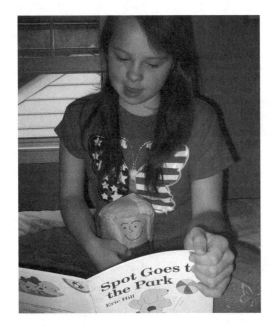

kids she wanted. She stated that she wanted four children. At the end of her experience, with huge black circles under her eyes, she quickly, and with no urging, wrote a huge zero under "number of children." To this day, she maintains that she wants no babies of her own, although she does like working with older kids.

In eighth grade health class, my daughter had to take care of a flour baby for two weeks. She had to lug it around everywhere she went or else arrange for a "babysitter" to watch it. She also had to keep a journal listing what she did with the flour baby each day. She really didn't learn much about how demanding a real baby is, since the "baby" let my daughter sleep through the night and didn't let out a peep if she ignored it while she was watching TV or forgot to "feed" it. She did get a general idea, though, that taking care of a baby is expensive, because one assignment was to go to the store to price a list of furniture, supplies, clothes, and food.

Teaching Activity: "Couple Interviews"

This activity will give your child and his or her partner a way to explore the variety of real reasons couples choose to become, or not become parents. Help your child identify two or three couples he knows who have chosen not to be parents, and two or three couples who have chosen the opposite path (are parents). These should be couples who truly made a conscious decision rather than experiencing "default" decision-making (e.g., got pregnant by accident, experienced infertility, or never really made a decision but instead pregnancy just "happened").

Encourage your child and his partner to interview these couples so they can gather information about how these decisions were made and the reasons behind their decisions. If your child has difficulty writing, use a video camera to tape the interviews to replay for discussion later. Below are some questions to begin the interview. Your son or daughter may have other ideas and questions as well:

Interview questions for couples with children:
- What kinds of things did you think about before you decided to have a child?
- What are 2 or 3 important reasons you both decided to have children?
- How did your life change after you had a child?
- Was being a parent like you thought it would be? What was the biggest surprise?
- What qualities do you think are needed to be a good parent?

Interview questions for childless couples:
- What kinds of things did you think about before you decided you didn't want to have a child?
- What are 2 or 3 important reasons you both decided not to have children?
- What things do you get to do because you don't have children?
- Was not having children like you thought it would be? What was the biggest surprise?

RESPONSIBILITIES OF PARENTING

Key Teaching Messages:

- Many people want to be parents; others don't want to be.
- Being a parent requires work, time, resources, and patience.
- People who choose to be parents should be able to provide:
  - ❏ Adequate home or shelter
  - ❏ Money for food and clothing
  - ❏ Education and an environment that helps the child grow and develop
  - ❏ Health care

Teaching Activity: "Facts & Myths about Being a Parent"

Use this activity to clarify facts and myths or misconceptions your son or daughter and his or her partner may have regarding parenthood, to share factual information, and to generate discussion about what it means to be a parent.

On two different index cards, write opposite words like "fact/fiction," "true/"false," "real/make believe," that make sense for your child or use symbols that might help illustrate these concepts. Type the statements below on a piece of paper, print them, and then cut them up into separate slips of paper so one phrase appears on each slip. Taking turns, have your child (and his partner) pick a slip of paper, read the statement, then determine whether the statement is a fact (true) or fiction (false). Use the information below to elaborate on fictional statements, encourage discussion, and explore feelings about being a parent.

- *Being a parent is hard work.*   FACT
  - What *work* is required if you have a child? (making meals and feeding the child, bathing him, changing his diaper/toilet training, taking him to doctor's appointments when sick and healthy, teaching him new things, helping with homework, talking with teachers, buying clothes, helping him understand appropriate behavior, etc.)
  - How do you think the *work* changes as the child gets older?
  - What do you think happens if the work is not done?
  - What do you think would be the hardest thing about being a parent?
  - Parents: Share your own experiences about the most difficult aspects of parenting.

- *As long as a couple is in love, they will be good parents.*   FICTION
  - Being with a person who loves and cares for you is important, but it takes much more to be a good parent. Besides love, parents need to provide basic things for their child(ren)—a safe place to live, food, clothing, schooling, medical care.
  - Beyond love, what other qualities are needed to be a good parent? (Patience, energy, skills to do the work of being a parent)

Teaching Activity: "How Would My (Our) Life Be Different?"

This activity is designed to be a concrete way to help your son or daughter and their partner understand specific ways everyday routines are altered when a child is in the picture.

On the computer or by hand, create a full-day schedule divided into one-hour increments. Begin the day at 6:00 AM and end with 10:00 PM. Leave writing room on the right of each hour (take a peek at a day planner if you need ideas for how to organize this on a sheet of paper). Label one of the pages "MY DAY," and the other "A DAY IN THE LIFE OF A PARENT" or other phrase that makes sense for your son or daughter. Make multiple copies of each of the final schedules.

On the "MY DAY" sheet, ask your son or daughter (and his or her partner) to track and make notations about what they are doing throughout the day. Have them do this for a weekday and one weekend day. Then help them identify a parent(s) who could complete the "A DAY IN THE LIFE OF A PARENT" schedule. Ideally, parents whose children are at different ages and stages will be most useful (infant, toddler, child, middle school, etc). After the schedules have been completed, place them side by side and compare and contrast differences.

- *Taking care of a child is the mother's job*   FICTION
  - Being a parent is a lot of work and can be stressful. It's always better if two people can share in the work of being a parent.
  - What kinds of work do you think you could do? Your partner?
  - What new skills would you need to learn if you decided to become a parent? Your partner?

- *Being a parent comes naturally*   FICTION
  - Most people don't know everything when they become parents and make mistakes along the way. There are many times when parents struggle with how to be a parent. During these times they have to learn new things. They might read books, take classes, or get help from others when they are struggling with the work of being a parent.
  - Parents: Talk about an aspect of parenting you struggled with and how you got through difficult times.
  - What kinds of things might you need help with?
  - Who could provide that help?

- *You aren't a real grown up unless you have children*   FICTION
  - Many grown ups are not parents.
  - What do you think it means to be grown up? (making decisions for yourself, taking care of yourself, keeping promises, being reliable, etc.)

- *Being a parent can be a fun and wonderful experience.*   FACT
  - What do you think you would enjoy most about being a parent?
  - Parents: Share your favorite aspects of parenting.

Parents with Intellectual Disabilities—How Do They Fare?

Families and professionals often want to know how well couples or individuals with intellectual disabilities do as parents. How many parents who have intellectual disabilities are successful? What contributes to a successful parenting experience? Although the number of families headed by a parent with a developmental or intellectual disability has increased during the past century, there is still very little research to help answer these questions. Poor record-keeping, differences in how disabilities are defined, and fragmented services make it difficult to acquire accurate data over time. Here are the few facts that are agreed upon:

- In a survey that was done in the mid-1990s, only 51 percent of parents with intellectual disabilities were currently living with their children (National Health Interview-Disability Supplement). This statistic is not necessarily due to parenting failure, but rather to strong system discrimination in Termination of Parental Rights (TPR) proceedings when the parent has an intellectual disability. For example, as of August of 2005, 37 states include having a "disability" as grounds for termination of parental rights.

- Parents with intellectual disabilities usually need and benefit from additional training and support. Common topics include:
  - Basic childcare
  - Safety
  - Nutrition
  - Problem-solving
  - Positive parent-child interaction
  - Behavior management

- There is evidence that integrated, coordinated service delivery models work best in supporting families headed by parents with intellectual disabilities. (This means that one agency serves the entire family but uses funds from several different programs.)

CONTRACEPTION

Couples should also be given information on contraception—specifically, what it is, how it is used, and reasons for using different methods. (See Appendix B-12 for the full range of contraception options and Chapter 5 for more information on pros and cons of contraceptive methods.) For example, many couples use birth control until they feel the conditions are right for raising a child (they have jobs that would help them be able to financially support a child, have a stable home, or are able to commit time that is needed to care for a child) or to help with spacing if more than one child is desired.

If past experience suggest that the couple will have difficulty with consistent contraceptive use, or if more reliable methods would not be good options due to health or medical issues, the couple should learn about options

Key Teaching Messages:

- Not all couples want to have children.
- Birth control methods (contraception) should be used when couples do not want to have children.
- There are many different types of birth control methods (contraception).

for permanent contraception. Laws related to sterilization vary from state to state. In most cases, physicians may only perform a sterilization procedure if the individual:

- is an adult (check with your state law for age);
- is his/her own legal guardian;
- can demonstrate that he or she truly consents to the procedure (can communicate that he or she understands what will happen and can describe the impact of the surgery on fertility); and
- was not coerced into the decision.

Sterilization laws that exist today are designed to prevent others from making decisions about sterilization on behalf of people who may not fully understand the implications of those decisions. If your adult child is moving in the direction of not wanting children, he will not only need understandable information about the procedure and its impact on fertility but will also need to convince his physician he is making an informed choice of his own volition.

"My decision to become sterilized was the last and only time I will ever make a decision based solely on the fact that I have a disability"— an adult male self-advocate.

References

Booth, T. & Booth, W. (2002). Men in the Lives of Mothers with Intellectual Disabilities. *Journal of Applied Research in Intellectual Disabilities 15:* 187-199.

Brown, R. I. (1995). Social Life, Dating, and Marriage. In L. Nadel & D. Rosenthal (Eds.) *Down Syndrome: Living and Learning in the Community.* New York: Wiley-Liss.

Cento, R. M., Ragusa L., et al. (1996). Basal Body Temperature Curves and Endocrine Pattern of Menstrual Cycles in Down syndrome. *Gynecological Endocrinology 10* (2): 133-37.

Edwards, J. (1988). Sexuality, Marriage, and Parenting for Persons with Down syndrome. In *The Young Person with Down Syndrome: Transition from Adolescence to Adulthood.* Baltimore: Brookes Publishing.

Field, M. & Sanchez, V. (1999). *Equal Treatment for People with Mental Retardation: Having and Raising Children.* Cambridge, MA: Harvard University Press.

Garcia, M. (1999). *Andy & Beth: A Love Story.*

The Inclusion of Disability as Grounds for Termination of Parental Rights in State Codes (Oct. 2006). *Policy Research Brief,* (Research and Training Center on Community Living, University of Minnesota)*17* (2).

Johannisson, R. et al. (1983). Down's Syndrome in the Male: Reproductive Pathology and Meiotic Studies, *Human Genetics 63* (2): 132-8.

Keltner, B. et al. (1999). Mothers with Intellectual Limitations and Their 2-year-old Children's Developmental Outcomes. *Journal of Intellectual & Developmental Disability 24* (1): 45-57.

Kettner-Pixa, U. (1999). Follow-up Study on Parenting with Intellectual Disability in Germany. *Journal of Intellectual & Developmental Disability 24* (1): 75-93.

Llewellyn, G. et al. (1999). Support Network of Mothers with Intellectual Disability: An Exploratory Study. *Journal of Intellectual & Developmental Disability 24* (1): 7-26.

Monat-Haller, R. (1992). *Understanding & Expressing Sexuality: Responsible Choices for Individuals with Developmental Disabilities.* Baltimore: Brookes Publishing.

National Center on Birth Defects and Developmental Disabilities, Centers for Disease Control and Prevention. www.cdc.gov/ncbddd/dd/ddmr.htm

Pietrzak, B. (1997). Marriage Laws and People with Mental Retardation: A Continuing History of Second Class Treatment. *Developments in Mental Health Law 17* (1 & 2).

Pradham, M, et al. (2006). Fertility in Men with Down syndrome: A Case Report. *Fertility and Sterility 86* (6).

Pueschel, S. (1988). *The Young Person with Down Syndrome: Transition from Adolescence to Adulthood.* Baltimore: Brookes Publishing.

Ross Roundtable Report: Caring for Individuals with Down Syndrome and Their Families (1995). Columbus, OH: Ross Products Division.

Sheridan, R. et al. (1989). Fertility in a Male with Trisomy 21. *Journal of Medical Genetics 26* (5): 294-98.

Tymchuk, A. et al. (1999). Parenting by Persons with Intellectual Disabilities: A Timely International Perspective. *Journal of Intellectual & Developmental Disability 24* (1): 3-6.

Van Dyke, D., McBrien, D., and Sherbondy, A. (1995). Issues of Sexuality in Down Syndrome. Down Syndrome Educational Trust: *Down Syndrome Research and Practice 3* (2).

Zuhlke, C. et al. (1994). Down Syndrome and Male Fertility: PCR-derived Fingerprinting, Serological and Andrological Investigations. *Clinical Genetics.*

Exploitation Prevention

Not long ago, I received a phone call from a distressed mother who had attended a workshop I had done a decade earlier. Her son had been fairly young at the time and she had believed, like most of us do, that there was plenty of time. She called me because she discovered that her son, now a teenager, had recently been sexually exploited by a neighborhood friend. What was disturbing to both of us was not that the exploitation had been perpetuated by his good friend, but that it had been going on for about a year. Her son never told her. The exploitation came to light one morning because, after mentioning the boy's name, the mother detected a subtle nonverbal cue from her son indicating a lack of enthusiasm. This made her think she needed to figure out what was going on. Later, she told me she hadn't thought anything could happen to her son because they lived in the country where her son was fairly isolated from others.

Most parents I speak with are keenly aware that individuals with developmental disabilities are more often sexually exploited than those without. How much more varies based on age, specific sampling methods used in research, and how abuse is defined. Some respectable estimates based on well-known research indicate the following:

- Regardless of age, race, ethnicity, sexual orientation, or class, women with disabilities are assaulted, raped, and abused at more than twice the rate that nondisabled women are (Sobsey, 1994; DisAbled Women's Network, 1998).
- For adults with developmental disabilities, the risk of being physically or sexually assaulted is likely 4 to 10 times higher than for other adults (Sobsey, 1994).
- Children with any kind of disability are almost twice as likely to be sexually abused (Petersilia, 1998).
- Women with developmental disabilities are more likely to be victimized more than once by the same person and more than half never seek assistance with legal or treatment services (Pease and Frantz, 1994).

Sexual exploitation is a broad term used to describe a wide range of sexual behaviors forced upon another person unwillingly. Although almost all researchers report a higher rate of sexual exploitation among individuals with developmental disabilities, they do not agree on the prevalence. One reason is that sexual exploitation is defined in a variety of ways, making incidence data highly variable and sometimes confusing. More recently the Centers for Disease Control and Prevention (CDC) has advocated that the term "sexual violence" be adopted to define and describe a range of illegal and exploitative sexual behaviors.

Categories of Sexual Violence (Centers for Disease Control)

Sexual harassment	■ Unwanted sexual talk, use of sexual language, or comments ■ Unwanted exposure to materials that are sexual in nature
Voyeurism	■ Staring at a person who is undressing or doing private things without their knowledge or permission
Exhibitionism	■ Unwanted exposure to a person's private body parts
Sexual assault	■ Forced attempts to touch or fondle genitals/private body parts ■ Attempted or forced acts of sexual intercourse (oral, anal, or vaginal)

Another factor that makes it difficult to get accurate data on sexual exploitation in people with cognitive disabilities is that most cases are never reported. Reasons for under-reporting are complicated and far-reaching. The fear that a person who is being abused experiences, particularly when the abuser is someone in an authoritarian or support role, cannot be underestimated. The victim may fear losing a relationship with the person, or may believe threats that she or a loved one will be in danger if she tells. Others feel that systems too often fail to incorporate guidelines and interventions that can assist in recognizing and responding to the unique needs of individuals with disabilities. For example, professionals may be unaware of the subtle signs and symptoms that may be present when abuse has occurred, or they may lack screening procedures that ensure safety.

Why Are People with Cognitive Disabilities More Vulnerable to Exploitation?

SOCIETAL ATTITUDES AND BELIEFS ABOUT PEOPLE WITH DISABILITIES

Attitudes that devalue individuals with disabilities within our society are critical factors contributing to increased risk of abuse (Sobsey & Doe 1991). The common belief that people with developmental disabilities are asexual, for example, makes it harder for others to recognize that abuse may be occurring. Research conducted by Dick Sobsey and Sheila Mansell (1990) showed that distorted perceptions and beliefs about individuals with developmental disabilities allowed offenders to rationalize and justify sexual abuse and exploitation with clients. Examples of attitudes these researchers found during interviews included beliefs that a person with a disability is less important, more vulnerable, and ignorant about what is happening and therefore less affected by the abuse.

UNIQUE ASPECTS OF THE DISABILITY

Characteristics of the disability itself also can make someone more vulnerable to exploitation. For example, people with Down syndrome who have difficulty with expressive language may have a harder time reporting or stopping abuse when it occurs. Even when people with disabilities report abuse, cases are often not investigated because the testimony and credibility of a victim who is not able to communicate in traditional ways are questioned (Griffiths, 2002). If someone has a physical impairment in addition to a cognitive disability, it is even more difficult for her to defend herself, resist the abuse, and escape from the offender.

SEXUAL ILLITERACY

Numerous studies have demonstrated that people with developmental disabilities have less information about sexuality than the general population. In one study comparing students with mild mental retardation with students of average intelligence (McCabe & Cummins 1996), the students with mild intellectual disabilities had more limited sexual knowledge and experience and more negative attitudes about sex, but had had more experiences with pregnancy, masturbation, and sexually transmitted infections. The participants with mild cognitive disabilities were also more likely to express positive feelings about sexual interactions that are normally considered exploitative and were more likely to think that having sex with anybody was acceptable. Other studies have found similar results.

Experts concur that information about sexuality—particularly facts about our bodies, sexual feelings, and rights to choose or not choose sexual partners—is an essential element of exploitation prevention programs for individuals with cognitive disabilities.

DEPENDENCY AND LEARNED COMPLIANCE

People with cognitive disabilities such as Down syndrome are often dependent on others for help with self-care and daily living tasks. This dependency increases the likelihood of abuse occurring. Marc Goldman (1994) found that people who rely on others for care are often more trusting and that the dependency and trust contribute to compliance and passivity. Being rewarded and praised for doing as authority figures ask increases the likelihood that the person will carry out requests that are inappropriate and exploitative in nature.

Given that the vast majority of sexual offenses are committed by people known to the victim—primarily caregivers or relatives—individuals with disabilities are increasingly vulnerable because they are exposed to larger numbers of caregivers over time.

ISOLATION

When people with developmental disabilities are isolated and segregated from the rest of society, the risk for exploitation increases. For example, abuse occurs within institutional settings two to four times more often than in the community (Rindfleisch & Bean 1988). The situation is not necessarily better for adults living in the community. If they lack friendships, romantic relationships, and have more limited opportunities for socialization, this can exacerbate feelings of loneliness. Lonely people may use less discretion in forming friendships, increasing their vulnerability. Reducing the factors that lead to isolation within service delivery systems is an important prevention strategy (Sobsey and Mansell).

Preventing Exploitation

The problem of sexual abuse and exploitation is complex and far reaching with no fast and easy solutions. There is still so much we don't know about what prevention strategies work. We do know what hasn't worked, however. Protecting and isolating individuals from the rest of society failed to result in safety and protection and instead created undesirable consequences. Many self advocates have shared their stories about life in institutions. These stories have motivated families and service providers to re-think the idea of separating and isolating groups of people from the rest of society for the purpose of protection. Keeping people with disabilities ignorant about sexuality information hasn't yielded great results either.

Current suggestions for preventing exploitation among individuals with cognitive disabilities are aimed at reversing some of the factors that contribute to increased vulnerability in the first place. They include:

1. Talk openly and honestly about sexuality at home. This will help your child feel that she can discuss sexuality with you and make it easier to communicate if concerns about abuse emerge.
2. Educate your child about her rights and help her learn how to express them through choice making and assertive communication. This decreases vulnerability.
3. Provide information about types of behavior that are inappropriate within specific types of relationships to help your child identify exploitation if it occurs.

Skill development and information are powerful tools. Those of us who work in the field of sexuality understand that people at the greatest risk for exploitation are those who are insulated, protected, or sheltered from what can happen. My philosophy and response to parental fears about exploitation never wavers: *the best way to help your child avoid exploitation is to give her the tools she needs to be empowered and educated.* The good news is that the same information and underlying philosophies that work toward promoting healthy sexuality (presented in previous chapters in this book) also help prevent exploitation.

Parental Roles and Responsibilities in Preventing Exploitation

Most experts agree that exploitation prevention requires comprehensive approaches that include educating parents, professionals, and individuals with developmental disabilities. But what specific contributions can families make toward preventing sexual abuse and exploitation? If your child is a minor or is nonverbal, you will need to act as his or her protector. In this role, knowing the basic and essential facts is important. When your daughter begins to date, or becomes more actively involved in the community, you will also need to share specific information about her rights so she can recognize and respond to abuse when and if it occurs. The remainder of this chapter is designed to prepare you for these roles.

**PARENTAL ROLE #1:
GET THE FACTS**

In order to help your child, you need to be informed and educated about what we know about exploitation. The following information is not meant to scare you, but rather make you aware of basic facts associated with sexual exploitation and individuals with developmental disabilities. Until your child has the skills and information she needs to become her own protector, you are her first line of defense, so educating yourself is critical.

WHO ARE THE OFFENDERS?

The majority of the time (over 90 percent), offenders will be people your child knows, trusts, and regularly encounters. Professionals and caregivers working in the field of disabilities, transportation providers, residential or support staff, personal care attendants, teachers, bosses, immediate family members, relatives, friends of the family, acquaintances, and neighbors are commonly identified in the literature as perpetrators. Facing this fact is tough, yet believing and acknowledging this is one of the most important realizations you face as you accept your role as protector and teacher.

In 1991, Dick Sobsey and Tanis Doe analyzed reports of sexual abuse involving individuals of all ages with a variety of disabilities. In this study, the perpetrators mirrored data we have on offenders in the general population: they were natural (16.8%) or step family (2.2%) members; acquaintances such as neighbors and family friends (15.2%); informal paid service providers such as baby sitters (9.8%); or dates (3.8%). A smaller percentage were strangers (8.2%). The remaining 44% of the cases involved perpetrators who had access to the victim as a result of disability services. For example, 28% were service providers (direct care staff members, personal care attendants, psychiatrists); 5.4% were specialized transportation providers; 4.3% were specialized foster parents; and 6.5% were individuals with disabilities. The researchers also noted that the abuse largely occurred in "disability" settings, or locations that were encountered because the individual had a disability. Other common characteristics of offenders:

- The vast majority of offenders are males. A smaller percentage of offenders are females.
- Offenders are opportunistic and often select professions or positions that will increase their access to vulnerable individuals.
- The majority of offenders have had multiple victims.
- People who exploit others lie and are often believed (Anne Salter).

The bottom line is that we often harbor stereotypes about people who offend and most of the time these imagined stereotypes are inaccurate. Individuals who offend are not suspicious-looking strangers but more often well-respected, well-liked individuals in the community.

**PARENTAL ROLE #2:
IDENTIFY
COMMUNITY
RESOURCES
AND SUPPORTS**

Most parents experience considerable anxiety about the possibility of abuse and consequently don't like to discuss it in any real detail. Locating local services within your community and understanding the role they play in preventing and responding to sexual abuse helps demystify things a bit and prevents denial. Encourage local parent groups you are connected with to help you get answers to your questions. Suggest they invite guest speakers from agencies to talk with your members about available resources in your state and communities.

Your local police department, sexual assault treatment center, or hospital may have an expert on staff who has experience working with child or adult sexual abuse and perhaps has expertise working with individuals who have developmental disabilities. Talk with guidance counselors at your child's school, or case managers. Here are some questions to ask that might be helpful:

- If my son or daughter reports an incidence of sexual exploitation, who should I call? What will they do? What does the process look like?
- Are there specialized clinical services available in our community if a person is sexually assaulted? What training have staff received in working with clients who have cognitive disabilities? How can we get services?
- What state and community experts offer information, training, and support? Many states have a key agency that acts as the designated resource for addressing exploitation issues. This agency may deal with broader issues such as violence and assault, but can also help with specific concerns about sexual exploitation. Often these agencies have comprehensive websites with lists of agencies in your state who can help. In addition to state resources, there may be specialized agencies located in larger metropolitan areas. Most disability agencies are also aware of increased needs for information among clients and families and can be helpful in providing support for families and self-advocates.
- Who provides sexual abuse prevention programming in our community? Are these programs adapted for participants with special needs? If not, are there other agencies with experience in this area?
- Are there specialized counseling and support services for individuals with disabilities who have experienced exploitation and need help with recovery?

EVALUATING CHILD SEXUAL ABUSE PREVENTION PROGRAMS IN YOUR COMMUNITY

Sometimes sexual abuse prevention programs are offered formally within the community. Many schools, for example, offer units on sexual abuse prevention in conjunction with general safety awareness programs. These programs can be single presentations sponsored by an outside agency or curriculum-based programs developed by the district and presented by school staff. Churches, Planned Parenthoods, or family support agencies might also offer instruction on sexual abuse prevention.

I still hear about outdated approaches for teaching about sexual abuse prevention. For example, decades ago sexual abuse prevention efforts focused solely on the *stranger danger* principle—the idea that strangers were inherently unsafe and that children should avoid them at all costs.

The stranger danger concept was long ago found to be ineffective as a sexual abuse prevention strategy. First, as mentioned earlier, studies repeatedly confirm that sexual exploitation is largely initiated by people who are known by the victim. Since most individuals know their abusers, it's not so much who the person is but rather what the person is *doing* that becomes the issue. If someone touches your child's body in inappropriate ways, shares sexually graphic pictures, or performs sexual acts with a minor child, it's illegal no matter who they are.

Second, most experts agree that the concept of "stranger" is too ambiguous and abstract, particularly for individuals with developmental disabilities. David Hingsburger often talks about the frequency of strangers moving in and out of the lives of people with developmental disabilities and reminds us that, from your child's perspective, a stranger is simply "a person they have not yet met."

Third, even though we tell our children not to talk to strangers, they often see us ignoring this rule. I remember when my daughter was about nine we passed an elderly woman during a walk to the library. We exchanged hellos, and after she had passed, my daughter asked who the person was. When I admitted I didn't know, she advised me to avoid speaking to strangers I didn't know. At that point I understood the flaw in assuming all strangers were dangerous and to be avoided.

Speaking with strangers is, in fact, a daily part of our lives. We converse with unfamiliar people at grocery stores, banks, department stores, and restaurants. Strangers help us get through our lives. Some experts agree that knowing how to speak with strangers and seek help when appropriate is actually a desirable skill to learn. In his book *Protecting the Gift: Keeping Children and Teenagers Safe and Parents Sane*, Gavin De Becker recommends we identify specific strangers our children *should* go to if they're lost or in need of help. His preferred choice? Women, ideally women who have children with them. He rationalizes that they're statistically less likely to hurt your child and will be more persistent and diligent about making sure your child is returned to safety.

Here are some things to consider as you evaluate sexual abuse prevention programs in your community:

1. *Does the program balance the positive aspects of sexuality with the hazards?*

Sexual abuse prevention programs are often a child's first formal introduction to sexuality, so care should be taken to prevent the dissemination of messages that create undue anxiety and fear about the body. Some *Good Touch/Bad Touch* programs, for example, offer narrowly defined definitions of good and bad touch. *Good touch* may be defined as touching involving non-genital parts of the body (hugs, etc.), while *bad touch* becomes associated with the genitals. This approach may unintentionally send messages that the genitals are somehow bad, making it difficult for your child to understand the positive aspects of pleasuring and need for sexual healthcare. Research has illustrated that children without disabilities who have been abused often misconstrue "bad touch" to mean they are a bad person for participating in the abusive behavior, liking the touch (genital touching can feel good no matter who is doing the touching), or enjoying the attention. The individuals with developmental disabilities I work with often have similar perceptions after experiencing an abusive situation.

2. *Does the program encourage and support parental involvement?*

Sexual abuse prevention programs have a greater impact when parents are educated and supportive of their role in promoting their child's safety. Any program your child is enrolled in should help you understand your roles and responsibilities in preventing exploitation, provide recommendations and resources for more information, and identify community resources you can turn to if you suspect your child has been or is being abused. Communities that understand the critical role parents play in keeping children safe will be more effective.

3. *Is the sexual abuse prevention program one component of a more comprehensive program?*

Abuse prevention programs are more effective when taught within the context of a comprehensive sexuality program. Multiple sessions presented and repeated throughout your child's schooling are more likely to balance information about the rights, responsibilities, joys, and pleasures of being a sexual person with the hazards and risks.

Important Components of Sexual Abuse Prevention Programs

Historically, sexual abuse prevention efforts have included subtle (and at times overt) messages suggesting that the child or other potential victim can or should take responsibility for her own safety. However, it is still quite uncommon for individuals with cognitive disabilities to report incidences of abuse. Experts are just now understanding the powerful and complex dynamics at work in these situations and how they contribute to underreporting. (For example, is it realistic to expect someone with a cognitive disability who requires assistance with self-care to know how to differentiate between appropriate and inappropriate touch?) Still, individuals with cognitive disabilities can benefit from prevention programs that include the following components:

■ **Body Rights**—Helping an individual understand that her body is her own and she has a say in how she shares it (or doesn't share it) are examples of "body rights" concepts. Modeling behaviors that acknowledge and reflect a respect for these rights (practicing what you preach) must also occur.

■ **Touching Rules for Private Body Parts**—People with cognitive disabilities are concrete thinkers and often do better with clear rules and limits. They need instruction about the private nature of the genitals as well as the few circumstances when others may need to see or touch them (for hygiene or health care—refer to Chapter 2.) As your child matures and becomes involved in dating and intimate relationships, the need for permission (consent) related to genital touching and sexual expression should be emphasized. (refer to Chapter 10).

■ **Assertiveness Skills**—Helping your son or daughter understand his or her right to say no or disobey when something is not right is an important skill. People learn this skill when they have opportunities to express opinions, make choices, and participate in decision-making that affects their lives.

■ **Feelings Training**—All of us need help learning how to identify and express feelings. Training that helps individuals identify and express a range of feelings and understand feelings commonly associated with healthy and abusive relationships is important (see Chapter 9).

■ **Telling**—Lessons centered around the importance of reporting when rules are violated should be included. Some curricula spend time helping the child identify "safe" people in her life she can talk to, who will listen and support her if she has concerns if her body rights are violated or if she feels unsafe.

DO SEXUAL ABUSE PREVENTION PROGRAMS WORK?

Research evaluating sexual abuse prevention programs has focused mainly on adults with mild to moderate cognitive disabilities. In these studies, participants have indeed demonstrated increases in knowledge and learned new self-protection skills. However, participants often had a harder time transferring new knowledge and skills to contrived testing situations. Experts point to the need for sustained training (repetition) and support in this area. Clearly, more research is needed to determine the effects of sexual literacy and skill development on sexual abuse prevention.

PARENTAL ROLE #3: **MAKE SEXUAL ABUSE PREVENTION AN ISSUE**

Thwarting sexual abuse and exploitation in individuals with cognitive disabilities requires collaborative efforts of the larger community. We now have a wealth of information about how predators work and the conditions that need to be present in order for them to victimize others. Schools and community agencies need to have systems in place that protect your child. Here are some ways you can bring the issue to the forefront:

Ask about Policies and Procedures. Most agencies have literature exploring staff roles and responsibilities in preventing, identifying, and responding to sexual exploitation of clients with cognitive disabilities. Yet, I am still amazed at how little staff and other professionals working in the field know about this as an issue. During a recent clinic visit, an adult patient with Down syndrome kept repeating a story about her "boyfriend" and what they did together in the basement. As I listened to the patient, the group home staff person who accompanied her seemed a bit too eager to dismiss anything she shared with me. ("That was a long time ago—remember?" Or, "She perseverates on things and won't let them go.")

This caregiver's easy dismissals combined with the unexplained symptoms that brought the patient to the clinic that day made me uneasy. I reminded the staff person about the incidence of exploitation among adults with developmental disabilities and asked her to pay close attention. She seemed amazed by my suggestion and admitted she had no idea this was a problem. I asked her to review her agency's policies regarding this issue so she could advocate on her clients' behalf (any and all of them) should she need to. She wasn't sure if her agency had policies, but said she would check (scary). In the end, the physician who performed the patient's physical exam identified sexual abuse as a possibility, amidst a long list of other health issues that needed to be explored. We reminded ourselves that perhaps we needed to be more vigilant about bringing the issue up with clients, support providers, and families.

My point is that people in the field who support and care for clients with disabilities need to be trained and knowledgeable about these issues. Here are some things you can ask as you screen agencies that may be providing services for your child:

- *What are your policies and procedures for identifying and responding to suspicious staff behavior and signs of abuse or exploitation in your residents?* Expect the provider to have a mandatory reporting policy as well as a clear plan for the safety of the individual with a disability. Most agencies that are licensed and accredited to provide care for individuals with developmental disabilities are required to have these policies in place (check mandates for your state). Agencies should have clearly written policies that identify examples of suspicious staff behaviors, require these behaviors to be reported to supervisors, and clearly spell out the consequences of sexual contact between staff and residents.

■ *How are staff trained and educated about these policies and procedures and handling allegations?* Remember, staff turnover in organizations that support or care for individuals with cognitive disabilities is a chronic problem. If training is only offered a few times a year, chances are that newer staff are not receiving information in a timely fashion.

■ *What kind of sexuality education is offered for clients they serve?* Helping individuals with cognitive disabilities recognize exploitation and know their rights is an important aspect of prevention. Your son or daughter needs to know what they can do and how to get help. These types of programs should be offered at least once a year, and ideally reviewed and repeated a few times a year.

■ *What staff screening procedures are in place?* Agencies supporting or caring for individuals with developmental disabilities should have strict procedures for performing background checks on people they hire and employ. Keep in mind that abusers who work in this field are often not charged, or may resign when concerns surface and move on to another agency. Still, screening procedures that include police checks should be in place.

■ *How are investigations of sexual abuse handled?* An outside agency—ideally the police—should be responding to and investigating allegations of abuse. When the agency itself handles investigations, or cases are transferred to an internal ombudsman, reporting becomes murkier and can interfere with an investigation, making prosecution less likely.

■ *When and if abuse occurs, what supports are offered to help clients recover?*

PARENTAL ROLE #4: PREPARING YOUR CHILD TO BE HER OWN PROTECTOR

Even though preventing sexual abuse is complex, research does suggest that sexuality education is one piece of the puzzle that can help reduce the risk of exploitation. The following strategies can be helpful in reducing the likelihood of exploitation. These topics can be taught at home and reinforced at school and in the community.

TEACH ACCURATE TERMS FOR PRIVATE BODY PARTS

If you want your child to feel comfortable talking about her body, she must have the vocabulary to discuss it. Using correct terms rather than words that are derogatory, babyish, or confusing helps to communicate respect for all parts of the body and encourages open communication. If exploitation does occur, using correct names for body parts enhances your child's credibility if the case is prosecuted and your child needs to tell her story.

TALK ABOUT BODY RIGHTS AND INSTILL A SENSE OF BODY OWNERSHIP

If your child is a minor, it is important to give her very specific information about circumstances when touch is okay. There are only two legitimate reasons why another person should be looking at or touching private parts of the body. These include activities related to 1) keeping the body clean (e.g., toileting, hygiene) or 2) keeping the body healthy (health care).

You could explain that if she needs help with going to the bathroom, bathing, or showering, her private body parts may be visible, but the person helping is only there to make sure the body gets clean, nothing else. Your child should know she has the right to tell the person to leave when he or she is done helping. If your child is nonverbal, teach her a sign or gesture to indicate she wants the person to leave or that she can complete the self-care task from here on. Share this information with people who are providing intimate care.

Key Teaching Messages:

- My body belongs to me.
- No one can make me share my body if I don't want to.
- If someone forces me to do sexual things, I should tell.

The only other time it is okay for a person to look at private parts of the body would be at the doctor's office during an exam. Remind your child that her health care professional (use his or her name) is responsible for making sure all parts of the body are healthy, private body parts too! If your doctor or nurse doesn't already do this, encourage him or her to ask before looking at or touching your child's body as a way of reinforcing the "your body is your own" message. Encourage health care professionals to reiterate and reinforce these concepts at every appointment.

If your child is older and independent with self-care, the above messages are still relevant. However, if she is an adult and involved in a relationship, messages related to her rights to set limits with her partner and decide what happens to her body are important as well (refer to Chapter 10).

As I've mentioned before, modeling is a critical component of teaching body ownership concepts. When body rights are respected and enforced in the home, your child will have an easier time understanding these concepts.

HELP YOUR CHILD READ, INTERPRET, AND RESPOND TO HER OWN INTUITIVE SIGNALS

As children with Down syndrome get older, some develop the capacity to recognize and respond to their own natural internal radar system that helps them know when experiences are dangerous, uncomfortable, or not quite right. Gavin De Becker, in his book *The Gift of Fear: And Other Survival Signals That Protect Us from Violence,* talks extensively about the natural alert system that works if we learn to pay attention and respond to cues our body gives us. Peg Flandreau-West, an Australian author, advocates teaching children (with or without disabilities) at young ages how to identify the physical body sensations that help warn us. She calls these signals *early warning signs* and describes them as cues our body gives us to help us know we are not feeling safe or that we need to be alert to what is happening.

Key Teaching Messages:

- My body gives me signals when I am feeling unsafe or need to be alert.
- My warning signals are _____.
- I should listen to and trust my body signals.
- If my body signals won't go away, I can talk about my signals with a safe person.

Because children and individuals with cognitive disabilities have more limited life experiences and less information, these warning systems are not always developed enough to be a source of protection. Back in the 1980s, Donna Fortin, a disability advocate here in Wisconsin, spent considerable time adapting these concepts of safety and an understanding of early warning systems specifically for individuals with cognitive disabilities with reportedly good results.

After receiving additional training on protective behaviors, I began incorporating these ideas into teaching I was doing for self-advocates with cognitive disabilities with some success. Frequently, the adolescents and adults I worked with were already aware of their own signals but did not understand the role they played in safety awareness. During a recent meeting, a group of self-advocates identified a list of *early warning signs* that included:

- sweaty palms,
- rapid heartbeat,
- hair standing up on back of the neck,
- shaky knees,
- sweaty armpits,
- goose bumps on the arms, or
- sick feelings in the stomach.

These physiological symptoms were associated with experiences like almost getting hit by a car, a dating incident, public speaking, going to a new job, and an assault.

Teaching Activity: "My Warning Signals"

Remind your child that her body sends her messages all the time. For example, when we are hungry, a growling tummy is a signal that helps us know it's time to eat or get something to drink. When our bodies smell, it's a signal we need to take a shower or bath. When we feel sick, it's a sign we may be ill and need to go to the doctor.

Explain to your child that our bodies also give us signals when we are in unsafe or stressful situations. Talk with your child about recent situations when she has felt scared or unsafe. For example, "Do you remember when we had that big thunderstorm and you were afraid?" Or, "you know how you were afraid to get your blood taken at the doctor?" Or, "Do you remember when you had to read your report in front of your class?" Most parents can identify situations that are stressful or create anxiety and fear in their own children. Use these situations to introduce and talk about signals your child's body sends. If she has difficulty with this, give her an example of something that happens in your own body when you are afraid. "When I get scared, like when I almost hit that car this morning, my heart beats faster and I breathe fast. What happens in your body?"

When your child is able to identify her own unique signals, use the body outlines in Appendix A to draw in illustrations that represent her signals. For example, drips under the arm for sweating, butterflies in the abdominal area for "butterflies in the stomach," etc. (If your child takes medication for anxiety or seems to experience high levels of anxiety most of the time, she might have more difficulty understanding this concept.)

A more recent pilot study evaluating a modified version of Flandreau-West's curriculum with adults with cognitive disabilities showed that the participants were able to comprehend these concepts and apply them in their daily lives. Clearly, more research is necessary, but the concept of empowering individuals to use their own body signals to recognize safe and unsafe situations is promising.

Key Teaching Messages:

- Most people are nice and will not hurt you.
- There are people who may try to do sexual things that are against the law.
- Most of the time people who try to do sexual things will be people you know and trust. Less often they are strangers or people you don't know very well.
- When someone tricks you or forces you to do sexual things you don't want to do it's called sexual abuse (or exploitation).
- Sexual abuse (or exploitation) is against the law.

DEFINE SEXUAL EXPLOITATION

Explaining sexual exploitation to your child is not easy, but if she is knowledgeable about abuse and laws that define sexual offenses, she'll be better prepared to identify illegal behavior when it occurs. Bringing up the subject can be awkward. You don't want to alarm your child, but at the same time you want her to be informed. Try to link instruction with a teachable moment or experience that makes sense.

Unfortunately, real life examples of sexual exploitation involving individuals with developmental disabilities occur with frightening regularity. A few years ago, an e-mail alert from my daughter's school was disseminated to district parents. The alert reported that an exhibitionist had approached a young child that morning on her way to school. Since the teachers and principal had spoken to students about the situation, this became an opportunity to bring up the subject at home with both of my daughters. We were able to talk about what the exhibitionist did and why it was illegal (private parts stay covered in public) and we also identified a range of other sexual behaviors that are against the law and should be reported.

Research indicates that, because of inexperience and sexual illiteracy, people with developmental disabilities tend to have difficulty identifying sexual exploitation when it is occurring. Being specific about what it looks like is important. See Appendix B-13 for a list of behaviors that are considered exploitive.

Teaching Activity: "What Is Sexual Exploitation?"

Although definitions for sexual exploitation vary somewhat from state to state, some common behaviors typically identified as sexual exploitation are listed in Appendix B-13. Use this worksheet to explain to your son or daughter the different types of exploitation and reasons they are against the law.

The Grooming Process: How Sexual Offenders and Predators Operate

Many families are surprised when they discover abusive situations involving their children. They ask themselves, "How could this have happened?" "Why didn't we know?" It's important to remember that people who repeatedly offend are quite skilled at grooming—a process that involves gaining emotional access to your child slowly over time. In Anna Salter's book, *Predators, Pedophiles, Rapists, and Other Sex Offenders*, she interviews offenders currently doing time in prison. Her book reveals their secrets, strategies, and techniques for gaining access to their victims, critical information when considering how to prevent sexual exploitation. Steps many offenders confessed to using include:

Image Boosting: Offenders frequently describe their intentional work and effort at improving their image. They make every attempt to appear as well-liked, respectable, do-no-harm citizens. They donate money, volunteer, and are often active participants in their community. They coach teams, run Scout troops, or do other work that helps others see them in a positive light. This effort to create what Salter refers to as a "double life" is a common step in the process of deception.

Accessing Victims: Predators have to identify places where they can access victims fairly easily, which is why sexual abusers often volunteer or work in child-centered organizations or professions. Schools, malls, playgrounds, day cares, church, parks, and video arcades are examples of kid-centered locations targeted by offenders. People with cognitive disabilities are most often abused during times when the person is in an isolated environment.

Victim Selection: Although there is no ideal victim profile (in other words, anyone can be victimized) predators often select and have an easier time winning over individuals who are vulnerable in some way. Frequently the most appealing targets are people who are lonely, whose emotional needs are not being met (they feel unloved, unpopular, or neglected), who have lower self-esteem or lack confidence, or have family problems. Predators may also select individuals who have a history of lying, or some other vulnerability that would interfere with their ability to report or be believed—which is one reason individuals with cognitive disabilities may be easy targets.

Emotional Grooming: Once the victim has been selected, the offender commonly begins showering the victim with some form of attention—showing favoritism to the child, writing letters, buying gifts, etc. Most will be quite charming and act interested in your child. Once trust has been established (often parental grooming needs to occur simultaneously), physical contact is introduced. Initial physical contact is usually not sexual, but incidental since this type of touching works to desensitize the victim. Eventually, the abuser introduces sexual touching.

Teaching Activity: "Secrets, Bribes, and Threats"

Abusers almost always use coercive techniques to get their victims to cooperate. Exposing your child to these techniques can help him or her recognize them if they occur. Explain that a person who is trying to get someone to do sexual things that are against the law usually has to coax him or her in some way. Use the worksheet in Appendix B-14 to provide specific examples of common techniques used by abusers.

Teaching Activity: "Okay? or Against the Law?"

This activity can be used to check your child's ability to compare and contrast healthy sexual behaviors with exploitative ones and to assess what she has learned after you've shared information about laws and techniques used by exploiters. Photocopy the list of experiences listed in Appendix B-15. Cut the worksheet up so there is one scenario on each slip of paper. Ask your child to read each situation (or read it to her) and then ask her to determine whether the behavior is okay (healthy or green light) or illegal (not okay or red).

ENCOURAGE ASSERTIVENESS AND APPROPRIATE NONCOMPLIANCE

Being able to make choices, independent from outside influences, is a basic premise for understanding that you have options, you have a say, you have the right to do or not do something. People with cognitive disabilities are often reinforced for obedience, however. This can create a dangerous tendency to always do as they are asked, placing them at risk for exploitation.

Encouraging your child *not* to comply in appropriate contexts is an important exploitation prevention skill. Your child will be more successful at understanding this if she has regular opportunities to make choices and decisions in her daily life. Being able to say "no" is another element of assertiveness. Review with your child the elements of an assertive "no" covered in Chapter 10.

TEACH HER TO TELL

It's a good idea to help your child come up with a list of individuals who would believe her if she reported difficult-to-hear, awful information. These are people your child would call if she's feeling uncomfortable about something that happened (experiencing early warning signs). Safe people are individuals who will listen to your child, believe her, and take action if necessary. Although you may be one of those "safe" people, you shouldn't be the only one. As I mentioned earlier, it is common for the abuser to be a family member, a professional, caregiver, or other individual your child knows and trusts. If you're the only designated "safe-to-tell" person and the abuser

Key Teaching Messages:

- Nothing is so bad it can't be talked about.
- If someone wants you to do sexual things that make you feel uncomfortable, say no, get away if you can, and tell someone.
- People I can tell are _____.
- If they don't believe me, I should keep telling until I am believed.

is Uncle Bob, it's entirely possible your child will not want to share this information with you.

Try to identify individuals who are accessible, interact with your child regularly, and can understand your child when she communicates. Teachers, job coaches, school social workers, health care workers, clergy, or family friends are all possibilities.

This list can be altered as your child moves in and out of different stages in her life.

Once you and your child have created a list of individuals, talk with these people to find out how comfortable they would be in a "safe person" role. You (or your child) can tell them this is part of an assignment for school, an independent living skills project, or something she is doing with her self-advocate group. Be clear about the expectations and responsibilities in this role. Pay attention to their voice or body language when they respond. Some people will choose not to participate and it's better to know that right up front rather than find out when your child is immersed in a scary situation and expecting assistance.

Teaching Activity: "Responding to Early Warning Signals"

Once your child has a body diagram that in some way depicts her own unique "early warning signs," make sure she knows what to do when these warnings are present and won't go away. Remind her that these body signals can come and go. For example, your child may notice these signals while giving a speech, on a carnival ride, or during a blood draw, but after these experiences are over, the signals usually go away.

Explain that when a person feels unsafe, warning signs may not go away until you *do* something. Encourage your child to talk with you or another safe person on her list when she notices these early warnings signs. Keep in mind that for individuals with cognitive disabilities these signals can surface in many different situations, for many different reasons. Your goals here are to help your child learn to identify her early warning signs, connect her early warning signs with specific situations or experiences, and understand what to do when early warning signs surface.

Revealing an abusive incident takes tremendous courage, but even when people with developmental disabilities report incidences of exploitation, they are often not believed. One reason is the prevalent and pejorative societal attitudes about people with cognitive disabilities and sexuality discussed earlier. Other times, those who are connected to the person being accused express powerful denial and disbelief. Some parents have concerns regarding their child's difficulty in separating events that have happened in real life from television shows or made-up stories, which creates doubt and confusion. Other parents recall times when their child shared information that was incomplete or out of context or misinterpreted events, so they may have trouble believing their child or view her as credible. It's important to remember that **people (with or without a disability) rarely lie about sexual abuse.**

Teaching Activity: "Safe People List"

Once your child has identified a list of "safe people" and has gotten their permission, write down their names and phone numbers. Make a safe people poster and hang it near the phone or put it in another area that is accessible.

Teaching Activity: "Fact or Fiction?"

Sometime during first grade, my daughter learned the difference between "fact" books and "fiction" books. These two words really made sense to her, and, over time, became a way for us to help her distinguish between her "pretend" world and "real" world. At some point my husband developed a game centered around helping her differentiate her "real world" from her "pretend" world. Before tucking her in at night, he would make five or six statements about her day. It became my daughter's job to decide if the statements were "fact" or "fiction." Statements would include real or made-up information about what she had for supper, things that we knew happened to her during the day or would be happening the next day, family information, etc. My husband started the game when we were having great difficulty getting accurate accounts about her day. The game helped her learn to differentiate real life from her pretend world and reinforced the importance of accurate reporting in less threatening aspects of her life.

To do this activity at home, identify vocabulary that will have meaning for your child. For example, words like "true" or "false," "real" or "make-believe" are other possibilities. If your child is nonverbal, create cards that illustrate differences between the two words and ask her to hold up the correct response as you create your own statements.

Beyond Prevention: Recognizing and Responding to Sexual Abuse

SIGNS AND SYMPTOMS

Reading the list below will be as disturbing and difficult for you to read as it was for me to write. Although this information is scary, it's important you have it for several reasons. First, sexual abuse and exploitation among individuals with developmental disabilities is dramatically underreported and symptoms that could indicate abuse in a nondisabled person are often attributed to something else or ignored when the person has a disability (Sobsey & Mansell, 1993). Second, most victims with developmental disabilities do experience emotional or behavioral consequences. Third, research suggests that the earlier abuse is reported, the less trauma the individual is likely to experience. My hope is that by sharing this list with you, earlier detection and prompt treatment and support can occur.

POSSIBLE PHYSICAL INDICATORS

Physical Indicators of sexual exploitation are usually the clearest, more obvious signs that abuse has occurred or is occurring. Physical symptoms can include:

- Difficulty walking or sitting
- Missing, stained, torn, or bloody underclothing
- Unexplained or unusual bruises, welts, bleeding, cuts, or scratches on the face, mouth, neck, chest, back, genital, thigh, or buttocks region.
- Genital pain or itching, inflammation, odor, or discomfort
- Sexually transmitted diseases in eyes, mouth, anus, or genitals
- Blood in urine or stool
- Pregnancy
- Unexplained stomach ulcers or abdominal pain
- Headaches or migraines
- Foreign objects in the genital, rectal, or urethral opening

POSSIBLE BEHAVIORAL INDICATORS

People with Down syndrome or other cognitive disabilities don't always have the verbal abilities to let us know what is happening. Instead, they may communicate that they are being sexually abused through changes in behavior. These changes can include:

- Depression or excessive crying spells
- Social withdrawal
- Aggression, or what seems to be inappropriate anger
- Regression or loss of living skills (not due to Alzheimer disease or lack of practice)
- Fearfulness, avoidance, or reluctance to be with specific people or in certain settings
- Sleep disturbances, nightmares, sleepwalking
- Resisting touch or physical exam
- Onset of self-destructive behavior (hair pulling, self-biting, head banging) hurting others, or poor sense of personal safety (substance abuse, indiscriminate sexual activity)
- Poor self-esteem, self-criticism
- Headaches
- Onset of compulsive, inappropriate sexual touching or other sexual behaviors or comments; new levels of sexual knowledge
- Lack of interest in hygiene or grooming
- Change in eating or sleeping patterns and habits
- Onset of new sounds (e.g., humming, screaming, groaning)
- Verbalizations or self-talk that suggest the person is being silenced or threatened ("Don't tell," or "I'll kill you")
- Regression to infantile behaviors (e.g., bed wetting, feces smearing)

Part of the difficulty in diagnosing sexual abuse is that often the signs and symptoms are subtle or easily attributed to a host of other health and medical problems or current life circumstances. For example:

- Loss of skills and regression could be related to depression.
- Experiencing the death of a loved one can lead to changes in behavior or depression-like symptoms.
- Obstructive sleep apnea, a common condition in individuals with Down syndrome, can lead to sleep disturbances, and lack of sleep can result in behavioral changes.
- Sexually inappropriate behaviors may be related to your child's lack of information and skill deficits rather than abuse.

You know your child better than anyone else. If a *combination of the above symptoms surface suddenly for unexplained reasons,* try not to exclude exploitation as one potential cause.

IF YOU SUSPECT ABUSE

If your child has not divulged that she has been abused, but has physical signs or symptoms that might suggest abuse is occurring, or you notice the types of behavioral changes listed above, you have a few options. First, you could speak with a professional at your local sexual assault treatment center or other agency that specializes in evaluating and treating sexual abuse. A physician or health practitioner who is familiar with your child might also be able to sift through potential health and medical issues that may be contributing to behavioral changes and determine whether abuse is a real possibility.

Be aware that doctors are less likely to diagnose sexual abuse in individuals with developmental disabilities. In one study, when clients with and without mental retardation exhibited similar symptoms, the clients with mental retardation were less likely to be diagnosed or were given a less severe diagnosis (Rindfleish & Bean, 1988; Lowry). Sometimes health professionals assume that the symptoms and behaviors are related to the disability itself rather than considering possible external causes.

HOW TO RESPOND IF YOUR CHILD REPORTS ABUSE

Hearing your child tell you that he or she has been exploited is never an easy experience. Try to remain calm and respect your child's safety and dignity. If she tells you in a place where others can hear, immediately move to a private place where you can talk. Ask basic questions such as, "Can you show me where he touched you?" or "Where on your body did he touch you?" This can help you clarify what is going on once allegations are made. After your child has shared key information, don't attempt to handle things on your own or pressure your child with additional questions. This can interfere with the investigation and influence reporting. Below is a list of important things you *can* do:

- *Believe your child.* No matter how old your child is, if she reports abuse, believe and support her. Remember, reporting abuse takes incredible courage, particularly when the abuser is known to the victim and her family. It is very possible the abuser has threatened your child's safety or the safety of other loved ones in her life if she tells, making your child fearful of what could happen to her or other family members.
- *Reassure your child that it is not her fault and that telling was the right thing to do.* It is common for individuals who have been sexually abused to blame themselves for what happened and, as a result, experience considerable shame and guilt. Praise

and support her willingness to tell with statements like: "I'm sorry this happened to you, but it was not your fault"; "Nobody deserves to be treated this way. I'm glad you told me"; "It takes a lot of courage to talk about this but I'm glad you shared this with me—now we can get help."

■ *Contact the authorities.* After authorities have been contacted, some victims experience relief that the secret is revealed and feel reassured that they will finally be protected from the abuser. Others become upset and even more afraid and anxious. Consider your own son or daughter's feelings to determine whether he or she should be present when you make the call. If your son or daughter is a minor, contact your local Child Protective Service Agency. If your child is an adult, contact the police. Police departments have a working relationship with both your county Child Protective Services (CPS) department or Adult Protective Services division and are required to report all investigations and allegations to them. They are also obligated by law to investigate any abuse that is reported.

INFORM AND PREPARE YOUR CHILD FOR WHAT WILL HAPPEN

Forensic Interview. Keep your child informed about the process. For example, a *forensic interview* is usually conducted after a report of abuse has been made. Let your child know that someone—a person from CPS, a police officer, or sometimes both—will be coming to hear her story and that she may have to tell it a few times. Professionals interviewing your child should conduct the interview in a place where your child feels safe and comfortable. Many agencies that work with children will videotape the interview or use other strategies to minimize the need for repeat interviews, reduce stress on the child, and avoid having the child encounter the abuser in court. Newer techniques for gathering information using visual tools, for example, often work better for children and adults with Down syndrome or other developmental disabilities. Unfortunately, many professionals responsible for investigating these cases are not trained in these techniques or have minimal experience working with individuals with intellectual disabilities.

Medical Exam. Depending on the type of abuse allegation, a *medical exam* may also need to be performed, especially if the incident occurred within the past few days (usually within 72 hours). During the exam, medical professionals try to gather concrete evidence that can be used in the investigation. Your child may also be tested for sexually transmitted diseases. Let your son or daughter know that the exam is needed to make sure his or her body was not injured when he or she was being abused. Following the exam, a medical report indicating the findings is sent to the law enforcement agency.

Based on evidence gleaned from the interview and medical exam, the police will determine whether there is enough evidence to prove that a crime has been committed. If there is sufficient evidence, the case will be referred to a district attorney who has the final say in whether or not prosecution can occur. Unfortunately,

What is a SANE Nurse?

Sexual Assault Nurse Examiners (SANE) specialize in providing comprehensive care to individuals (kids and adults) who are sexually assaulted. This profession requires training in gathering forensic evidence, observing criminal trial proceedings, providing expert testimony in court (because they are often subpoenaed), as well as preparation for providing quality, comprehensive care for individuals who are victims of violence. Many hours of clinical experience working with victims in sexual assault treatment facilities is also required. Not all SANE nurses have training in working with individuals with developmental disabilities but many states are now recognizing and responding to the need for additional training and support in this area.

Because SANE nurses have specific training in forensic medicine, they are more skilled and knowledgeable at working towards effective prosecution and getting offenders placed on national sex offender lists. These actions make it easier for agencies to identify and weed out offenders. If your son or daughter becomes a victim of sexual assault, be sure to ask for someone who is trained in this area.

these decisions may be made based on evidence, but also on your child's ability to speak or testify about the incident. The sad fact is that sexual abuse cases involving individuals with developmental disabilities are not often prosecuted. Reasons often cited are that the person with disabilities cannot share accurate information about what happened (e.g., due to limited verbal abilities or problems relaying the sequence of events or time concepts) or because there are questions related to consent (the offender may argue that the victim consented since she did not verbally or physically resist). Cases involving victims who have developmental disabilities also require considerable time and expertise. More often than not, charges end up being dropped, reduced, or pled out.

Common Aftereffects of Sexual Abuse

The effects of sexual abuse can vary widely depending on the nature of the incident, timing of the disclosure and the response, your child's skills and abilities for coping, and the types of intervention provided. In general, though, the aftereffects in people with and without cognitive disabilities are similar. They include:

BOUNDARY DIFFICULTIES/ SEXUAL INAPPROPRIATENESS

People who have been sexually abused may engage in sexually inappropriate behaviors, including: inappropriate touching of people's genitals; being overly seductive toward others; compulsive masturbation; or initiating sexual activity with younger children or peers (with and without disabilities).

Remember, these are behaviors that were probably modeled and taught by the abuser over time, so your child may believe this is how people normally interact with one another. Withhold permission for these behaviors and help your child relearn acceptable behavior. For example, if your child touches you on the genitals, say, "Stop, I am your dad and family members do not touch each other's private body parts." Then share a form of affection that is more appropriate—a hug, for example. If you notice increases in public masturbation, re-teach your child about privacy, what it means, and where it is okay to masturbate (see Teaching about Privacy—Chapter 3). If your child is initiating sexual contact with others who are younger or more vulnerable, understand that she may be trying to feel some control over another person in much the same way the abuser had some control over her. Increase your child's supervision and provide empathetic responses that can help your child understand reasons she may be doing this. In her book *Shared Feelings*, Diane Maksym uses the following explanation:

"I know you want to do the same things that were done to you with other kids. It's hard not to have that feeling. But it's not okay for you to do this anymore than it was okay for him to act this way with you. So I can't let you play alone with kids until you learn this."

ESCALATED FEAR AND ANXIETY

Many people who have been abused have a generalized fear of being harmed as well as specific fears about people or places associated with the abusive incident. Your child might show her fear and anxiety through nightmares, not wanting to be left alone with strangers, or concerns about safety. For example, she may refuse or aggressively protest participation in social activities or programs that she sees as threatening in some way. Crying, tantrums, or "freezing" (stopping of movement) are common ways this is demonstrated in people with and without disabilities.

Encourage your child to express these feelings in some way and let her know they are normal and understandable. You may have to create visual routines that help your child feel safe in her home—for example, locking doors, closing curtains, etc.

Our daughter was assaulted at her school. Following the incident, she refused to go back. We ended up switching her to a different school.

ANGER

Sometimes people are angry about what has happened and the consequences that ensue. They may express anger related to little things that happen, or towards people and life in general. If the individual loses some freedom or independence as a result of the abuse, she may be angry about that as well.

DEPRESSION

Symptoms of depression associated with sexual abuse in individuals with developmental disabilities are similar to those in the general population. These symptoms may include:

- irritability,
- withdrawal,
- self-injurious behavior,
- sleep disturbances,
- physical complaints (stomach pains).

Talk with your physician if you are concerned that your child is depressed and needs help in this area.

POST TRAUMATIC STRESS DISORDER (PTSD)

PTSD is a condition characterized by range of specific symptoms experienced by some individuals who have been exposed to a traumatic event. Common symptoms include:

- flashbacks (mentally reliving traumatic events or experiences),
- nightmares,
- avoidance of places or people associated with the traumatic event,
- increased agitation,
- physiological arousal (racing heart, rapid breathing).

Although there is still much to learn about PTSD and people with cognitive disabilities, they seem to have many of the same symptoms experienced by nondisabled people who have experienced trauma.

It's important to remember that the aftereffects of an abusive experience may emerge immediately afterwards, or at key developmental stages later on. For example, symptoms can be triggered anew once your child begins dating, becomes more independent, or shifts to a new living situation. Be open and respectful of the potential need to revisit interventions that help your child cope during these stages.

Helping Your Child Recover from Sexual Abuse

Dealing with the aftereffects of sexual abuse requires considerable energy, attention, and support. The list below identifies strategies that researchers have found to be helpful in assisting people with intellectual disabilities to recover from sexual abuse.

INDIVIDUAL THERAPY

People with developmental disabilities can benefit from treatment for abuse recovery or trauma. This is contrary to what many professionals believe, so you may have to advocate that your child receive treatment. Finding a professional who can work with your child may be your biggest obstacle. Call your local disability agency to locate professionals who have experience working with individuals with cognitive disabilities or who are recommended by other families. You might also try to find a professional who has interest in working with your child and then identify resources that might help prepare her for sessions. (Good starting points include Brian Chicoine and Dennis McGuire's book, *Mental Wellness in Adults with Down Syndrome* or David Pitonyak's website—www.dimagine.com.)

Initially, it may be helpful for a family member or other individual who understands your child well to share information with the therapist so he or she can alter and adapt therapeutic approaches to better fit the needs of your child (rather than expect her to communicate in more traditional ways). Information you might provide to help the therapist work more effectively with your child:

- *Unique Aspects of the Individual*—Orienting the therapist to your child's functioning levels is critical. Although many parents view IQ scores as an inaccurate (and sometimes offensive) reflection of their child's overall abilities and strengths, discussing your child's cognitive abilities can help the provider more easily adapt language and therapeutic techniques to your child's level of understanding. Providing specific information on expressive and receptive language abilities as well as communication styles is also helpful.

- *Characteristics of the Abusive Experience*—Professionals working with victims of abuse understand that different types of abusive experiences require different types of approaches. For example, if your child was abused by a family member, the dynamics of the situation change. If the abuse occurred over a long period or by multiple offenders, for example, different approaches may be necessary. Understanding unique aspects of the abuse experience can help the therapist work more effectively with your child.

- *Support System*—Identifying individuals in your child's life who provide care and support or have influential and meaningful relationships will be important. As the professional offers specific information and recommendations, those supporting your child may be called upon to model behaviors or reinforce information over time to improve your child's understanding. For example, if the therapist is working to help your child understand the concept of body rights and personal space, caregivers may need to model expected behaviors (e.g., asking permission before moving into your child's space when help is requested).

- *Preparation for Individual Therapy*—Most people with cognitive disabilities struggle with the language of feelings and how to express them, an important element of therapy (Ryan, 1996). Encourage the professional who will be working with your child to spend some preparation time helping your child understand the language of feelings and ways to express them. This can be done through use of pictures with facial expressions, games, mime, sign language, music, art, videotaping, computer programs, etc. (See Chapter 9 for ideas on teaching about feelings.)

Because many individuals with cognitive disabilities lack information about sexuality and relationships, assessing your child's knowledge prior to or early in the therapeutic process can be useful. Clearly, it may be difficult to talk about abuse if your son or daughter doesn't understand what it is. Body rights and boundaries in relationships are examples of other basic concepts she may need to learn before moving forward.

Our daughter was assaulted by her brother when she was six. It was horrible and ugly. The sexual encounters took place in our home when we were here. The police became involved because she talked about it at school rather than telling us. We had to hire a lawyer and go to court. She was seen at the sexual assault center at our Children's Hospital and I was told to take her to our pediatrician. I sat and cried as they took this tiny girl and examined her through a microscope. We went through a lot of therapy for this incident. Our son had extensive therapy, as did our family. It was very hard to find a therapist for our daughter. There are not a lot of therapists who deal with young children with disabilities who have been abused.

OTHER TYPES OF THERAPY

When a victim of abuse has a cognitive disability, he or she is often more isolated and may have a more limited support network, which can place a significant burden on immediate caregivers or family members. Some larger communities offer specialized support groups for individuals with cognitive disabilities who have been abused. The social support provided in these groups can help your son or daughter feel less isolated. Not all individuals with a cognitive disability are candidates for group therapy. Rely on the professional(s) who is working with your child to give you guidance regarding when and if group therapy is advisable.

Sometimes victims of abuse may benefit from therapeutic techniques that allow people to express themselves without words. Music, art, or dance are often natural outlets for expressing emotions for people whose verbal abilities are more limited. Music therapy and art therapy are also used to help people without disabilities explore and express their feelings.

SURROUND YOUR CHILD WITH SAFE, FUN, NURTURING RELATIONSHIPS

Individuals in crisis need to feel safe and supported during this difficult time. Encourage people who have caring, loving, supportive relationships with your child to do things that are fun and exciting with her. Let your child take the lead in selecting the individuals she wants to interact with and the activities she feels most comfortable doing.

EXERCISE

Many people who have been sexually abused experience increased anxiety, which can result in a constant state of arousal. Movement, especially activities that increase heart rate, can help to reduce stress and reduce symptoms associated with anxiety and agitation.

HELP YOUR CHILD SHARE HER STORY WHEN SHE IS READY

Talking about the experience can be therapeutic for a victim of abuse. When your son or daughter is ready, encourage him or her to talk about the experience. At a recent conference for self-advocates, a young woman with Down syndrome had the courage to share her story in order to help others become more aware of their own safety. Here is the story she shared at the conference in her own words:

"I would like to tell you about a couple of relationships that I thought were good but turned out not to be good. I moved into my own apartment on April 24th of this year. When I moved into my apartment, I got to know different people. They talked to me and that's how I got to have a relationship with most of the people in the apartment complex.

"This new friend had an organ and I have a piano and we thought we would play together. I was excited about that. Then we had a cookout. That was fun, joking around and being together. We also played some games and cards. Then I asked him to come to church sometime and watch me lector. He was excited to hear me read. Then, only ten days after I was in my own apartment, the relationship made a complete turn-around.

"On a Thursday afternoon, he asked me to help him with his groceries so I was nice enough to help. While there he decided he wanted to make lunch. Before lunch he showed me a magazine with pictures of boys and girls naked and having sex. Then he talked about peeling some carrots and cucumbers, so he said, you can go in my bathroom and take a vegetable, put it inside of you, and make it go

up and down. He then said after you are done, I will take the vegetables and eat them. I played dumb and kept asking what he meant. After that he took off the light and went to his bedroom and laid on the bed and said, "_____, I am ready for you to come in bed with me." I got scared and I cried. I saw Jesus, because I am so religious, and he led me out of the room. I just could not let Jesus down.

"Jesus gave me the strength to tell my mom, dad, my priest, my landlord, plus my sister-in-law. I called the police and they talked to him. That is all they did. They did not take action. I feel, in my heart, he needs to be in jail. I also told the manager of our apartment complex and the Apartment Board about the incident. They have told each of us to stay away from each other."

Interestingly, both the young woman and her mother credited her participation in sexuality education classes in middle and high school for helping her know what to do during this experience. Both mother and daughter agreed that the freedom to talk about the experience played an important part in her recovery process.

References

Baladarian, N. (1991). Sexual Abuse of People with Developmental Disabilities. *Sexuality and Disability 9* (4): 323-335.

Ballan, M. Parents as Sexuality Educators for Their Children with Developmental Disabilities. *SIECUS Report 29* (3): 14-19.

Benson, B. (1995). Psychosocial Interventions Update: Resources for Emotions Training. *The Habilitative Mental Healthcare Newsletter 14* (3).

Blanchett, W.J. & Wolfe, P.S. (2002) A Review of Sexuality Education Curricula: Meeting the Sexuality Education Needs of Individuals with Moderate and Severe Intellectual Disabilities. *Research and Practice for Persons with Severe Disabilities 27*: 42-57.

DeBecker, G. (1999). *Protecting the Gift: Keeping Children and Teenagers Safe (and Parents Sane).* New York: Dell Publishing.

Fortin, D. (1998). *Living Safely for People with Special Needs Based on the Protective Behaviors Process.* Madison: Wisconsin Committee to Prevent Child Abuse.

Furey, E. (1994). Sexual Abuse of Adults with Mental Retardation: Who and Where. *Mental Retardation 32* (3): 173-80.

Griffiths, D. et. al (2002). *Ethical Dilemmas: Sexuality and Developmental Disability.* Kingston, NY: National Association for Dual Diagnosis.

Haseltine, B. & Miltenberger, R. (1990). Teaching Self Protection Skills to Persons with Mental Retardation. *American Journal of Mental Retardation 95* (2).

Hingsburger, D. (1995). *Just Say Know: Understanding and Reducing the Risk of Sexual Victimization of People with Developmental Disabilities.* Eastman, Quebec: Diverse City Press.

Khemka, I. et. al (2005). Evaluation of a Decision-Making Curriculum Designed to Empower Women with Mental Retardation to Resist Abuse. *American Journal on Mental Retardation 110* (3): 193-204.

Lowry, M.A. (1997). Unmasking Mood Disorders: Recognizing and Measuring Symptomatic Behaviors. *The Habilitative Mental Healthcare Newsletter 16:* 1-6.

Lowry, M.A. (1998). Assessment and Treatment of Mood Disorders in Persons with Developmental Disabilities. *Journal of Developmental and Physical Disabilities 10:* 387-406.

Ludwig, S. & Hingsburger, D. (1989). Preparation for Counseling and Psychotherapy: Teaching about Feelings. *Psychiatric Aspects of Mental Retardation Reviews 8* (1).

Lumley, V. & Miltenberger, R. (1997). Sexual Abuse Prevention for Persons with Mental Retardation. *American Journal of Mental Retardation 101* (5): 459-72

Lumley, V. et al. (1998). Evaluation of a Sexual Abuse Prevention Program for Adults with Mental Retardation. *Journal of Applied Behavioral Analysis 31* (1): 91-101.

Maksym, D. (1990). *Shared Feelings: A Parent's Guide to Sexuality Education for Children, Adolescents and Adults Who Have a Mental Handicap.* Ontario: G. Allan Roeher Institute.

Mansell, S., Sobsey, D., et al. (1998). Clinical Findings among Sexually Abused Children with and without Disabilities. *Mental Retardation 36* (1): 12-22

Mansell, S. & Sobsey, D. (2001). *The Aurora Project: Counseling People with Developmental Disabilities Who Have Been Sexually Abused.* Kingston, NY: NADD Press.

McCabe, M., Cummins, R., et al. (1994). An Empirical Study of the Sexual Abuse of People with Intellectual Disability. *Sexuality and Disability 12* (4): 297-305.

McCarthy, M. & Thompson, D. (1997). A Prevalence Study of Sexual Abuse of Adults with Intellectual Disabilities Referred for Sex Education. *Journal of Applied Research in Intellectual Disabilities 10* (2): 105-124.

Muccigrosso, L. (1991). Sexual Abuse Prevention Strategies and Programs for Persons with Developmental Disabilities. *Sexuality and Disability 9* (3): 261-71.

National Clearinghouse on Child Sexual Abuse and Neglect Information. IN FOCUS: The Risk and Prevention of Maltreatment of Children with Disabilities, February 2001.

Pitonyak, D. (2005). *Supporting a Person Who is Experiencing Post Traumatic Stress Disorder (PTSD).* www.dimagine.com.

Rappaport, S., Burkhardt, S., and Rotatori, A. (1997). *Child Sexual Abuse Curriculum for the Developmentally Disabled.* Springfield, IL: Charles Thomas Publisher.

Reynolds, L. *People with Mental Retardation and Sexual Abuse.* www.TheARc.org/faqs/Sexabuse.html.

Rindfleish, N. & Bean, G. J. (1988). Willingness to Report Abuse and Neglect in Residential Facilities. *Child Abuse and Neglect 12*: 509-20.

Roeher Institute (1992). *No More Victims: A Manual to Guide the Police in Addressing the Sexual Abuse of People with Mental Handicap.* North York, Ontario: Roeher Institute.

Ryan, R. (1996). *Handbook of Mental Health Care for Persons with Developmental Disabilities.* Denver: The Community Circle Publications.

Salter, A. (2003). *Predators, Pedophiles, Rapists, and Other Sex Offenders: Who They Are, How They Operate, and How We Can Protect Ourselves and Our Children.* New York, NY: Basic Books.

SIECUS Report (2000). *Sexual Abuse,* October/November: 28-34. New York, NY: SEICUS.

Sobsey, D. & Doe, T. (1991). Patterns of Sexual Abuse and Assault. *Sexuality and Disability 9* (3): 243-59.

Sobsey, D. , Gray, S., et al. (1991). *Disability, Sexuality, and Abuse: An Annotated Bibliography.* Baltimore: Paul Brookes Publishing.

Sobsey, D. & Mansell, S. (1990). The Prevention of Sexual Abuse of People with Developmental Disabilities. Edmonton, Alberta: J.P. Das Developmental Disabilities Centre.

Chapter 12—Framework for Teaching Exploitation Prevention Skills

Concepts	Key Messages	Goal Behaviors
Names for private body parts	■ All body parts have names ■ Girls have a vulva, clitoris, breasts ■ Boys have penis, testicles, scrotum ■ Both boys and girls have nipples, butt	■ Uses correct names for private body parts
Body rights	■ My body is private and belongs to me ■ No one should touch private parts of my body except for health reasons or to help me keep my body clean (child message) ■ I can refuse any sexual behavior that makes me feel uncomfortable (teen or adult who is dating) ■ Others have these same rights	■ Recognizes violations of body rights ■ Respects body rights of others
Identify body warning signals	■ My body gives me signals when I am unsafe or need to be alert ■ My warning signals are _____ ■ I should listen and trust my body signals ■ If my warning signals won't go away, I can talk to my safe person	■ Identifies own early warning signals ■ Talks to safe person(s) re: warning signals
Assertiveness	■ If others are touching me in ways I don't like, I can say no, get away if I can, and tell my safe person	■ Assertively says no to unwanted or inappropriate touch
Define exploitation	■ Most people are nice and will not hurt others ■ There are people who may try to do sexual things that are against the law ■ Most of the time people who try to do this will be people you know and trust ■ Less often they are strangers or people we don't know very well ■ When someone tricks or forces you to do sexual things you don't want to do it's called sexual abuse (or exploitation) ■ Sexual abuse (or exploitation) is against the law	■ Recognizes exploitation when it occurs
Reporting	■ Nothing is so bad it can't be talked about ■ If someone wants you to do sexual things that make you feel uncomfortable, say no, get away if you can, and tell someone ■ People I can talk to are _____ ■ If they don't believe me, I should keep telling until I am believed	■ Reports unwanted or exploitative touch

CHAPTER 13

Sexuality Education in Schools

βy the time your son or daughter approaches adolescence, you've done some significant work creating a foundation of information, attitudes, and values from which to build as he or she moves into adulthood. Hopefully, your child has some familiarity with the basic foundational concepts identified earlier in the book and you've been able to coach him through various experiences that have contributed to informal learning. But let's face it, most teens grow weary of harping parents who won't let up, especially during adolescence. Taking advantage of formal learning opportunities offered through schools is another way to continue learning about sexuality.

The quality and comprehensiveness of sexuality education in American schools varies considerably from state to state and district to district. Although most states

Defining Terms

States often use specific terminology to describe their approach to sexuality education. In the United States, there are two popular categories of sexuality education programs:

Comprehensive Sexuality Education—These human growth and development programs begin presenting information in kindergarten and continue through twelfth grade. They cover a broad category of topics, allowing students to learn factual information and develop skills over time. They encourage young people to postpone or delay sexual activity until they are older **and** to practice safe sex if and when they do become sexually active. Content generally includes information regarding a range of sexual behaviors, contraception, and disease prevention methods.

Abstinence-Only—These programs emphasize abstaining from all sexual behaviors until marriage and do not include information about contraception or disease prevention. (The assumption is that sexual contact will not occur until marriage, so information about pregnancy and disease prevention is unnecessary.)

have developed sexuality education laws, few actually mandate programming. (To view laws for your state, go to www.siecus.org/policy/states/index/html.) More often, state laws *encourage* programming, and then within the law they identify other qualities, characteristics, and content deemed important. For example, New Jersey is one of the few states that requires schools to provide comprehensive (K-12) sexuality education. North Dakota offers very little guidance at all on what should be taught within school classrooms. Other states recognize the impact of STDs and HIV/AIDS on public health and do require that these topics be covered in certain grades. A nationwide survey

Who Decides What Gets Taught in American Schools?

State Influences	District Influences	Roles & Responsibilities
State Legislators		■ Decisions regarding funding sources for sexuality education ■ Acceptance of federal funds may influence flavor of sexuality education in districts across the state ■ Write or modify laws that influence: ❏ Mandates ❏ Type of program (K-12, Abstinence–Only-Until-Marriage, other) ❏ Content ❏ Teacher training requirements ❏ Parental notification
State Department of Instruction		■ Help interpret sexuality education laws for school districts in state
	Teachers	■ Provide primary input on materials, resources, and content ■ Curricula implementation
	School Board/District Administrators	■ Approve human growth and development and sexuality curricula
	Human Growth & Development Committees (some states)	■ Advisory role to district curriculum developers ■ Preview materials to ensure they reflect community mores, values
	Parents	■ Provide feedback (positive or negative) on district sex ed. programming ■ Advocacy

conducted in 2002 of 300 principals in the United States indicated that the majority of public schools at the secondary level (95 percent) provide some form of sexuality education. Most administrators (58 percent) described their school-based sexuality programs as comprehensive, while about one-third (34 percent) say their school's key messages are more abstinence-based.

It's important to remember that even when mandates do exist, they are generally not viewed as relevant or applicable to students with cognitive disabilities. Only one state, California, makes any reference at all to sexuality education needing to be accessible to people with disabilities.

Common Components of School Sexuality Education Law

PARENT NOTIFICATION

School districts understand that some parents have strong feelings about, or can be uncomfortable talking with their child about, sexuality. For this reason many state laws include parental notification requirements within their sexuality education laws. If this provision is listed in your state law, it means you will be contacted ahead of time and then can choose whether or not you wish to have your child participate in sexuality classes. Notification can occur a variety of ways. Many districts schedule orientation sessions so parents can discuss content, preview videos, and become better prepared to have follow-up discussions at home. At the middle school level, you might simply receive a letter that provides an overview of topics and dates the material will be covered.

If you're in a state that does not require parental notification or are unsure about what your district offers, speak with your child's principal or homeroom teacher. They should be able to give you basic information about topics that are covered. If you decide that content offered within your district will not be beneficial, many states include "opt-out" policies, meaning you have the right to withdraw your child from the classroom. Some districts provide an alternative activity, unrelated to sexuality instruction.

HUMAN GROWTH AND DEVELOPMENT COMMITTEES

When school sexuality programs are offered, some state laws dictate that school boards create a subcommittee of community representatives who can assist, advise, or direct district staff on content and evaluate appropriateness of teaching materials for the district. Some laws are very specific about the types of individuals who should be included on the committee so diverse perspectives are represented. In Wisconsin, for example, Human Growth and Development Committees must include "parents, teachers, school administrators, pupils, health care professionals, members of the clergy, and other residents of the school districts." These committees function mainly in an advisory capacity.

CONTENT

Topics taught within schools' sex education curricula vary considerably based on state laws, and decisions being made at the local level. For example, twenty-one states require schools to provide instruction on both sex education and HIV/STDs. Other states require districts to teach about abstinence; some, both sexual education and abstinence. Even when state policy dictates specific content, considerable latitude exists at the local level.

Example: Sexuality Topics Integrated in

Grade Level	Concepts

Kindergarten	■ Physical health
	  ❏ five senses
	  ❏ awareness of personal health habits
	■ Safety Rules
	  ❏ role of community helpers
	■ Mental Health
	  ❏ feelings about/for others
	  ❏ friendships/ Getting along with others

Grade One	■ Physical Health
	  ❏ health habits
	  ❏ growth & development
	■ Safety
	  ❏ playground
	  ❏ home & school
	  ❏ community
	■ Family Life
	  ❏ uniqueness of individuals
	  ❏ importance of family to well being
	■ Mental Health
	  ❏ value of friendships
	  ❏ being cheerful and cooperative
	  ❏ need for limitations

Grade Two	■ Physical Health
	  ❏ senses
	■ Mental Health
	  ❏ self-esteem
	  ❏ relationships with others

Grade Three	■ Physical Health
	  ❏ growth & development
	■ Mental Health
	  ❏ emotions
	  ❏ cooperation
	  ❏ respect

Grade Four	■ Physical Health
	  ❏ senses
	■ Mental Health
	  ❏ sharing
	  ❏ leaders & followers

Grade Six	■ Protective Behaviors
	  ❏ definitions related to sexual assault/harassment
	  ❏ facts & myths about sexual assault
	  ❏ reporting—who, what, when, where, how
	  ❏ safety on the Internet

School Health Education (Grades K-9)

(Grade Six continued) ■ Human Growth & Development
- ❑ puberty: physical & emotional changes
- ❑ hygiene
- ❑ male & female reproductive systems
- ❑ reproduction: pregnancy, birth, & multiple births

Grade Seven ■ Self Responsibility - Decision Making

Grade Eight ■ Human Growth & Development (review)
- ❑ anatomy review
- ❑ reproduction
- ❑ physical & emotional changes of puberty

■ Friendship & Dating
- ❑ communication
- ❑ peer pressure
- ❑ friendships vs. dating
- ❑ dating pressures
- ❑ friendships without dating
- ❑ avoidance of situations in which personal values and standards are likely to be violated
- ❑ responsibilities of males & females in relationships

■ Protective Behaviors
- ❑ the law: sexual harassment & sexual assault
- ❑ unwanted touch
- ❑ protecting oneself
- ❑ where to go for help
- ❑ consequences of harassment in schools

Grade Nine ■ Family relationships
- ❑ role of family
- ❑ ways to make a family strong
- ❑ changes in family (separation, divorce, death)
- ❑ dealing with family crisis
    - domestic violence
    - emotional, physical, sexual abuse
    - cycle of violence

■ Friendships/dating relationships
- ❑ communication skills
- ❑ peer pressure and refusal skills
- ❑ sexual decision making skills
- ❑ setting limits and dating rights
- ❑ healthy vs. unhealthy relationships

■ HIV/STDs
- ❑ how they are transmitted
- ❑ where to go for testing
- ❑ responsibilities of sexual behavior
- ❑ abstinence as prevention
- ❑ resources available for someone engaging in risky behaviors

■ Birth Control
- ❑ medical & psychological effects of current birth control methods

■ Personal Safety
- ❑ difference between flirting and harassment
- ❑ consequences of sexual harassment

According to a Kaiser Foundation study conducted in 2000, most general education students attending public schools (89 percent) receive sexuality education sometime between seventh and twelfth grade. Classes are typically co-ed and integrated within other classes (e.g., Health Education, Family and Consumer Education).

What Gets Covered When?

Percentage of 7th-12th grade students who say their most recent sexuality education class covered:

The "Core Elements"

HIV/AIDS	97%
STDs	93%
Basics of reproduction	90%
Abstinence	84%

Other Topics

Birth Control	82%
Abortion	61%
Homosexuality	41%

Safer Sex and Negotiation Skills

Dealing with pressure to have sex	79%
Emotional Issues & consequences of sex	71%
Getting tested for HIV/AIDS & STDs	69%
How to use condoms	68%
Talking with parents about sex	62%
How to use & get birth control	59%
What to do if you or friend has been raped	59%
How to talk with partner about birth control & STDs	58%

Other Common Questions about School Sexuality Education

WHO TEACHES SEXUALITY EDUCATION IN SCHOOLS?

Decisions regarding who actually teaches sexuality education are made at the local level, which means the professional designated to implement programming can vary based on your child's grade level and whether or not your child is in an inclusive or segregated classroom. Sexuality education provided in school is almost always a component of school health education, so the professionals who teach school health education may also be teaching segments of the curricula that address sexuality issues.

At the elementary school level, district nurses, guidance staff, or classroom teachers are often responsible for introducing early sexuality education topics. In middle school, physical education and/or health teachers often provide instruction. In high school, sexuality information may be included in health classes, or within elective courses such as Family and Consumer Education courses or Child Development. If your child spends most of his time with students who have cognitive disabilities, sex education (if it's offered) will likely be taught by your child's special education teacher, a speech therapist, guidance counselor, or school nurse. In some districts, groups of teachers are identified as "experts" and responsible for teaching sexuality education as well as coordinating other efforts that support quality instruction (e.g., staff training, involvement in district advisory committees, curriculum development, etc.).

WHOSE VALUES ARE TAUGHT?

Most professionals in this field agree that it's impossible to teach sexuality education without also communicating value messages. For example, values that underlie many sexuality programs include the assumptions that relationships should not be exploitative or that most teens are not emotionally ready to become parents. In the late 1990s, the Sexuality Information and Education Council of the United States (SIECUS) recognized that values were in fact an important component of sexuality education and published a list of what they deemed *universal values* that should be inherent in quality, comprehensive sexuality programming.

An important aspect of training and preparation for individuals who teach sexuality education (for students with and without disabilities) is that they have ample op-

Universal Values

- Sexuality is a natural and healthy part of living.
- All persons are sexual.
- Sexuality includes physical, ethical, spiritual, psychological, and emotional dimensions.
- Every person has dignity and self-worth.
- Individuals express their sexuality in varied ways.
- In a pluralistic society like the United States, people should respect and accept the diversity of values and beliefs about sexuality that exist in a community.
- Sexual relationships should never be coercive or exploitative.
- All children should be loved and cared for.
- All sexual decisions have effects and consequences.
- All persons have the right and obligation to make responsible choices.
- Individuals and society benefit when children are able to discuss sexuality with their parents and/or other trusted adult.
- Young people explore their sexuality as a natural process of achieving sexual maturity.
- Premature involvement in sexual behavior poses risks.
- Abstaining from sexual intercourse is the most effective method of preventing pregnancy and STD/HIV.
- Young people who are involved in sexual relationships need access to information about healthcare services.

From **Guidelines for Comprehensive Sexuality Education, Kindergarten- 12th Grade**, 2nd Edition (1996), Sexuality and Information and Education Council of the United States (SIECUS), www.siecus.org, 212-819-9770. Used with permission.

portunities to evaluate and reflect on personal feelings and values about a wide range of sexual issues. Educators who have not had this training are often more uncomfortable and are more likely to infuse personal values into content rather than adhere to more pluralistic, universally accepted values. Considering the still quite prevalent laundry list of myths and misconceptions about sexuality and people with cognitive disabilities, (see Chapter 1—Getting Started), well-trained instructors are critical.

Values awareness training allows potential instructors to:

- explore their own attitudes, feelings, and values about a range of sexuality topics and issues;
- recognize diverse perspectives on sexual behavior;
- recognize their personal values and attitudes about the students they serve.

Because we live in a diverse society, value conflicts are inevitable. A colleague of mine told me about a conversation she had had with a mom whose teenage daughter with Down syndrome was now in high school and pretty proud that she could walk home independently after school. The mother, also proud, informed the teacher. The teacher advised her to talk to her daughter about wearing pants to school rather than dresses, believing pants would reduce the chances that she would be exploited en route from school to home. The antiquated idea that dressing a certain way invited exploitation angered the parent.

Sometimes when there are conflicts over values, both the parent and professional viewpoints have merit. For example, a parent I know was upset when she discovered that the school was allowing her son to masturbate in the bathroom located in the special education classroom at school. The mother believed that masturbation was inappropriate during the school day and was more acceptably performed at home. She didn't want her son to learn that he could masturbate any time he wanted as long as he was in private. She felt there were times and places that were appropriate and school wasn't one of them. She asked the teacher to share these messages rather than encourage private masturbation time at school. For her part, the teacher viewed these urges as completely natural and had, over the years, observed many of her students expressing an increased interest and curiosity about the body during this phase of puberty.

After a discussion with the mother, the teacher agreed to provide some brief educational sessions focused on body changes, including spontaneous erections and ejaculation. The teacher shared some resources with the mother so she could explain masturbation to her son and communicate clearer guidelines and expectations for behavior at home. The mom also agreed to work on increasing private time at home for her son, something she had forgotten was important in a maturing adolescent. In this example, the parent and professional worked together to resolve differences.

SEXUALITY EDUCATION IN SPECIAL EDUCATION

While state and local officials influence sexuality programming for the larger student population, *standards, guidelines, and directives influencing sexuality instruction for students with cognitive disabilities are virtually nonexistent.* As a result, there is great diversity in availability, comprehensiveness, and quality of programming for students with cognitive disabilities. Various reasons for reduced access to sexuality education are commonly cited. Some believe that yearly differences in student characteristics and abilities make it difficult to follow one or two homogenous curricula even within one district. In other districts, specialized instruction for students with cognitive disabilities was discontinued after more inclusive practices were embraced. Others argue that educational priorities for students with cognitive disabilities are driven by the Individualized Education Program and sexuality is not often included or identified as something that could or should be addressed.

Even when teachers are motivated to provide sexuality education, they often lack information about resources or do not have the support that is necessary to provide quality instruction. Some parents and professionals still have difficulty recognizing people with developmental disabilities as sexual human beings who have greater needs for information (rather than less). This denial interferes with advocacy efforts.

Characteristics of Sexuality Education for Students with & without Developmental Disabilities

Students with Cognitive Disabilities	General Student Population
■ Typically smaller groups (8-10 ideal) ■ Individualized instruction more common	■ Standard classroom size (15-30)
■ 1-2 learning objectives per session	■ More material covered in short periods of time
■ Slower-paced, more repetition	■ Rapid pace, less repetition
■ Content focused on common problems and issues for people with developmental disabilities	■ Advanced content (see Sexuality Topics table for content)
■ Teaching materials more often graphic and concrete (use of drawings, illustrations, models, etc.)	■ Fewer visuals ■ Use of activities that sometimes require abstract thought processes

If you believe your child will benefit from sexuality education geared more toward the needs of students with cognitive disabilities, communicate your goals and be prepared to work with school personnel. As a parent, you can:

- Identify learning goals you have for your child.
- Share home approaches for dealing with sexuality issues or behaviors.
- Identify teaching strategies that work well for your child.
- Share stories and struggles so teachers can integrate examples into teaching sessions, improving relevance for your child.
- Communicate your personal values to others supporting your child.
- Identify sexuality education materials and resources for students with cognitive disabilities.

Professionals supporting your child have an important role in teaching sexuality education as well. Often they have access to materials designed specifically for people with disabilities that are cost prohibitive for most families. They can develop alternative teaching techniques for addressing sexuality issues, help you identify resources within the community, and supplement and reinforce sexuality teaching in environments outside of the home.

Preparing Your Child for Sexuality Education in School or Community

Regardless of whether your district provides sexuality education within regular or special education classes, you'll need to be proactive to prepare your child to participate. Here are some things you can do:

FIND OUT IN ADVANCE WHAT CONTENT IS COVERED

Because children with cognitive disabilities often have less information than their peers, I advise parents to review content that will be covered in advance. If parental notification is included in your state statute, you'll receive basic information ahead of time. Otherwise, you can speak with your child's teacher for grade-specific content or the Director of Curriculum Instruction for a broader district overview of what topics are covered when. If they're unable to answer questions, they should be able to identify key district personnel who can help.

Understand that many school administrators and teachers routinely deal with a vocal minority of parents or community members who do not support school sexuality education or agree that topics they are covering are appropriate. As a result, school personnel may be wary of requests for detailed information about district programming. Communicate your goals up front so they understand why you are trying to gather information. For example, let them know you want your child to participate in sexuality education and would like to know what will be covered so you can prepare him and make him feel comfortable in the classroom. If videos are used, ask if you can preview them to be sure you and your child are on the same page. Ask about activities and assignments so you'll know what to expect. Help school personnel see the advantages of working with your child ahead of time. Your efforts can help your child participate more actively in sessions, improve comprehension, and provide opportunities for repetition and reinforcement outside the classroom.

PREPARE YOUR CHILD FOR WHAT HE WILL SEE AND HEAR

Once you have a better understanding of content to be covered, explore your child's current level of knowledge related to the topic and introduce or review key information that can help make the presentation more understandable. For example, if conception and pregnancy will be discussed, ask your child if he knows (or remembers, if you've discussed this before) how a woman gets pregnant. Use pictures in the back of the book to review male and female anatomy, sexual intercourse, conception, and pregnancy.

Check in with your child during and after instruction. Speaking with your son or daughter afterwards can help you assess what he or she learned, clarify his or her perspectives, and provide opportunities to promote your own values around sensitive topics. One mother told me that her daughter participated in an inclusive sexuality class on date rape at her school. During the session, students watched a video that profiled a young woman and events that lead to her actual rape. During a follow-up discussion at home, the mother discovered that her daughter believed the girl in the video deserved to be raped because she had made the boyfriend angry. She reminded her daughter that *nobody* has the right to hurt, rape, or assault another person even if they *are* angry. They ended up talking about a whole range of issues including healthy ways to handle angry feelings and ways to tell if a relationship is unhealthy. I shudder to think of the messages this girl may have retained if her mother had not been able to help her process the video.

> *When my daughter was in 4th grade, our district offered a preview night for parents so we could watch the puberty video ahead of time. The video they used had a fairly complex story line about two friends who were interested in learning about menstruation after one of the girls got her first period. The brief section of the video that talked about menstruation was rather abstract, but I decided I wanted my daughter to participate with her peers and prepared her as best as I could. After she saw the movie, we talked about it. When I asked her if she remembered what the movie was about, she told me, "two girls who giggled a lot."*

STRIVE FOR A BALANCE

When parents and professionals make decisions about what content is appropriate, students with cognitive disabilities sometimes inadvertently end up with information slanted toward the negative side. For example, many parents I speak with want their child to participate in school health classes or sexuality programs that address exploitation prevention because of the increased incidence of abuse among people with disabilities. Or, some educators and parents figure that if their child sits in on some gruesome sessions on the perils of getting a sexually transmitted disease, it may scare him into not wanting to date at all! (We have known for a long time that using fear to change sexual behavior is ineffective for people with or without disabilities.)

It would be unfair for your child to only hear about the risks, dangers, and negative consequences of experiencing relationships. Make sure he also has opportunities to understand the positive, healthy, and pleasurable qualities of being with others.

Advocating for Sexuality Education

In the event your district is not currently providing sexuality education and you feel strongly about its importance, here are some things you can do to advocate for formal opportunities for sexual learning:

Be Specific about What You Want. Simply asking school personnel to provide sexuality education is vague, too general, and may not be productive. Remember, sexuality education is broad and includes a whole range of topics. It's more helpful to focus on specific skills and information that would be beneficial for your child. If other students are receiving similar content, your child has the right to receive the same information in understandable ways. One mother I know included her daughter with Down syndrome in the regular human growth and development program at school but recognized she needed extra help understanding how to use pads. Her teacher was able to elicit help from the district nurse, who developed some individualized instruction. In this case the school was helping other girls learn how to handle periods and body changes, so it was appropriate for the parent to request modified programming for her daughter.

Be Involved. Recognize that getting what you want may mean digging in and helping out. One mother, after becoming frustrated with the lack of sexuality education for her daughter, spoke with a member of her district's Human Growth and Development committee. The representative invited her to attend a meeting, where she came prepared to talk about her daughter's needs and then distributed a list of specialized resources that might be useful for students with cognitive disabilities. District staff were grateful for the work she had done and ended up allocating money to purchase specialized resources for the district. Later she was asked to become a member of the committee and helped secure opportunities for teacher training when it became obvious that teachers wanted and needed support in this area. Her involvement improved her district's ability to respond to needs of students with cognitive disabilities.

Be Creative. In an era of tight budgets and frugal spending, it's not always economical, efficient, or even necessary to develop a comprehensive sexuality program. I often advise professionals to think about programs that already exist but could be enriched, improved, or strengthened by adding a sexuality component. One district I worked with had a longstanding career exploration program in which students with cognitive disabilities participated in various job experiences during their final years of high school. Because some of the students were behaving inappropriately on the job, they supplemented existing classroom instruction with sexuality information that supported their program goals, one of which was enhancing employability. They added relationships education, appropriate social skills in the workplace, privacy training, and exploitation prevention information with an emphasis on sexual harassment laws. These modifications helped reduce inappropriate behaviors and increased the students' preparedness to function in the workplace. Other natural places to infuse sexuality education into existing school programs include social skills, life skills, peer mentor, or guidance groups.

Being creative may also mean looking beyond the school environment and advocating for programming in other ways. Sheltered workshops, disability agencies, job training sites, self-advocacy groups or other programs your child participates in may be able to initiate or augment existing programs with sexuality topics. Often the sexuality programs I am asked to do are started by groups of parents or professionals who are simply listening and responding to the needs of the individuals and families they serve.

Recognize and Respect Best Practices. It's important to recognize that not all professionals are comfortable teaching or addressing sexuality issues in students with cognitive disabilities.

I have met health teachers, Planned Parenthood educators, and other professionals who are skilled and comfortable teaching sexuality topics to regular students, but become apprehensive, anxious, and uncomfortable working with students who have cognitive disabilities. Without appropriate training, educators run the risk of being insensitive to the unique needs and circumstances of students with cognitive disabilities and offering instruction that may be too sophisticated and complex, thereby decreasing relevancy and comprehension for students.

Other educators may have good skill, comfort, and knowledge working with students with cognitive disabilities, but have little training or experience addressing sexuality issues.

Either of these two scenarios can result in instruction that focuses on teacher comfort rather than student needs. Because sexuality in our culture is such a sensitive and difficult topic for many people, I strongly advocate that educators receive some type of specialized training that addresses the unique aspects of providing sexuality education for students with cognitive disabilities. (See the "Teaching Materials for Professionals" in the Resources.)

Avoid Reinventing the Wheel. During the past few decades, many good resources for teaching students with cognitive disabilities about sexuality have been developed. Although no one curricula will work for every student, they can provide good starting points for a wide range of students. Refer to pages 317-20 for a list of available resources.

References

Berne, L. & Huberman, B. (2000). Lessons Learned: European Approaches to Adolescent Sexual Behavior and Responsibility. *Journal of Sex Education and Therapy 25* (2-3): 189-99.

Blanchett, W. & Wolfe, P. (2002). A Review of Sexuality Education Curricula: Meeting the Needs of Individuals with Moderate and Severe Intellectual Disabilities. *Research and Practice for Persons with Severe Disabilities 27* (1).

Couwenhoven, T. (2001). Sexuality Education: Building on the Foundation of Healthy Attitudes. *Disability Solutions 4* (6).

Hoff, T. & Greene, L. (2000). *Sex Education in America: A Series of National Surveys of Students, Parents, Teachers, and Principals.* Menlo Park, CA: Kaiser Family Foundation.

SIECUS Guidelines for Comprehensive Sexuality Education, Kindergarten -12th Grade, 2nd ed. (1996). New York, NY: Sexuality Information and Education Council of the United States.

SIECUS. Issues & Answers: Fact Sheet on Sexuality Education. www.siecus.org.

CHAPTER 14

You've Postponed This 'til Now

You may have turned to this chapter because something happened—an incident, a conversation, an observation—that helped you realize that your child needs more information and assistance on her journey to becoming a sexually healthy adult. You are not alone if your child has somehow arrived at adolescence (or even adulthood) and you are just now grasping how little he or she knows and understands about sexuality. This chapter was designed to provide you with models and templates for approaching situations that inevitably come up in the area of sexuality.

PLISSIT: A Model for Determining How Much Intervention Your Child Needs

When issues and concerns related to sexuality arise for children with cognitive disabilities, parents may be paralyzed by discomfort, making it difficult for them to guide and assist their child through the situation. The PLISSIT model is a useful way to think about the *level of need* your child may have and help you determine the *type of support* that may be necessary. It can also help parents clarify their own role in responding to these needs.

The PLISSIT model was developed by Jack Annon, a sex therapist who found that the majority of clients he worked with really needed less complicated interventions in order to resolve issues and concerns related to sexuality. The model can be visualized like this:

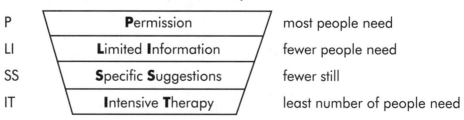

P	**P**ermission	most people need
LI	**L**imited **I**nformation	fewer people need
SS	**S**pecific **S**uggestions	fewer still
IT	**I**ntensive **T**herapy	least number of people need

PERMISSION

The first level of the model is the most basic but important component. Annon found that most people who came to him had been denied the right to learn, talk, or explore their own attitudes and feelings about a particular issue related to sexuality and consequently were experiencing some type of internal struggle. Let's face it, there is much discomfort about sexuality, but anxieties can often be resolved or managed once people understand that their feelings are normal and experienced by others. Permission at this most basic level means that you recognize your child is a sexual human being with similar feelings, desires, and needs that all of us have and experience.

Because your child is a sexual human being, you'll want to share information, answer questions, and respond empathetically to her feelings and concerns. Listening and talking about sexuality helps your child know that her feelings and desires are normal and healthy and validates her humanness. When your child is given permission to explore all aspects of who she is, she has a better chance at becoming a sexually healthy adult. When we choose to ignore or deny our child's sexuality, we run the risk of finding ourselves in situations like that of the mother who attended one of my sessions and voiced her concerns about her daughter's preoccupation with masturbation. When I asked her how she had addressed the issue so far, her message was loud and clear. She had told her daughter masturbation was wrong, against their religion, and was not something she allowed in her home.

Most professionals have numerous examples of what happens when normal and healthy sexual responses and needs are denied, repressed, ignored, or punished. Generally, they lead to bigger problems like lowered self-esteem, unhealthy ideas about what's okay and not okay, unhealthy attitudes, and inappropriate behaviors. Indeed, this mother's inability to recognize masturbation as normal and healthy prevented her from offering limited information about appropriate places for masturbating (in her mind, there were no appropriate places). As a result, her daughter continued to masturbate at inappropriate times and places.

Of course, giving permission *does not* mean blanket approval for any or all sexual attitudes and behaviors. One of your roles as a parent is to teach and model healthy attitudes and respectful boundaries within the context of societal norms and family values. This model can be used to help you determine when permission should be withheld (not allowed). For example, sexual activities or behaviors that are harmful (for your child or another person), nonconsensual, or illegal should be immediately curtailed. Offering limited information about the reasons why a behavior is wrong and consequences that could result if it is repeated is not only appropriate but necessary. Sometimes parents fail to withhold permission and allow inappropriate sexual behavior to continue because:

- They use a different set of behavioral standards for their child who has a disability than they would for their other children.
- They're not sure their child has the capacity to learn to be appropriate.
- They don't have the knowledge or skills to respond.
- They are not sure what healthy or "typical" sexuality looks like
- They are tired or just plain burned out.
- They hope their child will "grow out" of the behavior.

One parent emailed me seeking information about sexual harassment cases involving individuals with developmental disabilities. Her adult son with Down syndrome had recently been fired from his job for sexual harassment (due to inappropriately touching a coworker). The mother understood her son's intent was not malicious but rather innocent, so the family chose to pursue legal action, believing his firing was unjustified. What the family may not have understood was that in sexual harassment cases the *impact* the message has on the receiver is far more important than the *intentions* of the sender. In this example, rather than withholding permission for the behavior and sharing limited information about boundaries with their son, especially in the work environment, the family allowed inappropriate affection to continue with dire consequences.

Allowing inappropriate sexual behavior to continue unchecked teaches your child that the behavior is, in fact, acceptable. Over time, this can lead to your child developing more challenging behaviors that require increasingly complex solutions. For example, during a workshop, one mother told me that her daughter had a habit of grabbing male crotches. Men who knew her (family and friends) joked about it and had learned over time to keep their distance. Men who did not know her, however, were very often unexpectedly surprised. The crotch-grabbing behavior was clearly nonconsensual, as it violated the rights of others. Rather than withhold permission for the inappropriate behavior, over time her family had accepted it as "just something she did." They generally ignored the crotch-grabbing incidents, which essentially gave her permission to continue.

LIMITED INFORMATION

In addition to needing permission, Annon found that many individuals also need limited information or basic facts that address specific sexuality concerns or questions. Giving your child limited information can mean imparting new information or simply dispelling myths. Teaching about ways to handle spontaneous erections during puberty and identifying appropriate places to masturbate are examples of interventions you might provide at this level. Much of this book, in fact, was designed to help you perform at this level of the model.

YOUR ABILITY TO GIVE YOUR CHILD PERMISSION AND LIMITED INFORMATION

Not all parents are capable of giving permission or limited information using the PLISSIT model. Although I believe it's important for parents to view their child's sexuality as a healthy and positive aspect of who they are, I also recognize that not all parents can or want to do this. Your attitudes and beliefs about sexuality have been shaped by a lifetime of cumulative experiences and reading this book is unlikely to change all that. However, if you are interested in accepting your role as primary sexuality educator for your child, it may be helpful for you to understand how your own attitudes, knowledge, and behavior can affect your ability to give your child the support and information she needs. Examples of traits that support and healthy sexuality are listed in the chart on the next page.

SPECIFIC SUGGESTION AND INTENSIVE THERAPY

In fewer instances, children may need specific suggestions or intensive therapy, the bottom levels of the model. The bottom two levels of the model almost always require assistance from professionals who have more advanced skills and training in counseling, behavior modification, or evaluation and assessment. Specific suggestions are typically recommendations for helping an individual address sexual needs. For example:

- A young man was taken to the emergency room after staff at a group home realized he had injured himself while masturbating unsafely. I was later called in to provide specific suggestions on safe masturbation techniques.

Traits That Affect Your Abilities to Provide Permission and Limited Information

	Traits that make it easier to provide permission & limited information	Traits that make it harder to provide permission & limited information
Attitudes	■ You view sexuality as positive aspect of being human ■ You are reasonably comfortable with a wide range of sexuality issues ■ Your child sees you as approachable ■ You recognize a wide range of diverse attitudes	■ You view sexuality as a burden or negative aspect of your child's life ■ Your child sees you as unapproachable
Knowledge	■ You are familiar with common developmental issues in sexuality ■ You offer accurate information about topic being addressed ■ You have a good understanding of societal norms and expectations	■ You provide little information about sexuality ■ You have limited awareness of societal norms
Behaviors	■ You address your child's needs at her own level ■ You talk openly and honestly about sexuality ■ You positively reinforce question-asking and curiosity about sexuality ■ You model healthy behavior ■ You use teachable moments to reinforce sexual learning	■ You refuse to discuss sexuality issues ■ You use shame and guilt to shape behavior

- A young woman who experienced a sexual assault needed intensive therapy to help her address feelings that were surfacing as a result of the abuse.
- After a teen exhibited sexually aggressive behavior at school, a local behaviorist was able to conduct an assessment to assist the family in managing her inappropriate and difficult sexual behaviors.
- Couples who are sexually active may need specific suggestions regarding the importance of consent, privacy, protection, and pleasuring from someone who is trained in educating individuals with cognitive disabilities.

As a parent, your work in supporting healthy sexuality will involve use of the top two levels of the model, Permission and Limited Information. These two levels can be used to address a wide range of sexual issues and concerns. Below is a process for thinking about the steps involved in using the Permission and Limited Information components of the model.

A Step-by-Step Process for Sharing Limited Information

As you may remember from Chapter 1, children with disabilities often experience altered scripts for learning about sexuality. These scripts include less information, negative attitudes, and fewer opportunities for socialization. Consequently, recognizing and then addressing needs for information is often the key to helping your child work through situations or issues involving sexuality. The following process can be a guide for preparing yourself to share information with your child.

STEP #1 BEGIN WITH THE MOST IMMEDIATE NEED

Usually, parents can identify their child's needs informally by observing her interacting with others in natural environments. Paying attention is typically all that is needed. We overhear our child's conversations with peers or see him or her do things which help us recognize information or skills that might be helpful. Some common examples of needs include:

- Your child touches her genitals while out in public.
- You notice your son's body has started to mature and develop.
- Your preadolescent daughter comes downstairs only partially dressed during an adult party.
- Your child hugs peers, adults, and strangers indiscriminately.
- The school calls to report that your child is touching others inappropriately on the bus.
- Your teenage daughter wants a boyfriend.
- You walk in on your teenage daughter and her boyfriend engaged in intimate affection.

Whatever the issue, rather than launch into an immediate teaching session, try to evaluate how much your child knows or understands about the issue at hand. It's common to make assumptions or interpret events and experiences through our own eyes rather than explore our child's perspective. Gathering insights from your child before jumping to conclusions improves your ability to develop meaningful, relevant goals.

STEP #2 PREPARATION

Some situations will require minimal preparation and you will be able to respond quickly with little thought or consideration. For instance, you notice your child fidgeting with her genitals during a trip to the store and remind her she is in a public place where others can see. You quickly and quietly review rules and continue shopping. Or, when you are in the middle of a conversation with a friend, your daughter blurts out the fact that she has her period. Your response is fairly simple and direct. You might quietly acknowledge you understand she is excited about getting her period but that it's private. Many times quick responses and corrections are all that is needed to handle these situations or inappropriate behaviors.

Other situations are more complicated and the element of surprise forces you to take time to process what has happened and figure out an appropriate response. You may want to evaluate your own feelings, find the right words, and formulate messages that accurately convey your personal attitudes and values about a particular topic. Or you may need to locate resources that can help you prepare to teach. Questions that can help with preparation include:

- What actually happened?
- What does your child already know and understand?
- What new information might be helpful (knowledge deficit)?
- What skills may be necessary to teach (skill deficit)?
- Are there values (rules) I feel strongly about and want to communicate?
- Are there resources (people or materials) that might be helpful to you?

STEP #3 SET A GOAL

Once a clear need has been identified and you feel adequately prepared, set a goal for what you would like to accomplish. Try to be clear, specific, and formulate goals that communicate behaviors you want to see (rather than eliminate). Here are some examples of teaching goals:

- Use a menstrual pad independently.
- Masturbate in private.
- Plan a date.
- Use a condom correctly.
- Identify appropriate topics to talk about with peers.
- Respond assertively to peer pressure.
- Use appropriate affection with authority figures.

Sometimes more than one goal may need to be addressed simultaneously. For example, a boy who had always hugged peers in the past began getting into trouble when his hugs became more intense as he approached puberty. School staff were concerned that he was using the contact for sexual gratification and threatened to slap him with a sexual assault charge if he continued. In this instance, both the family and school created more than one goal. They wanted the boy to greet his peers appropriately and learn about body changes, specifically spontaneous erections. To work on these goals, the teacher introduced a puberty education unit to cover information about erections and other physical changes that were happening to his body, as well as more age-appropriate greeting skills. Over time, slow and gradual improvement was made and their goals were accomplished.

STEP #4 TEACH

Select Concrete Teaching Strategies. Individuals with Down syndrome and other cognitive disabilities learn more effectively when concrete teaching methods are used. Remember your goal and the change you are trying to create. Are you sharing information or attempting to teach your child a skill? Learning how to greet authority figures is a skill, so selecting a teaching method that will help your child learn and practice the skill will be most effective. Keep in mind that no one teaching technique is better than another. In fact, using a combination of methods over time is most effective. Consider your child's own strengths and weakness as you choose a teaching technique.

Collaborate. Including key people who support and influence your child is a critical component of the teaching process. If your goals involve transfer of learning from home to other settings, you are more likely to succeed if you working with support people.

Troubleshooting—What Are You Trying to Teach?

Goal	Teaching Techniques
Change Attitudes—You want to identify ranges of viewpoints, encourage empathy, support positive feelings about sexuality. For example, You want your child to: ■ feel okay about body changes during puberty ■ be less fearful about pelvic exams ■ feel good about herself and her disability ■ respect feelings of others	■ field trip/tours ■ games ■ discussion ■ exercises, structured experiences ■ simulations
Knowledge Acquisition—You're helping your child develop new knowledge, link new learning with existing understanding, assimilate new learning into everyday life. For example, You want your child to: ■ identify ways the body changes during puberty ■ understand how a woman gets pregnant ■ differentiate between public and private	■ slides ■ diagrams ■ photos ■ videos ■ anatomically correct dolls ■ realistic models ■ realistic drawings ■ demonstration ■ field trips
Skill Development—you're helping your child develop and practice doing something. For example, You want your child to: ■ use a pad correctly ■ clean up after wet dreams ■ refuse unwanted advances ■ close the door when privacy is desired ■ take a shower independently	■ role play ■ improvisation ■ pantomime ■ demonstration ■ videotapes of skills being performed by others ■ modeling ■ drill ■ simulation

STEP #5 EVALUATE LEARNING

Once you've completed your teaching sessions, identify ways to determine whether your child understood what was taught and your teaching was successful. If your goals are clear, figuring out a way to evaluate if your child is accomplishing those goals will be easier. Ways to check learning include asking questions, playing board games, having your child identify pictures, or observing her in natural environments. (See Chapter 3 for other ways to assess learning.)

STEP #6
PROVIDE
REPETITION &
REINFORCEMENT

Most people are uncomfortable talking and teaching about very personal things such as erections, sexual expression, or masturbation, so we tend to talk about them as little as possible. It is, however, a rare occasion when a person with a cognitive disability is able to grasp information and apply it in her daily life after a single teaching session. For example, your child learns good manners, self-care, and skills needed for independence over time, little by little, with ongoing coaching and support. Sexuality concepts will be no different. Look for teachable moments when new learning can be repeated and reinforced.

A psychiatrist once gave me an insight into my exasperation with my daughter's need for repetition. He told me typical children require 10 to 20 repetitions to "get something." He guessed my daughter needed 1,000 to 2,000 repetitions.

Permission and Limited Information in Action

CASE EXAMPLE #1:
FLIRTATIOUS
BEHAVIOR

A few summers ago my daughters were cast as townspeople in our local community theater summer production of *The Music Man*. They had a wonderful time learning choreography and songs, rehearsing, and interacting with a diverse group of cast members. During the cast party following the final performance, all participants received a commemorative folder with photos, an individual award, and various other mementoes. Most of the awards were generic—"Best Smile," " Best Dancer," "Best Voice," etc.

Imagine my dismay when my fifteen-year-old daughter with Down syndrome brought home the "Biggest Flirt" award! She was, in fact, quite proud of her award, even though she had no idea what it meant. I had never sat down and taught my daughter how to flirt. Her knowledge and experience with flirting happened through informal learning. Knowing she is a great visual learner, I suspect much of her skill came from watching her teenaged peers work their magic in the hallways at the high school. Nevertheless, this situation became an opportunity for me to put the PLISSIT model into action.

PERMISSION TO FLIRT?

I have to admit my initial reactions to the award were negative. With time, however, I reminded myself of the benefits of understanding how to let your interests be known and that flirting is, in fact, a desirable skill, especially if you want to find a partner, begin a romantic relationship, and date. I did want that for my daughter. However, I also wanted her to understand the complexities and nuances between innocent flirting and sexual harassment.

PLAN FOR SHARING LIMITED INFORMATION

STEP #1—IDENTIFY NEED

After some questioning, my daughter admitted she had no idea what flirting meant or why she had been perceived as a flirt.

STEP #2 – PREPARATION

This was one of those situations I did not feel prepared to address on the spot. I needed to do some research and frankly was not sure at all how I was going to approach the subject. This whole process really took very little time, but I spread it out over a few days. In preparation for teaching, I:

- Conducted an Internet search to gather ideas for words I could use to explain flirting. Then I simplified those words to make them understandable for my daughter.
- Reviewed some sexuality curricula I had in my office (not specific to people with developmental disabilities) to look for pictures or images I could use to make the concept visual. I didn't find anything.
- Thought about messages I wanted to communicate related to the topic. For example, it's okay to flirt with peers, not adults or teachers.
- Spoke with some of her female peers and a few adults I knew who were also in the production to see if I could gather specific information on why she was given the award. They were not helpful.

STEP #3—SET GOAL

After preparing myself, I was able to identify four goals for my daughter's information session. I wanted her to be able to:

- Understand reasons people flirt.
- Identify specific actions typically interpreted as flirting.
- Evaluate whether her flirting was welcome or unwelcome.
- STOP flirting if it was unwelcome.

STEP #4—TEACH

A few nights later when she was relaxing in her room, I asked if I could talk to her about her award. Our discussion revolved around these key messages:

- Flirting is "a way we let others know we are interested in them."
- We talked about reasons why people flirt. For example, I mentioned it can be a way of letting someone know you want to go out or that you think they are cute.
- I demonstrated the behaviors other people probably interpreted as flirting. They included things like standing too close to people and using a flirty voice (I did demonstrations of flirty voice vs. regular voice, normal personal space vs. flirting space).
- I asked her who she thought it was okay to flirt with and her response was appropriate—"her friends." I agreed, but we did review who it was not appropriate to flirt with—adults, teachers, coworkers, coaches, etc.
- Flirting is okay if the other person likes it, but I reminded her that not everyone does like it (this was new information and she seemed surprised to know this).
- I showed her ways she could tell if people liked or did not like the flirting. (They didn't like it if they turned away, walked away, or did not respond, for example.)
- If words or gestures get no response or a negative response, she needed to stop. I reminded her that continuing to flirt with people when they don't like it makes them feel uncomfortable. I emphasized reading the signals was important.

Step #5—Evaluate Learning

I evaluated her understanding of flirting mainly through:

- *Use of Media*—My daughter loves to go to the movies, and often examples of "flirting" came up in movies or on television. During these moments she could identify behaviors that were indicative of flirting and could determine if the flirting was wanted or unwanted based on the other person's responses (eye contact, body movements, etc.).
- *Teachable Moments*—Interestingly, once she understood the concept of flirting she was able to label it. During a conversation we were having about gym class one day, she interjected a side comment about a male friend who was supposed to be working out and instead was "flirting" with the girls. When I asked her what exactly he was doing, she described his behaviors and was right on. This helped me know she was understanding the basic essentials of flirting.

Step #6—Repetition and Reinforcement

I planned to reinforce my daughter's learning by:

- Reviewing key concepts prior to social events (e.g., asking her "What are signs people may or may not like flirting?" and "What do you do if you notice these signs?");
- Using media to identify examples of flirting and interpret whether the flirting was wanted or unwanted (and in some cases appropriate or inappropriate).

CASE EXAMPLE #2: INAPPROPRIATE HUGGING

Recently a mother called the clinic to discuss ways she could help her son become more discriminatory about affection. Ryan (not his real name), a seventh grader, still greeted everyone with a hug, including teachers, physicians, or any other adult he encountered. Concerned about her son's vulnerability and increased risk of exploitation, the mother was interested in helping her son learn more age-appropriate greeting skills.

PERMISSION TO HUG INDISCRIMINATELY?

Although permission had been given to hug indiscriminately in the past, both parents now recognized it was time to begin withholding permission to help their son become more age appropriate.

PLAN FOR SHARING LIMITED INFORMATION

Step #1—Identify Need

Ryan needed to learn more age-appropriate skills for greeting authority figures.

Step #2—Preparation

- Ryan's mom called the clinic as one step in her preparation process.
- She had already discussed her concerns with her son's teacher and the school guidance counselor.
- She and her husband had attended a recent support group meeting in order to gather ideas from other families with children

Ryan's age, anticipating other families may have experienced similar problems.

- In the process of talking with others, the *Circles* curriculum was mentioned as a resource, and the mother wondered if I was familiar with it. (*Circles*, by Leslie Walker-Hirsh, is a color-coded visual system for helping individuals with cognitive disabilities learn about varying levels of intimacy and appropriate affection within different relationships. See the Resources.) I gave her the name of an agency that made it available to both families and professionals.
- Ryan's mom later went to the agency to preview the resource and gather ideas for how she could use the concept at home with her son at home.

Step #3—Identify Goal

The goal was clear for Ryan's parents—they both wanted their son to stop hugging adults indiscriminately. They therefore needed to choose a substitute behavior for their son to use instead. They decided they wanted Ryan to use verbal greetings with known and new authority figures.

Step #4—Teach

Since the inappropriate hugging was occurring both at school and in the community, the parents communicated their goal with Ryan's teacher. A collaborative plan for both school and home was developed.

Home Education Plan:
- Borrow CIRCLES from library.
- Create modified CIRCLES map with pictures and appropriate greetings to hang on fridge.
- Demonstrate appropriate verbal greetings for Ryan to use with authority figures (replacement behavior).
- Role play every morning before school and other social situations for two weeks.
- Praise Ryan whenever he used new greetings in community settings.

School Education Plan:
- Ryan's parents and teacher identified appropriate greetings for Ryan to use with teachers and other authority figures at school.
- The teacher communicated with other key staff the parents' goals for Ryan and praised him for using verbal greetings.
- The guidance counselor used the CIRCLES curriculum with Ryan and other special education students.

Step #5—Evaluate Learning

Ryan's parents evaluated their son's learning by:
- observing him in the community with authority figures and verbally reminding or redirecting him as needed.

- following up with Ryan's teacher during parent-teacher conferences a month later to discuss progress at school. At that time, Ryan had made significant progress with occasional regressions.

STEP #6—REPETITION
To help reinforce Ryan's learning:
- His parents continued role playing prior to community outings for another month.
- They continued to praise him when he used appropriate greetings in community settings.

The PLISSIT Model and People with Cognitive Disabilities

As a sexuality educator, I was introduced to the PLISSIT model early in my career as a tool for thinking about a variety of need levels that people experience. As I gained more experience working with individuals with cognitive disabilities and the parents and professionals who supported them, I began to see the discrepancies in how sexuality issues in people with cognitive disabilities were viewed. In short, the behaviors of people with disabilities were more often interpreted as abnormal or atypical. For instance, a young man with limited language skills who was hugging his female classmates in middle school was labeled a "sexual predator" by his principal and referred for psychological testing and therapy (intensive therapy) in lieu of being offered social skills instruction (limited information). An adult male with Down syndrome who lived alone and often visited the play area of his neighborhood park was assumed to be a pedophile without appropriate testing and evaluation.

Are there people with cognitive disabilities who are sex offenders, predators, or deviant? Absolutely! However, most of the time the presence of altered scripts in the lives of people with cognitive disabilities (see Chapter 1) requires us to begin with the basic idea that our child is a sexual human being who needs permission to be sexual as well as understandable information that can help support healthy sexuality. Using the PLISSIT model described in this chapter, you will very likely be able to help your child learn the information and skills she needs to enable her to behave more appropriately.

References

Blasingame, G. (2001). *Developmentally Disabled Persons with Sexual Behavior Problems.* Oklahoma City, OK: Woods 'N' Barnes Publishing.

Griffiths, D. et al. (1989). *Changing Inappropriate Sexual Behavior: A Community-Based Approach for Persons with Developmental Disabilities.* Baltimore: Brookes Publishing.

Kempton, W. (1993). *Socialization and Sexuality: A Comprehensive Training Guide for Professionals Helping People with Disabilities that Hinder Learning.* Philadelphia: Planned Parenthood Southeastern Pennsylvania.

Lucyshyn, J. et al. (2002). *Families & Positive Behavior Support: Addressing Problem Behavior in the Context of Families.* Baltimore: Brookes Publishing.

Maksym, D. (1990). *Shared Feelings: A Parent Guide to Sexuality Education for Children, Adolescents, and Adults Who Have a Mental Handicap; A Discussion Guide.* North York: Ontario: G. Allan Roeher Institute.

Ryan, R. (1996). *Handbook of Mental Health Care for Persons with Developmental Disabilities.* Denver: The Community Circle Publications.

Appendix A

Teaching about the Body

A-1

Pre-pubertal Female

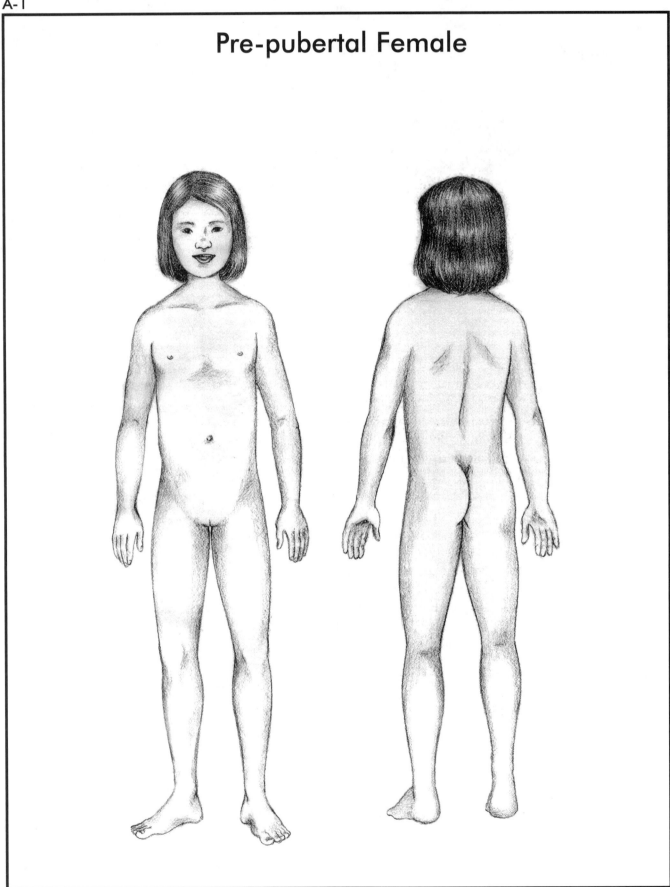

A-2

Pre-pubertal Male

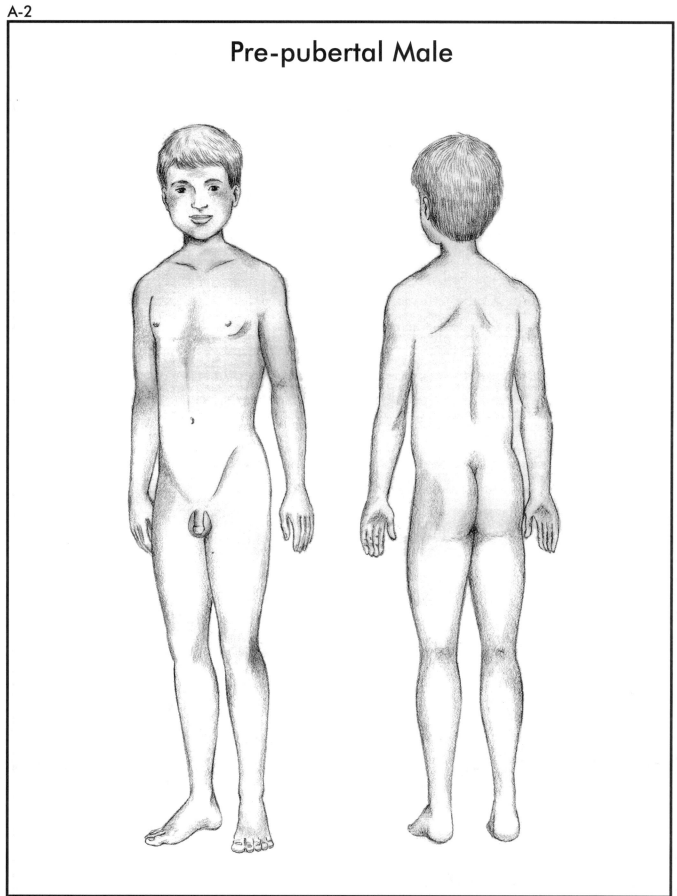

A-3

Post-pubertal Female

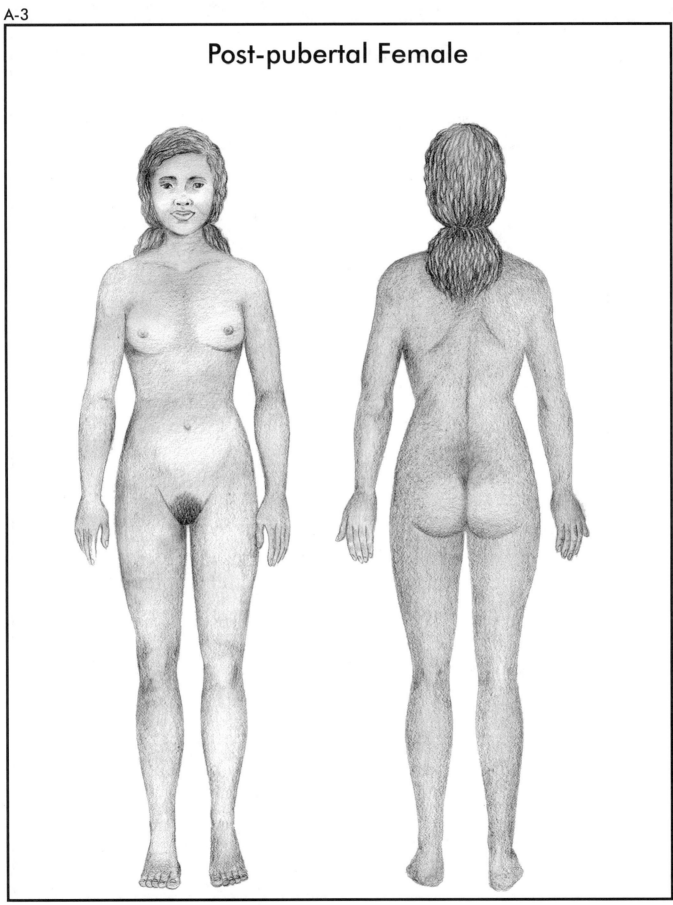

A-4

Post-pubertal Male

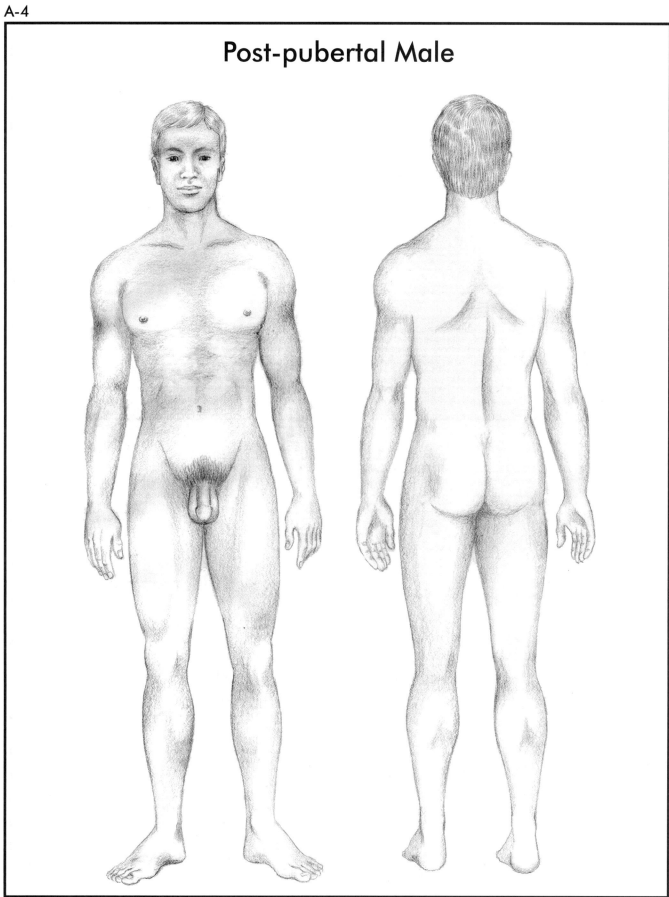

A-5

Female Body Outline

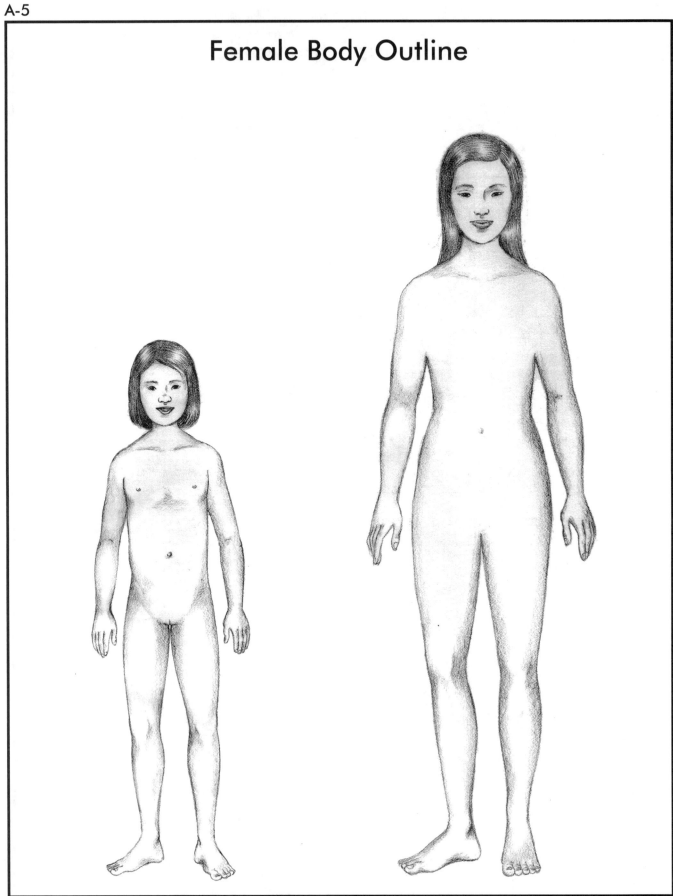

Male Body Outline

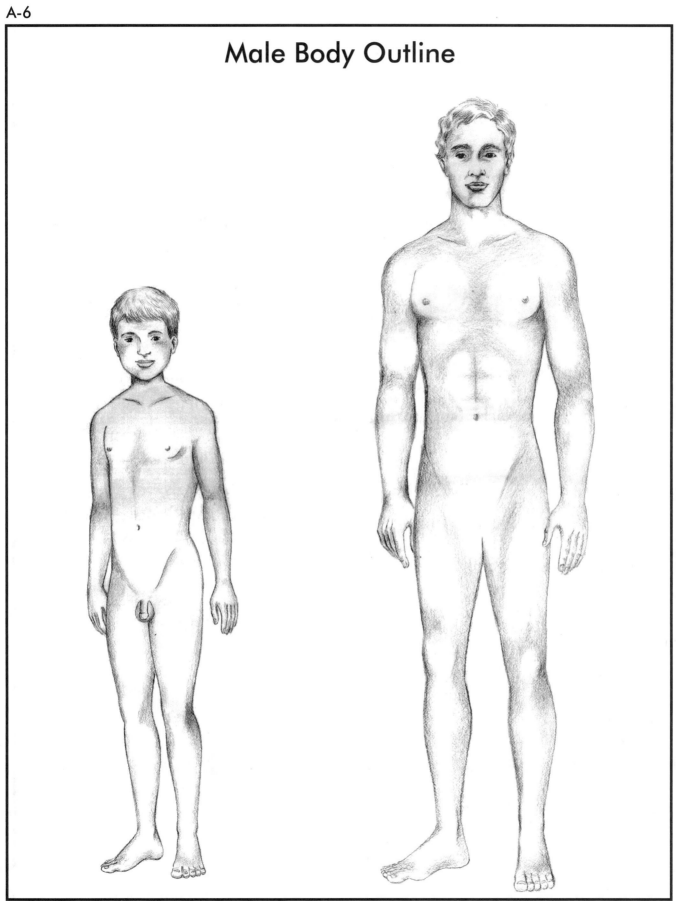

Private Body Parts (Female)

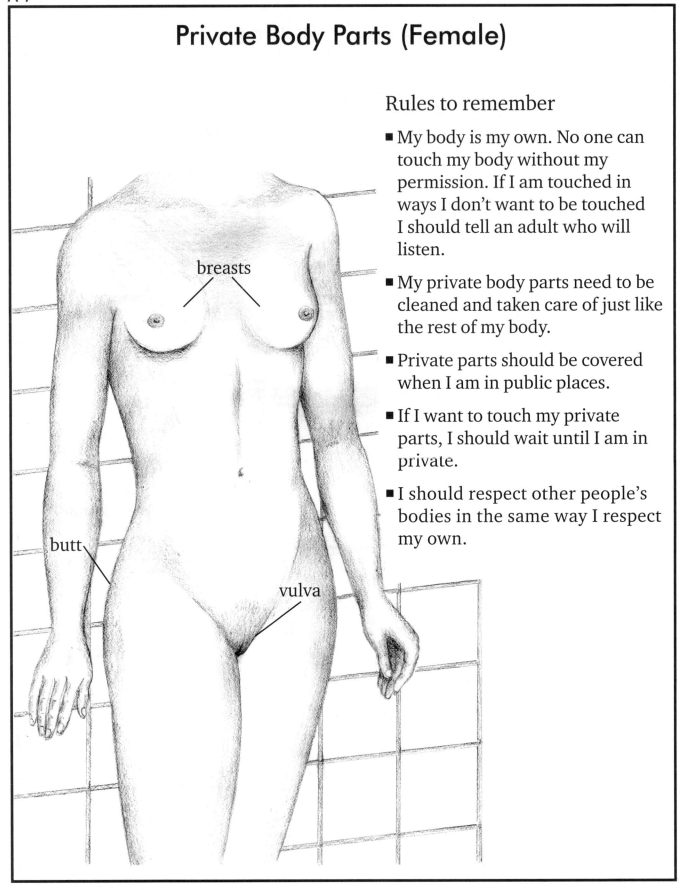

breasts

butt

vulva

Rules to remember

- My body is my own. No one can touch my body without my permission. If I am touched in ways I don't want to be touched I should tell an adult who will listen.

- My private body parts need to be cleaned and taken care of just like the rest of my body.

- Private parts should be covered when I am in public places.

- If I want to touch my private parts, I should wait until I am in private.

- I should respect other people's bodies in the same way I respect my own.

Private Body Parts (Male)

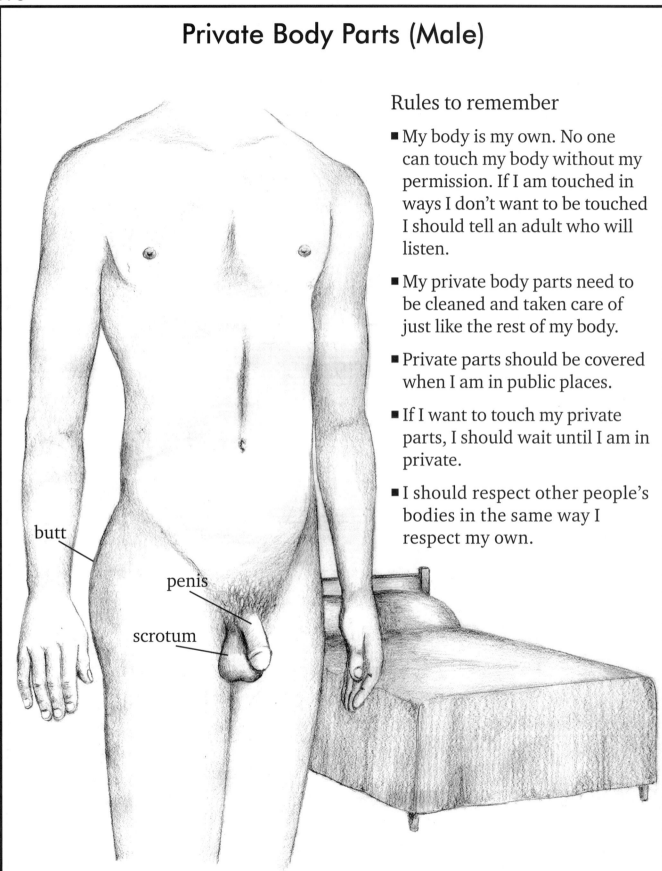

butt

penis

scrotum

Rules to remember

- My body is my own. No one can touch my body without my permission. If I am touched in ways I don't want to be touched I should tell an adult who will listen.

- My private body parts need to be cleaned and taken care of just like the rest of my body.

- Private parts should be covered when I am in public places.

- If I want to touch my private parts, I should wait until I am in private.

- I should respect other people's bodies in the same way I respect my own.

Puberty Progression (Male)

- A time when your body changes from looking child-like to more adult-like

- These changes happen on the outside and inside of your body

- These changes are normal and happen to everyone

- Your body will change at its own speed. Some boys will change early, others later

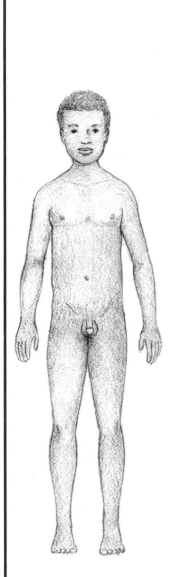

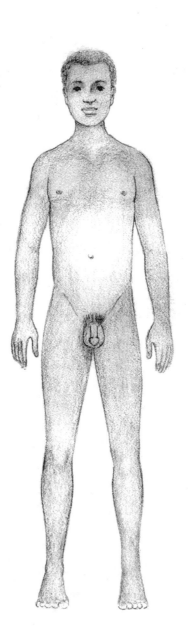

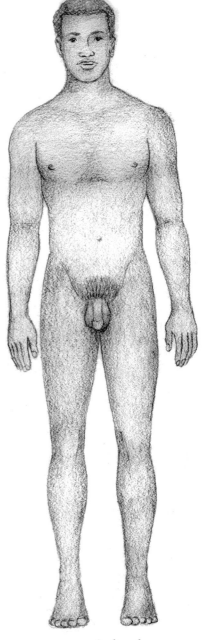

boy's body

man's body

A-10

Puberty Progression (Female)

■ A time when your body changes from looking child-like to more adult-like

■ These changes happen on the outside and inside of your body

■ These changes are normal and happen to everyone

■ Your body will change at its own speed. Some girls will change early, others later

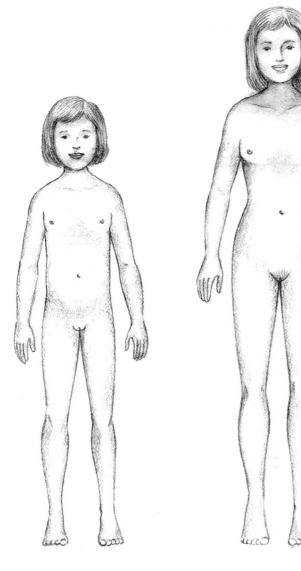
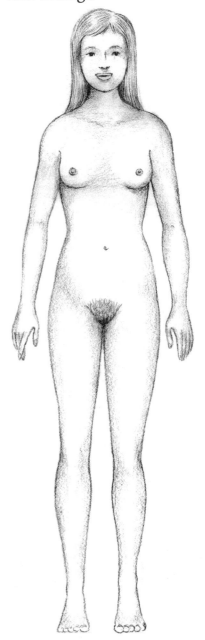

girl's body   woman's body

A-11

Inside Body Parts (Male)

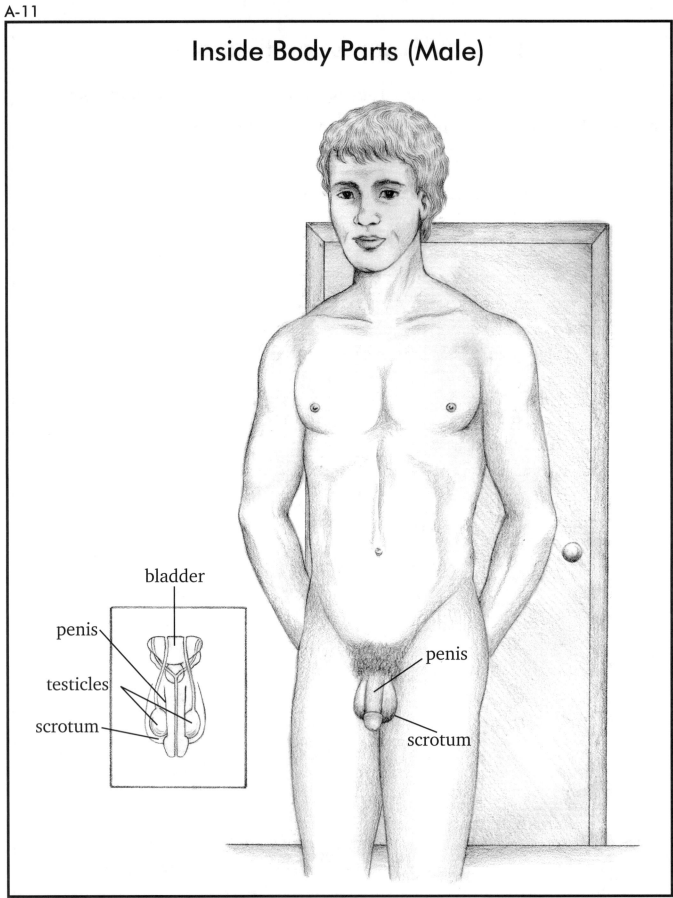

bladder

penis

testicles

scrotum

penis

scrotum

A-12

Facts about Erections

- Sexy thoughts and feelings can make blood flow to your penis

- Blood flowing to the penis is what causes the penis to get harder and longer

- Erections are more common during puberty

- Erections are normal and happen to all males

- Erections are private

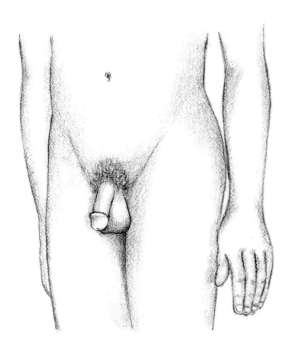

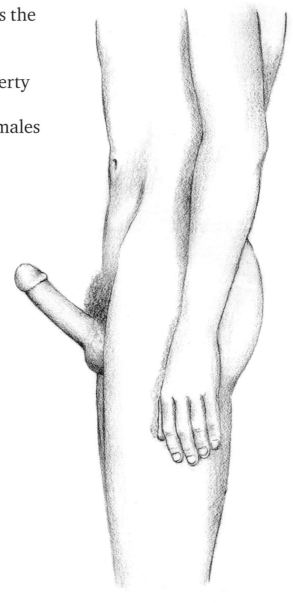

A-13

Facts about Ejaculation

- An ejaculation is when white sticky stuff called semen comes out of the penis

- During puberty, ejaculations can happen while you sleep. These are called "wet dreams."

- Wet dreams are normal and happen to all boys.

- Ejaculations also happen after rubbing the penis (masturbation).

- After ejaculating, the penis can be cleaned with a wet cloth, towel, or by bathing.

- Ejaculations are private.

ejaculation

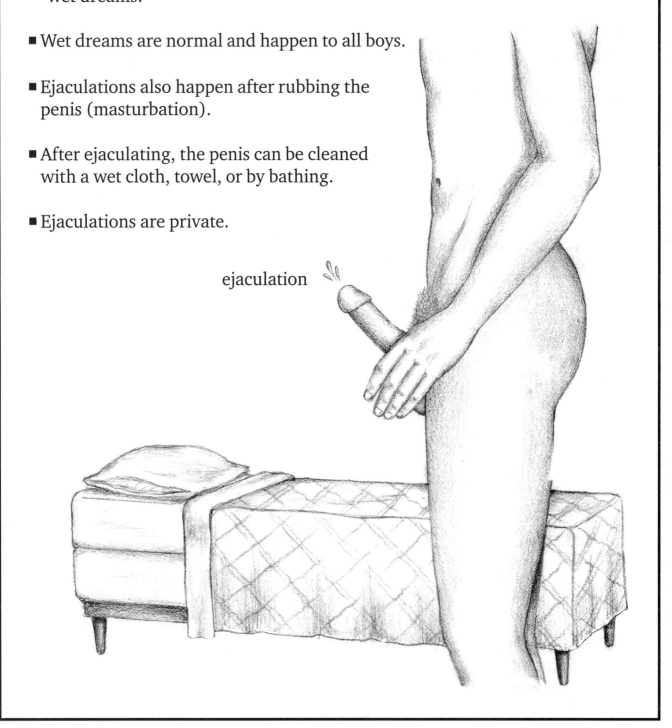

Outside Body Parts (Female)

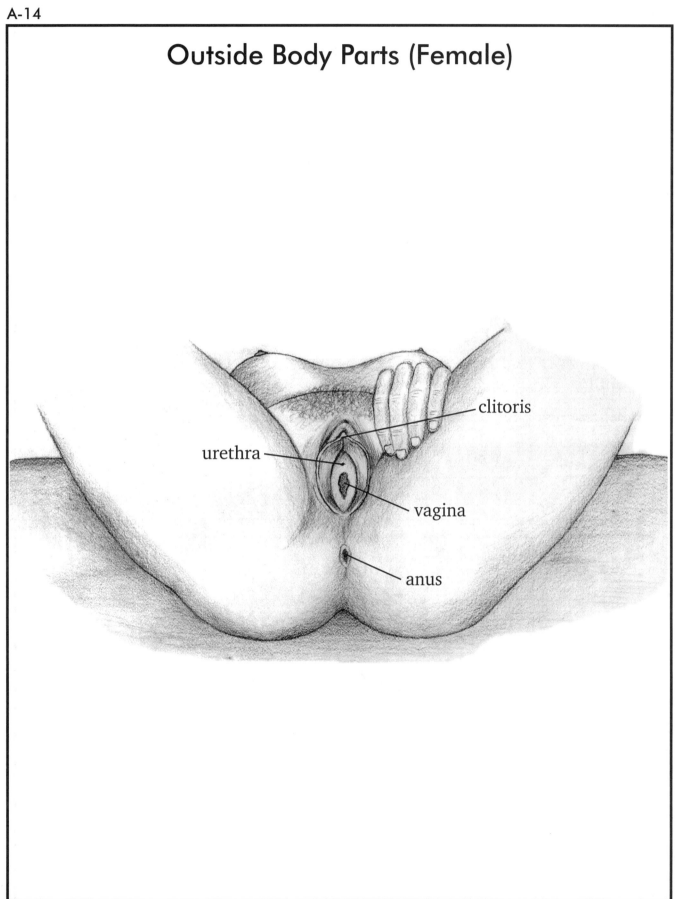

A-15

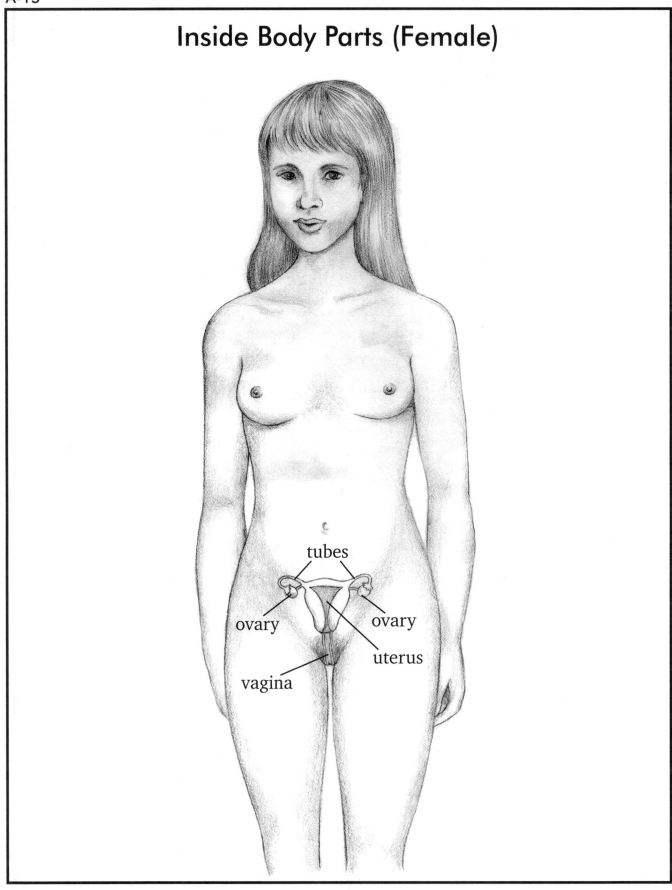

Inside Body Parts (Female)

tubes

ovary

ovary

uterus

vagina

A-16

Facts about Menstruation

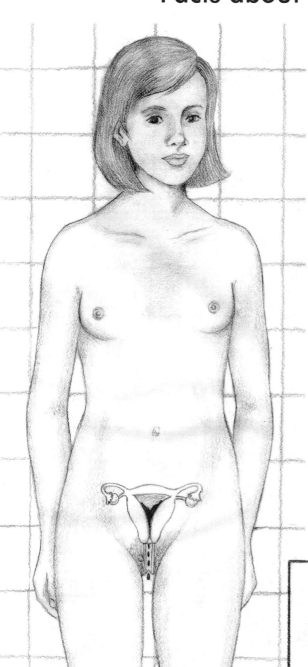

- Menstruation is when blood comes out from inside the body from an opening between your legs (vagina).

- Menstruation is also called "having a period."

- Period blood is a sign your body is healthy and working as it should.

- Periods come every month and will last from 4 to 7 days.

- Menstruation is private.

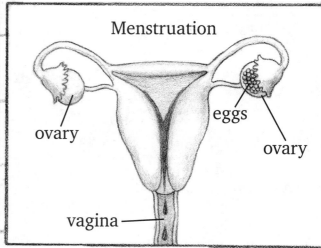

Menstruation

ovary

eggs

ovary

vagina

A-17

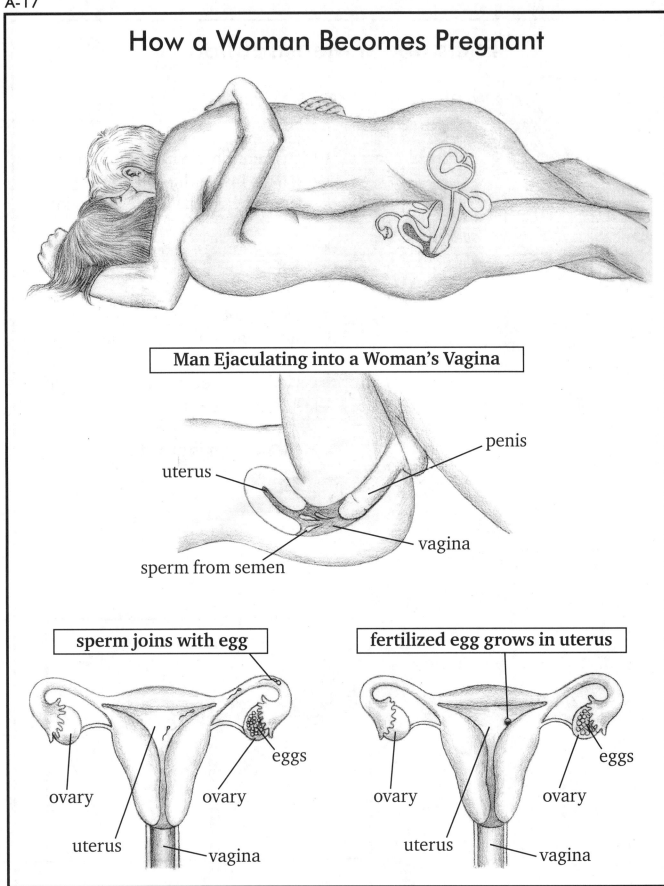

How a Woman Becomes Pregnant

Man Ejaculating into a Woman's Vagina

penis

uterus

vagina

sperm from semen

sperm joins with egg

ovary

eggs

ovary

uterus

vagina

fertilized egg grows in uterus

ovary

eggs

ovary

uterus

vagina

A-18

Pregnancy and Birth

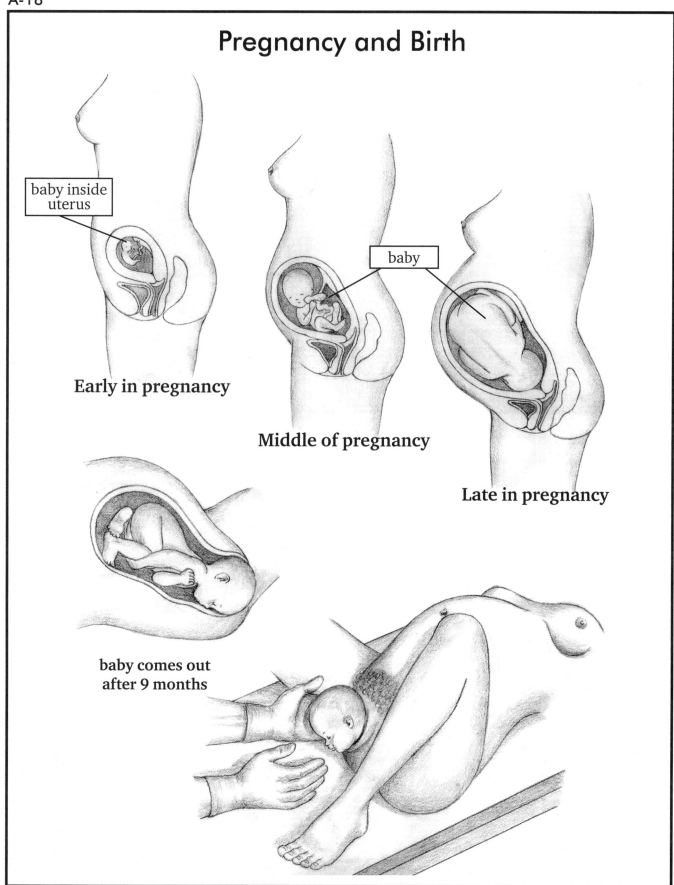

baby inside uterus

Early in pregnancy

baby

Middle of pregnancy

Late in pregnancy

baby comes out after 9 months

Appendix B

Other Teaching Materials

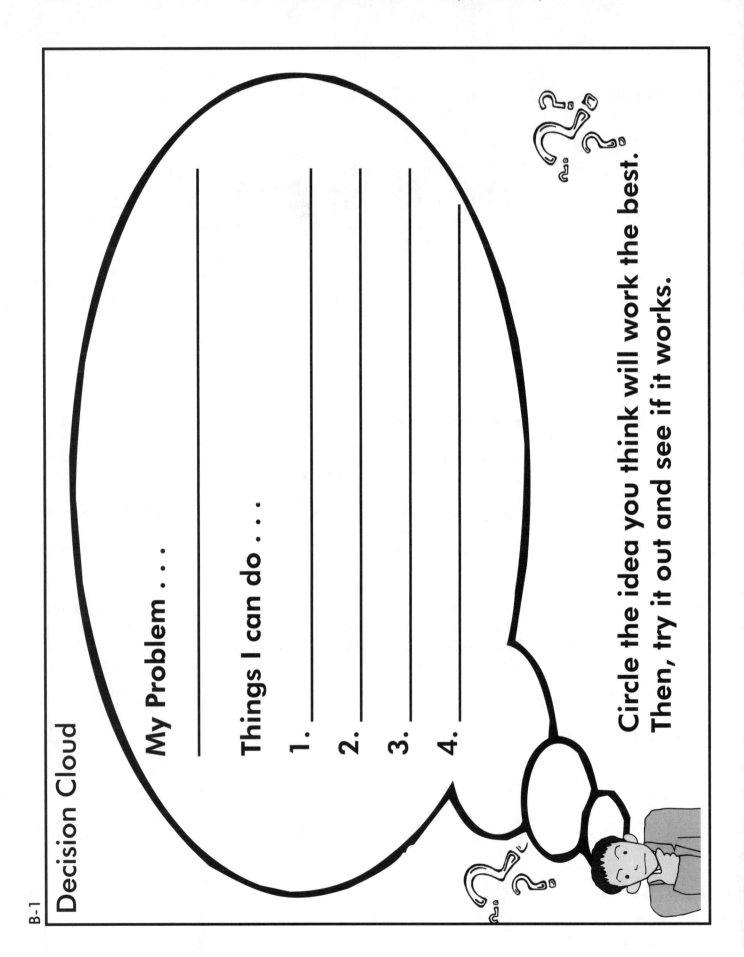

B-1

Decision Cloud

My Problem . . . .

Things I can do . . . .

1.

2.

3.

4.

Circle the idea you think will work the best.
Then, try it out and see if it works.

B-2

Public & Private Illustration

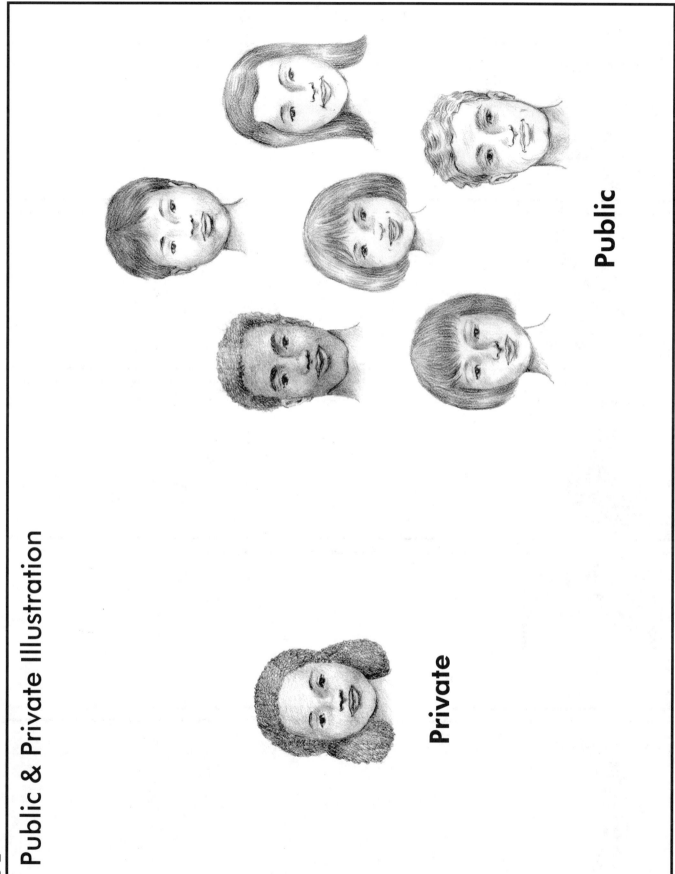

Public

Private

B-3

People in My Life

My Family

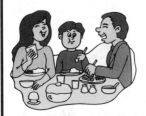

My Friends

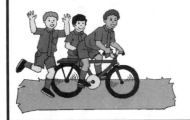

Sweetheart

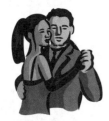

Paid Helpers

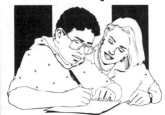

Strangers

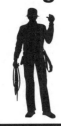

B-4

Okay Touch

My Family

My Friends

Sweetheart

Paid Helpers

Strangers

B-5

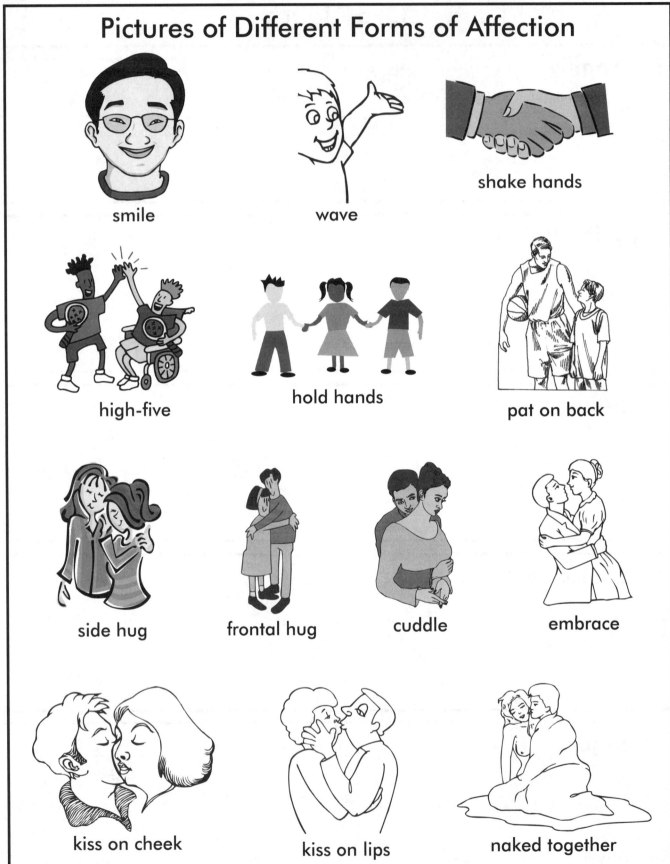

Pictures of Different Forms of Affection

smile

wave

shake hands

high-five

hold hands

pat on back

side hug

frontal hug

cuddle

embrace

kiss on cheek

kiss on lips

naked together

B-6

Guide to Teaching about Relationships

Relationship Type	Possible Definitions	Role	Touch
Family	■ Group of people who provide love and support	■ Provides food, place to live, medical care, love	■ Wide range ■ No sexual touching
Friend	■ Someone who has similar interests ■ Someone I enjoy being with and who enjoys being with me ■ Someone who sticks up for me ■ Someone who respects me ■ Someone who is honest (doesn't lie) ■ Someone who keeps promises	■ Shares hobbies and interests ■ Goes places with me ■ Talks to me and hangs out with me	■ Similar to what same-age peers use ■ No sexual touching
Romantic (Sweetheart)	■ Someone I have sexual feelings for ■ Someone who has sexual feelings for me ■ Someone I am dating ■ Not everyone has a sweetheart	■ Share hobbies and interests ■ Go places together ■ Talk and hang out together ■ Touch and affection ■ Sharing and intimacy	■ Varying levels of affection ■ Sexual touching with permission
Personal Helpers/ Paid Helpers	■ Someone who is paid to help or assist me	■ Supports me in specific ways ■ Teaches me (teacher) ■ Helps me do my job better (job coach) ■ Teaches me how to play a sport (coach) ■ Takes care of me in the hospital (nurse) ■ Makes sure I'm healthy (doctor) ■ Takes me to work (driver)	■ Verbal greeting ■ Limited touching ■ No sexual touching
Community Helpers	■ People who are paid to help others (not just me)	■ Supports others (not just me) in specific ways ■ Keeps communities safe (police) ■ Transports people (bus driver) ■ Helps me find things at the store (clerk)	■ Verbal greetings
Strangers	■ People I do not know	■ None	■ No touching

B-7

Getting Together with Friends Worksheet

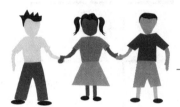

1. Who can I ask? _____ _____
_____

2. What could we do?

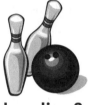  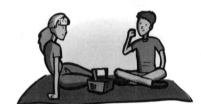

bowling?   movie?   picnic?   _____ other?

3. How will I ask?   by phone? in person?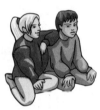

4. When will we go? _____ _____
                    day?   time?

5. How much will it cost? 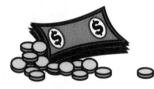 $ _____

6. How will we get there?

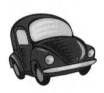 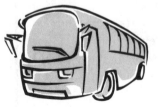 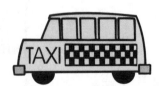

car?   bus?   taxi?   _____ other?

B-8

Planning a Date Worksheet

1. Who can I ask? 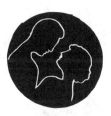 _____

2. What could we do?

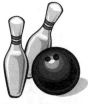   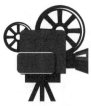   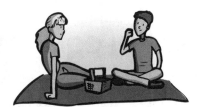   _____

bowling?   **movie?**   **picnic?**   **other?**

3. How will I ask?   by phone?   in person?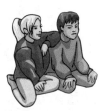

4. When will we go? _____ _____

day?   time?

5. How much will it cost? 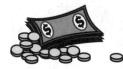 **Who will pay?**

$ _____   _____

6. How will we get there?

          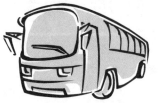   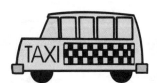

_____

car?   **bus?**   **taxi?**   **other?**

B-9

Ingredients of a Healthy Relationship

1. There is MUTUAL INTEREST.

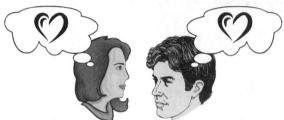

2. You have THINGS IN COMMON.

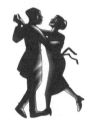 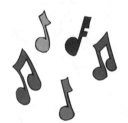 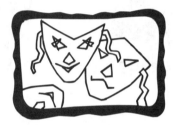

3. You have gotten to know each other slowly over TIME.

 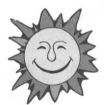 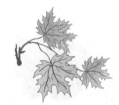 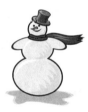

4. BOUNDARIES are respected.

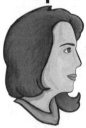 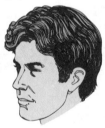 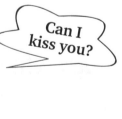

5. There is SHARED POWER in the relationship.

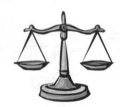

GREEN LIGHT = HEALTHY RELATIONSHIP

Keep the relationship going if:

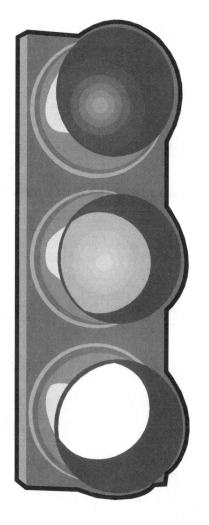

- You both like to do the same kinds of things.

- You say nice things to each other.

- You take turns making decisions.

- Your feelings and ideas are valued.

- The person says nice things about you to others.

- You feel comfortable being yourself when you are together.

- You can share personal thoughts and feelings even if you disagree.

- Your relationship develops slowly over time and you take time to get to know & trust each other.

- Your partner hears "NO" and stops.

- You respect and support each other.

- You feel happy, safe, and loved.

B-11

RED LIGHT = UNHEALTHY RELATIONSHIP

Stop the relationship if:

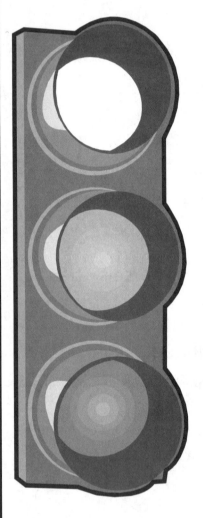

- The person puts you down (says bad things about your clothes, body, or looks).

- The person makes all the choices.

- The person tells you how to act and dress.

- The relationship moves too fast.

- The person wants to keep secrets.

- The person wants to keep you away from family and friends.

- The person hits you and says he or she is sorry.

- The person gets mad when you spend time with others.

- The person pushes you to have sex or do sexual things you don't want to do.

- The person refuses to use birth control.

- There seems to be lots of anger, fear, or jealousy in your relationship.

B-12

Contraceptive Methods—A Guide for Parents

FEMALE CONTRACEPTIVE METHODS

Hormonal Methods	How It Works	Other Information
ORAL CONTRACEPTION		
Combined (COC's)—Pills containing various levels of synthetic estrogen and progesterone are taken around the same time daily for 21 days followed by 7 days off.	Suppresses or stops ovulation, thickens cervical mucus, causes atrophy of endometrium	▪ Highly dependent on user—95% when used correctly ▪ Can reduce menstrual symptoms ▪ Reduces risk of endometrial and ovarian cancer (uncertain effect on breast cancer)
Progestin-only Pills (POP's, Minipills)—Pills containing varying and lower levels of synthetic progestin are taken at the same time every day.	Some suppression of ovulation, thickens cervical mucus, some atrophy of endometrium	▪ Highly dependent on user—95% when used correctly ▪ Fewer side effects than COC's ▪ Irregular bleeding is common side effect ▪ No cancer protection
Extended Contraceptive Regimen (Seasonale™)—pills containing hormones taken continuously for 84 days, followed by 7 days off.	Suppresses or stops ovulation, thickens cervical mucus, causes atrophy of endometrium	
Emergency Contraceptive Pills—A specific regimen of combined OCP's taken within 72 hours of unprotected intercourse.	Disrupts hormonal cycle resulting in delayed ovulation or anovulation (no ovulation)	
Hormone Patch (Ortho Evra)—Patches containing hormones are placed on lower abdomen, upper outer arm, buttocks, or upper torso (excluding breast) and changed every week x 3 wks. Then one week patch-free for withdrawal bleeding.	Steady release of hormones leads to suppression of ovulation, thickening of cervical mucus, atrophy of endometrium	▪ 98% or better effectiveness ▪ Initial, minor changes in bleeding pattern during first 2 mths, then comparable to COC's ▪ May be headaches, breast tenderness, mood changes, nausea (similar to COC's) ▪ Application-site reactions—mainly first 2 mths. ▪ May be less effective in women over 198 lbs.
Vaginal Ring (Nuva-Ring)—Flexible, transparent, one-size-fits-all doughnut-shaped ring that delivers daily doses of estrogen and progestin. The ring is inserted by the user into the vagina and worn for 3 weeks, then removed and discarded. After one week off, a new ring is inserted.	Steady release of hormones prevents ovulation, thickening of cervical mucus, atrophy of endometrium	▪ 99% or better effectiveness rate ▪ No fitting necessary ▪ If ring is removed from vagina for longer than 3 consecutive hours, backup method needed x 7 days ▪ May be headaches, increases in vaginal discharge, vaginitis, coital problems, or device expulsion

continued on next page

continued from previous page

Method	How it works	Notes
3-month shot (Depo-Provera™)—Injection of progestin in buttocks or arm by health care professionals once every 3 months (12 weeks).	Suppresses or stops ovulation, thickens cervical mucus, causes atrophy of endometrium	■ Almost 100% ■ Major changes in bleeding pattern (after initial irregularity, for most women, menses stops) ■ May be headaches, breast tenderness, mood changes, acne ■ Concerns re: impact on bone density ■ Weight gain likely (often more significant in women with DS)
Subdermal implant (Implanon™)—Single progestin-containing capsule is inserted by skilled health care professional under skin of inner upper arm. Good for up to 3 years. Must be removed by professional.	Suppresses or stops ovulation, thickens cervical mucus, causes atrophy of endometrium	■ Almost 100% ■ Wound concerns (infection, bruising, scarring) ■ May be changes in bleeding pattern (less bleeding, amenorrhea) ■ Some weight gain likely
INTRAUTERINE DEVICES (IUDS)		
Plastic devices containing copper or crystallized hormones are inserted into the uterus by professional. Removed and reinserted after 1, 5, or 12 yrs (depending on brand). Patient checks strings regularly.	Thickens cervical mucus, inhibits sperm survival and capacity	■ Almost 100% ■ May be changes in cramping/bleeding pattern ■ Small risk of headaches, acne, breast tenderness, and mood changes ■ Risk of perforation or infection (at time of insertion) or expulsion
SURGICAL METHODS		
Tubal Ligation—Permanent surgical procedure involving cutting, blocking, or cauterization of fallopian tubes.	Blocks tubes and prevents fertilization	■ Usually performed on adults only (21 or older) ■ Physician must be convinced woman is consenting to procedure
BARRIER METHODS		
Diaphragm—Dome-shaped, custom-fitted rubber cup that holds spermicidal jelly or cream is inserted into vagina before intercourse. Device rests on pubic bone to stay in place.	Creates physical barrier that blocks the cervix; cream or jelly used with it kills sperm	■ Effectiveness highly dependent on user—80% typical use*; 94% perfect use**
Cervical Cap—Soft, deep rubber cup that holds spermicidal jelly or cream and fits snugly over cervix. Device is inserted before intercourse and can remain in up to 48 hrs.	Creates physical barrier that blocks the cervix; cream or jelly used with it kills sperm	■ Effectiveness highly dependent on user as well as on whether user has had children (e.g., effectiveness can be reduced if vagina has been stretched during birth process)

Methods	How It Works	Other Information
Cervical Sponge—Small, one-size-fits-all pillow-shaped device with concave dimple is moistened with water (to activate spermicide) and inserted into vagina (dimple side up) before intercourse. This over-the-counter method is good for 24 hours and must remain in place 6 hrs. following intercourse.	Creates physical barrier that blocks the cervix; cream or jelly used with it kills sperm	▪ Same as for cervical cap, above
Female Condom—Soft, loose-fitting, lubricant-lined polyurethane sheath with 2 flexible rings. The inside ring is inserted and rests on the pubic bone to anchor condom. Outside ring is external and partially covers labia.	Creates physical barrier that blocks the cervix	▪ Highly dependent on user—79% typical*; 94% perfect use**

MALE CONTRACEPTIVE METHODS

Methods	How It Works	Other Information
Male Condom—A thin sheath placed over the penis during intercourse.	Prevents passage of semen	
Vasectomy—Permanent surgical procedure involving cutting, blocking, or cauterization of vas deferentia.	Prevents passage of sperm into man's seminal fluid.	▪ Usually performed on adults only (21 or older) ▪ Physician must be convinced male is consenting to procedure

*Typical use refers to failure rates for women whose use is not consistent or always correct.
**Perfect use refers to failure rates for those whose use is consistent and always correct.

References:

Alexander, N. (2002). New Methods of Delivering Hormonal Contraception. *Conversations in Counseling 4* (1). *Contraceptive Update,* November 2002.

Hatcher, R. et al. (1998). *Contraceptive Technology.* New York: Ardent Media.

Mangan, S. et al. (2002). Overweight Teens at Increased Risk for Weight Gain While Using Depot Medroxyprogesterone Acetate. *Journal of Pediatric Adolescent Gynecology 15:* 79-82.

Special Report: An Overview of the Hormonal Patch, Monthly Injection, and Vaginal Ring (October 2002). *OB/GYN Special Edition.*

Greydanus, D. et al. (2001). Contraception in the Adolescent: An Update. *Pediatrics 107* (3).

B-13

Sexual Behaviors That Are Against the Law

What it's called	What is it?	It's against the law because:	If this happens you should:
Indecent Exposure	• When someone shows you their private body parts in public • Showing other people your private body parts in public	• Bodies are private • Private body parts should be covered in public places	• Leave immediately • Tell a safe person
Incest	• When family members have sex together	• Families show they love each other in nonsexual ways	• Tell a safe person

Sexual Harassment	• Unwanted sexual talk, touch, or behavior in school or at work
	• Can include:
	  □ sexual comments, words
	  □ dirty jokes
	  □ showing sexual pictures
	  □ inappropriate touching
	  □ staring
	  □ moving into another person's personal space
	  □ asking others to do sexual things
		• This kind of behavior can make people feel unsafe or uncomfortable
		• There is no permission; it's unwanted
			• Tell the person to stop
			• Understand that schools and work have laws that protect people against unwanted sexual conduct
			• At work, tell a supervisor
			• At school, tell a teacher or principal

Child Sexual Abuse	■ Sexual contact between an adult and a child under the age of consent (check your state law—usually between 16 and 18, but as low as 14 in a few states)	■ Adult taking advantage of child ■ The law says children don't have the ability to say yes to having sex with an adult	■ Tell a safe person
Sexual Assault	■ Sexual contact that is not wanted ■ Can include: 　□ showing private body parts 　□ touching private body parts (with mouth or hands) 　□ kissing	■ There is no permission; it's unwanted ■ Person is afraid to say no	■ Tell a safe person
Rape	■ You are forced to have sex by someone who uses: 　□ weapons 　□ bribes or threats 　□ physical force	■ It's never okay to force a person to do sexual things when they don't want to	■ Tell a safe person
Date Rape	■ Someone you know or are dating forces you to have sex using: 　□ weapons 　□ bribes or threats 　□ physical force 　□ drugs or alcohol	■ No one can force you to have sex. It should be your decision ■ Even in dating relation-ships, both people must agree to have sex	■ Tell a safe person

B-14

Ways People May Try to Take Advantage of You

➤ **THEY USE SECRETS**

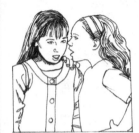

A SECRET is something you keep to yourself (in your head) and don't tell others. People who want to take advantage of you will ask you to keep secrets about the sexual things they do because they know what they are doing is wrong! Secrets might sound like this:
- "What we did today is a secret. You can't tell anyone."
- "What we do together is special and just between us."

IF A SECRET INVOLVES SEXUAL THINGS, TALK TO A SAFE PERSON!

➤ **THEY USE BRIBES**

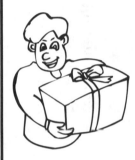

A BRIBE is when a person gives you gifts, money, treats, or special time together to persuade you to do something you don't want to do. Someone might use bribes to get you to do sexual things with them. Bribes might sound like this:
- "If you take your clothes off, I'll take you to the movies."
- "I'll buy you something special if you touch my penis."
- "We can get a special treat if you do what I tell you to do."
- "I have some gifts I can give you after we're done with our game."
- "If you have sex with me, I'll give you money."

IF THIS HAPPENS TO YOU, SAY "NO," LEAVE, and TELL A SAFE PERSON!

➤ **THEY USE THREATS**

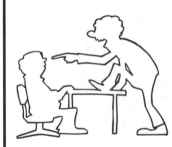

A THREAT means a person will try to scare you into doing something you don't want to do. Normally you might say no, but you're too afraid. Threats might sound like this:
- "If you tell, I will hurt you."
- "If you tell, I will hurt your parents."
- "Even if you told someone, they would never believe you because you're retarded."
- "If you tell, I'll kill you."

IF THIS HAPPENS TO YOU, LEAVE IF YOU CAN, and TELL A SAFE PERSON!

B-15

Okay? or Against the Law?

 ■ Chris and Lori have been dating for two years. They both like to spend private time hugging and kissing. Okay or against the law?

 ■ Maria is waiting at the bus stop for her bus. While she is waiting a man opens his coat and shows her he has no clothes. He leaves quickly. Okay or against the law?

 ■ A coworker where John works brings pictures of naked women and makes him look at them during breaks. It makes John nervous. Okay or against the law?

 ■ Another student (coworker) grabs Nigel's arm to help him get up after tripping and falling. Okay or against the law?

 ■ Jim and his uncle spend the weekend together doing fun things. Jim's uncle buys him presents and takes him to the movies. Later, when they are alone, Jim's uncle wants Jim to touch his penis. Okay or against the law?

 ■ During a slow dance, a man asks Leah to dance. Once they begin dancing, he grabs her breasts and touches her vulva. Okay or against the law?

 ■ Tamara's best friend's father has died. When Tamara sees her friend at the funeral, she gives her a big hug. Okay or against the law?

 ■ Ellen's boss gives her a big hug and kiss because she is doing such a nice job at work. Okay or against the law?

Resources

Organizations Specializing in Sexuality Information & Education

American Association of Sexuality Educators, Counselors,
and Therapists (AASECT)
P.O. Box 1960
Ashland, VA 23005-1960
804-752-0026
www.assect.org

AASECT's mission is to promote an understanding of human sexuality and healthy sexual behavior. They are the only U.S. agency providing certification for professionals in the field of sexuality. A list of professionals and their interests and specialties for each state can be found on their website.

Canadian Federation for Sexual Health
1 Nicholas St., Suite 430
Ottawa, ON K1N 7B7
613-241-4474
www.ppfc.ca

A national network affiliated with the International Planned Parenthood Federation which advances sexual and reproductive health and rights in Canada and abroad. Website includes information written for parents as well as teens and young adults.

Planned Parenthood Federation of America
www.plannedparenthood.org

Many Planned Parenthood affiliates have educators trained to design and implement sexuality programming for diverse audiences, sometimes including individuals with intellectual disabilities. To check resources for your state, go to the national website above and enter your state abbreviation. You may have to ask for specific information related to programs available for families and individuals with intellectual disabilities.

Rainbow Support Group
New Haven Gay & Lesbian Community Center
P.O. Box 8914
50 Fitch St.
New Haven, CT 06532
303-387-2252
Contact: John D. Allen

The only support group in the U.S. that focuses on addressing the unique needs of individuals who are gay, lesbian, bisexual, or transgender and also have intellectual disabilities. The original group began in New Haven, but other groups, based on this same model, continue to form around the country.

Sexuality Information and Education Council of Canada (SIECCAN)
850 Coxwell Ave.
Toronto, Ontario M4C 5R1
416-466-5304
www.sieccan.org

Canada's nonprofit educational organization dedicated to promoting education about all aspects of sexuality and supporting the positive integration of sexuality into people's lives. Not a disability-specific organization, but the website has online resources and links.

Sexuality Information and Education Council of the United States (SIECUS)
130 West 42nd St., Suite 350
New York, NY 10036-7802
212-819-9770
ww.siecus.org

SIECUS is a national organization providing information and advocacy on sexuality education issues, sexual health, and sexual rights. Their site is not specific to individuals with intellectual disabilities but does have parent newsletters and bibliographies.

Disability Organizations

The ARC of the United States
1010 Wayne Ave.
Silver Spring, MD 20910
800-433-5255
www.thearc.org

Best Buddies
100 SE Second Street, Ste. 2200
Miami, FL 33131
305-374-2233
www.bestbuddies.org
    Best Buddies is a program designed to match people with intellectual disabilities one-to-one with nondisabled peers in middle, high school, college, and work environments.

Canadian Down Syndrome Society
811 14th Street NW
Calgary, AL T2N 2A4
Canada
www.cdss.ca

Disability Solutions
14535 Westlake Drive, Ste. A-2
Lake Oswego, OR 97035
503-443-2258
www.disabilitysolutions.org

National Down Syndrome Congress (NDSC)
1370 Center Dr. Ste. 102
Atlanta, GA 30338
800-232-NDSC (6372)
www.ndsccenter.org

National Down Syndrome Society
666 Broadway
New York, NY 10012
800-221-4602
www.ndss.org

TASH
1025 Vermont Ave., Floor 7
Washington, DC 20005
202-263-5600
www.tash.org

Publications for Parents

SEXUALITY EDUCATION FOR CHILDREN WHO HAVE SPECIAL NEEDS

Drury, John, Hutchinson, Lynne, and Wright, Jon. *Holding On Letting Go: Sex, Sexuality and People with Learning Disabilities.* London: Souvenir Press, 2000.

Discusses general information about sexuality from the perspective of parents and professionals as well as strategies for working together on issues.

Maksym, Diane. *Shared Feelings: A Parent Guide to Sexuality for Children, Adolescents, and Adults Who Have a Mental Handicap.* Toronto: The G. Allan Roeher Institute, 1990 (www.roeher.ca).

General information on sexuality issues and approaches for handling sexuality education in the home.

Schweir, Karin Melberg and Hingsburger, David. *Sexuality: Your Sons and Daughters with Intellectual Disabilities.* Baltimore: Brookes Publishing, 2000.

General information on sexuality issues and approaches for handling sexuality education in the home.

Talk to Me: A Personal Development Manual for Women and Girls with Down Syndrome, and Their Parents. Parramatta, NSW, Australia: Down Syndrome Association of NSW, 1999.

A curriculum designed to help parents of teens and adults with Down syndrome teach their child. A section designed to prepare parents for teaching accompanies actual worksheets that can be used during teaching sessions. Although the title implies females are the target audience, most of the content is relevant for males too. The section designed for the young adults covers feelings, self-esteem, friendships and dating, public and private, body changes, masturbation, relationships, intercourse, and sexual assault. Can be downloaded for nonprofit use from www.dsansw.org.au.

EXPLOITATION PREVENTION

De Becker, Gavin. *The Gift of Fear and Other Survival Signals That Protect Us from Violence.* New York, NY: Dell, 1997.

De Becker, a sought-after crime investigator, discusses predictable patterns and behaviors frequently used by criminals and offenders.

De Becker, Gavin. *Protecting The Gift: Keeping Children and Teenagers Safe (and Parents Sane).* New York, NY: Dell, 1999.

The logical sequel to *The Gift of Fear*, this book contains many helpful ideas for parents in their role as protector and teacher.

Hart-Rossi, Janie. *Protect Your Child from Sexual Abuse: A Parent's Guide.* Seattle, WA: Parenting Press, 1984.

This parent book is designed to accompany the children's book *It's My Body.* The guide includes facts about sexual abuse, a guide for reading the book with your child, and nice reinforcement activities that can be taught at home.

Hingsburger, David. *Just Say Know: Understanding and Reducing the Risk of Sexual Victimization of People with Developmental Disabilities.* Richmond Hill, Ontario: Diverse City Press, 1995.

A great book that focuses on what can be done to prevent exploitation in individuals with developmental disabilities.

No More Victims: A Manual to Guide Family and Friends in Preventing the Sexual Abuse of People with a Mental Handicap. Toronto: G. Allan Roeher Institute, 1992.

A training manual that explores factors that put people with disabilities at risk, identifies symptoms of abuse, and discusses appropriate responses and preventative measures.

Salter, Anna C. *Predators, Pedophiles, Rapists, and Other Sex Offenders: Who They Are, How they Operate, and How We Can Protect Ourselves and Our Children.* New York, NY: Basic Books, 2003.

The author interviews people who exploit and shares insights on how they work to exploit others.

HYGIENE AND SELF-CARE

Baker, Bruce and Brightman, Alan. *Steps to Independence: Teaching Everyday Skills to Children with Special Needs.* Baltimore: Paul Brookes Publishing, 2004.

Includes basic template for teaching skills for self-care, toilet training, home care, and managing behavior that interferes with learning.

Wrobel, Mary. *Taking Care of Myself: A Hygiene, Puberty and Personal Curriculum for Young People with Autism.* Arlington, TX: Future Horizons, 2003.

This book is essentially a social stories curriculum for teaching about body changes, appropriate sexual behavior, and encouraging independence with hygiene and self care. Great ideas for creating teaching tools using Boardmaker© and Picture This© picture symbol programs.

PREPARING FOR PUBERTY

Gillooly, Jessica B. *Before She Gets Her Period: Talking with Your Daughter about Menstruation.* Glendale, CA: Perspective Publishing, 1998.

Designed to help parents prepare their daughters for puberty and menstruation.

STAGES OF SEXUAL DEVELOPMENT

Engel, Beverly. *Beyond the Birds and the Bees: Fostering Your Child's Healthy Sexual Development in Today's World.* New York, NY: Pocket Books, 1997.

A nice resource for understanding what typical sexual development looks like from birth to adolescence.

Haffner, Debra. *From Diapers to Dating: A Parent's Guide to Raising Sexually Healthy Children.* New York, NY: Newmarket Press, 2000.

Covers stages of sexual development birth- puberty.

Haffner, Debra. *Beyond the Big Talk: Every Parent's Guide to Raising Sexually Healthy Teens.* New York, NY: Newmarket Press, 2001.

Covers physical and psycho-sexual issues from puberty through adolescence.

Publications for Children, Teens, and Self-Advocates

BODY RIGHTS, OWNERSHIP, AND EMPOWERMENT

Freeman, Lory. *It's My Body*. Seattle: Parenting Press, 1982.

A good introduction to body rights. Encourages children to recognize touches that feel good and say no to those they don't want. The key message "your body is special and belongs to you" is emphasized. A Spanish version, *Mi Cuerpo is MIO,* is also available.

Freeman, Lory. *Loving Touches.* Seattle: Parenting Press, 1986.

A simply illustrated book about the need for touch throughout life and feelings associated with healthy touch. Geared toward younger children.

Girard, Linda Walvoord. *My Body Is Private.* Morton's Grove, IL: Albert Whitman, 1984.

A young girl, Julie, discusses the word private and her understanding related to things, her body, and body parts. The story includes her family rules and discussions related to her rights and what to do when those rights are violated.

Kleven, Sandy. *The Right Touch: A Read-Aloud Story to Help Prevent Child Sexual Abuse.* Bellevue, WA: Illumination Arts Publishing Company, 1997.

A mother helps her son understand the difference between healthy affection and problem touching. Emphasizes paying attention to body warning signs and reporting.

Payne, Lauren Murphy. *Just Because I Am: A Child's Book of Affirmation.* Minneapolis: Free Spirit Publishing, 1994.

A simple book that encourages appreciation of individual uniqueness. Includes empowering messages about the body, feelings, boundary awareness, touch, and feeling safe.

Spelman, Cornelia. *Your Body Belongs to You.* Morton's Grove, IL: Albert Whitman & Company, 1997.

This book, written by a social worker, is designed to help children understand their touching rights. The book balances messages regarding the need we all have for healthy affection with our right to determine who touches us. Includes multicultural drawings.

PRIVATE BODY PARTS/GENDER DIFFERENCES

Anatomically Correct Dolls: Teach-A-Bodies

This company carries a line of handmade dolls and puppets that are anatomically complete. For more information contact them at 956-581-9959 or on the web at www.valleyonline.com/tabdolls

Body Diagrams: RECAPP (Resource for Adolescent Pregnancy Prevention)

Drawings of anatomically correct male and female bodies with detached bathing suits that can be cut out to cover private parts can be downloaded off the web site: www.etr.org/recapp/freebies/learningactivity200206.htm

Brown, Marc and Brown, Laurie Krasny. *What's the Big Secret: Talking about Sex with Girls and Boys.* New York, NY: Little Brown and Company, 2000.

An easy-to-read storybook with animated drawings for young children that help distinguish differences between boy and girl bodies. The book discusses societal rules related to talking, looking, touching and being touched, and reproduction.

Schoen, Mark. *Bellybuttons Are Navels.* New York, NY: Prometheus Boks, 1990.

A story about two young children discovering their body parts while bathing together. Useful for helping children understand differences between boy and girl bodies and identifying correct names for genitals.

Stinson, Kathy. *The Bare Naked Book.* Toronto: Annick Press/Firefly Books, 1988.

A good introduction to teaching all body parts, including the genitals. Realistic illustrations highlight a specific body part on each page.

CONCEPTION AND REPRODUCTION

Cole, Joanne. *How You Were Born.* New York, NY: HarperTrophy, 1994.

Actual photographs describe conception, fetal development, and birth.

Gordon, Sol and Judith. *Did the Sun Shine Before You Were Born?* New York, NY: Prometheus Books, 1992.

This book designed for young children explains facts about sex, reproduction, and the birth process in clear and concise language within the context of families.

PUBERTY

Gravelle, Karen and Jennifer. *The Period Book: Everything You Don't Want to Ask but Need to Know.* New York, NY: Walker and Company, 1996.

A more advanced book for females that covers "changes you can see" and "changes you can't see" but includes information on tampon use, first pelvic exams, and how to handle common problems.

Harris, Robie. *It's Perfectly Normal: Changing Bodies, Growing Up, Sex, and Sexual Health.* Cambridge, MA: Candlewick Press, 1996.

A comprehensive book that uses colored, animated illustrations to address male and female puberty, reproduction, birth, sexual orientation, decision making, and staying healthy. Parents may want to read this with their child.

Mayle, Peter. *What's Happening to Me?: An Illustrated Guide to Puberty.* Lyle Stuart, 1981.

A humorous approach to male and female puberty. Mostly cartoon pictures with a few realistic drawings on body changes.

Schaefer, Valerie Lee. *The Care and Keeping of You: A Body Book for Girls.* Middleton, WI: Pleasant Company Publications, 1998.

This American Girl "head-to-toe" advice book addresses female puberty changes, hygiene issues, self-esteem, fitness, sleep, and emotions. Lots of color pictures (cartoon) and easier text makes it fun reading for girls with lower reading levels. Includes empowering messages about the body.

Siegel, Peggy. *Changes in You.* Richmond, VA: Family Life Education Associates, 1991.

The only resource written specifically for girls and boys with cognitive disabilities, this book uses realistic drawings and straightforward language to explain the physical, emotional, and social changes of puberty. Separate books are available for males and females. For sale at www.specialneeds.com.

Out of Harm's Way: A Safety Kit for People with Disabilities Who Feel Unsafe and Want to Do Something About It. Toronto: G. Allan Roeher Institute, 1997. www.roeher.ca.

A unique tool for helping self-advocates examine places they live, work, study, and play. It helps them define what is an unsafe environment, services, or relationships. Suggestions for changing their surroundings are included.

Royal College of Psychiatrists. *Books Beyond Words* (series). www.rcpsych.ac.uk/publications/bbw

Books Beyond Words are books especially designed for teaching people who cannot read; they include books designed to teach about caring for the body and reproductive health for males and females.

Wrobel, Mary. *Taking Care of Myself: A Hygiene, Puberty and Personal Curriculum for Young People with Autism.* Arlington, TX: Future Horizons, 2003.

This book is essentially a Social Stories curriculum for teaching about body changes, appropriate sexual behavior, and encouraging independence with hygiene and self care. Great ideas for creating teaching tools using Boardmaker© and Picture This© picture symbol programs.

Making Connections: A Humorous Look at Dating By and For Persons with Disabilities Choices. Choices, Inc. & American Film Video, 1995. Available from www.specialneeds.com.

People with cognitive and physical disabilities act out dating experiences resulting from a video dating service and then others discuss what they have learned from the film.

McKee, Lyn, Kempton, Winifred, and Stiggall-Muccigrosso, Lynne. *An Easy Guide to Loving Carefully for Women and Men.* 4th ed. Haverford, PA: Winifred Kempton Associates, 2002.

This book can be used as an advanced sequel to the above *Changes in You* book. It is designed to help people with developmental disabilities understand how pregnancy occurs (includes drawings of vaginal intercourse) and describes how to prevent pregnancy and sexually transmitted diseases. Methods of contraception, including abstinence, are discussed, as are male and female reproductive health exams, sexual orientation, and alternate lifestyles. Nicely illustrated and ideal for individuals who are thinking about becoming sexually active.

Talk to Me: A Personal Development Manual for Women and Girls with Down Syndrome, and Their Parents. Parramatta, NSW, Australia: Down Syndrome Association of NSW, 1999.

A curriculum designed to help parents of teens and adults with Down syndrome teach their child. A section designed to prepare parents for teaching accompanies actual worksheets that can be used during teaching sessions. Although the title implies females are the target audience, most of the content is relevant for males too. The section designed for the young adults covers feelings, self-esteem, friendships and dating, public and private, body changes, masturbation, relationships, intercourse, and sexual assault. Can be downloaded for nonprofit use from www.dsansw.org.au.

Teaching Materials for Professionals

COMPREHENSIVE
SEXUALITY
EDUCATION
CURRICULA
(MULTIPLE TOPICS)

Brekke, Beverly. *Sexuality Education for Persons with Severe Developmental Disabilities.* Santa Barbara, CA: James Stanfield Company (www.stanfield.com; 800-421-6534).

Designed for students with more limited cognitive abilities these slides address parts of the body (male and female), menstrual hygiene, social behavior, and reproductive exams.

Kempton, Winifred. *Life Horizons I & II.* Santa Barbara, CA: James Stanfield Company (www.stanfield.com; 800-421-6534).

The most comprehensive slide series and teaching script on sexuality designed for people with cognitive disabilities. Part I focuses on the physiological and emotional aspects and includes sections on parts of the body, sexual development, human reproduction, birth control, and STDs. Part II emphasizes the moral, social, and legal aspects of sexuality and covers self-esteem and relationships, dating skills and learning to love, marriage and other lifestyles, and parenting. Parts I & II are each sold separately.

Kempton, Winifred. *Socialization and Sexuality: A Comprehensive Training Guide for Professionals Helping People with Disabilities that Hinder Learning.* Haverford, PA: Winfred Kempton Associates, 2003.

An everything-you-need- to-know training guide for professionals interested in implementing sexuality education programs.

Rodgriguez Rouse, Geraldine and Pence Birth, Carol. *Socialization and Sex Education: Life Horizons Curriculum Module.* Santa Barbara, CA: James Stanfield Company (www.stanfield.com; 800-421-6534).

Designed to be used with the Life Horizons slide series by Winifred Kempton, this curriculum offers supplemental classroom and group activities. Published by James Stanfield Company (www.stanfield.com; 800-421-6534).

Stangle, Jane. *Special Education: Secondary Family Life and Sexual Health (FLASH).* Family Planning Publications, Seattle-King County Department of Public Health (sections of this resource can be previewed or downloaded from their website—www.metrokc.gov/health/famplan/flash/index.htm—scroll down to Special Education).

A teacher-friendly curriculum that provides student lessons on teaching relationships, public and private, communication, body changes, feelings, reproduction, STDs, birth control, and exploitation prevention. Geared toward high school students.

PUBERTY

Janet's Got Her Period. Santa Barbara, CA: James Stanfield Company, 1990.

This training manual provides extensive background information, a video, and instructional curriculum for teaching menstrual hygiene to young woman who have moderate or severe cognitive disabilities.

Siegel, Peggy. *Changes in You.* Santa Barbara, CA: James Stanfield Company (www.stanfield.com ; 800-421-6534).

A pricey visual teaching program for teaching preadolescents about physical, emotional, and social changes that accompany puberty. Includes laminated drawings with optional teaching scripts on the back of each picture. Comes with teacher's guide and male and female *Changes in You* books.

HYGIENE AND SELF-CARE

First Impressions Can Make a Difference. Santa Barbara, CA: James Stanfield Company (www.stanfield.com; 800-421-6534).

A four-module video series that addresses male and female hygiene, grooming, dress, and attitude using humor and exaggeration. Modules can be purchased separately or as a package.

Wrobel, Mary. *Taking Care of Myself: A Hygiene, Puberty and Personal Curriculum for Young People with Autism.* Arlington, TX: Future Horizons, 2003.

This book is essentially a social stories curriculum for teaching about body changes, appropriate sexual behavior, and encouraging independence with hygiene and self care. Great ideas for creating teaching tools using Boardmaker© and Picture This© picture symbol programs.

MASTURBATION

Hingsburger, David and Haar, Sandra. *Finger Tips: Teaching Women with Disabilities about Masturbation through Understanding and Video.* Richmond Hill, Ontario: Diverse City Press (www.diverse-city.com).

A video and teaching program for adult females with developmental disabilities that models safe and appropriate masturbation.

Hingsburger, David. *Hand Made Love: A Guide for Teaching About Male Masturbation Through Understanding and Video.* Richmond Hill, Ontario: Diverse City Press (www.diverse-city.com).

A video and teaching program for adult males with developmental disabilities that models safe and appropriate masturbation.

ANATOMY AND REPRODUCTIVE HEALTH

The GYN Exam Handbook: An Illustrated Guide to Gynecologic Examination for Women with Special Needs. Santa Barbara, CA: James Stanfield Company, 1991.

Videos and pictures that help explain pelvic exams.

Let's Talk about Health: What Every Woman Should Know. North Brunswick, NJ: ARC of New Jersey, 1994. (908-246-2525).

A video for teaching women with developmental disabilities about gynecological exams, breast exams, and mammograms.

Life Size Instructional Body Chart Kit.

Available to purchase from Planned Parenthood of Minnesota/South Dakota: www.ppmsd.org/store/viewproduct.asp?ec_products=84 (click on Store, then Curriculum).

Testicular Self Exam (TSE) and Breast Self Exam (BSE) Models.

Designed to make learning how to do self examination easier. Can be purchased at egeneralmedical.com/familyhealth.html.

SOCIAL SKILLS,
RELATIONSHIPS,
AND DATING

Baker, Jed. *Social Skills Training for Children and Adolescents with Asperger's Syndrome and Social-Communication Problems.* Shawnee Mission, KS: Autism Asperger Publishing Company, 2003.

Teaching curricula that includes 70 lesson plans for teaching common social skills. Categories of skills fall under basic conversational skills, cooperative play skills, friendship management, emotions management, developing empathy, and conflict management.

Being with People: An Eight Part Video Series to Teach Essential Social Skills to Special Needs Students. Santa Barbara: James Stanfield Company (www.stanfield.com).

A people-skills program that includes instruction geared towards being with friends, housemates, a date, or authority figures.

McGinnis, Ellen and Goldstein, Arnold. *SkillStreaming: New Strategies and Perspectives for Teaching Prosocial Skills.* Champaign, IL: Research Press, 2003-2005.

These kits are designed to teach social skills for different developmental levels—early childhood, middle schoolers, and adolescents. Each kit includes assessment forms, training manual, and social skill cards that can be used with learners. Social skills cards can be purchased separately.

Siperstein, Gary and Rickards, Emily Paige. *Promoting Social Success: A Curriculum for Children with Special Needs.* Baltimore: Paul Brookes Publishing, 2004.

An excellent and comprehensive teaching curricula that includes detailed lesson plans for facilitating skill development in the areas of understanding feelings and actions, noticing and interpreting social cues, problem-solving in social situations, and friendships.

Walker-Hirsch, Leslie. *Circles I: Intimacy and Relationships*. Santa Barbara, CA: James Stanfield Company (www.stanfield.com).

A well-respected program that uses videos and vignettes to teach students about social distance (how close to stand to others, depending on intimacy), changing relationships, and relationship-building skills. Appropriate for students from middle school through adulthood.

Young Adult Institute/National Institute for People with Disabilities Network. *Relationship Series.*

A comprehensive (and expensive) video series for adults that includes a friendship series (differences between strangers, acquaintances, and friends, becoming acquaintances and friends, and being a friend), boyfriend/girlfriend series (starting a special relationship, building a relationship I like, and having a good relationship), and sexual relationship series (enjoying your sexual life, working out problems, and sexual acts that are against the law). Available through YAI: www.yai.org; 212-263-7474.

EXPLOITATION PREVENTION

Hingsburger, David. *Just Say Know: Understanding and Reducing the Risk of Sexual Victimization of People with Developmental Disabilities.* Richmond Hill, Ontario: Diverse City Press, 1995.

A great book that focuses on what can be done to prevent exploitation in individuals with developmental disabilities.

Hingsburger, David and Harber, Mary. *The Ethics of Touch: Establishing and Maintaining Appropriate Boundaries in Service to People with Developmental Disabilities.* Toronto: Diverse City Press, 1998.

Addresses issues of privacy, touch, affection and boundaries for those providing direct care for individuals with cognitive disabilities.

No-Go-Tell! Santa Barbara, CA: James Stanfield Company.

A program designed for children with special needs ages 3-7 by experts who work with children with disabilities. The curriculum package includes pictures, anatomically correct dolls, and lesson plans.

No More Victims: Manual for Counselors and Social Workers. Toronto: G. Allan Roeher Institute (www.roeher.ca), 1992.

This resource discusses factors that put people with developmental disabilities at risk of sexual abuse, describes symptoms of abuse, and outlines appropriate responses and preventative measures.

Safety Awareness for Empowerment (SAFE). Madison, WI: Waisman Center's Healthy and Ready to Work Project (2005). (Available from: www.waisman.wisc.edu/hrtw/Publications.html)

An all-inclusive curricula designed to teach personal safety and prepare teenagers and young adults for life in the community. Numerous sections of this curricula address issues related to sexuality including feelings, relationships, rights to privacy, tactics used by exploiters, safe dating, and exploitation prevention.

SEXUAL ORIENTATION/ GENDER

Allen, John D. *Gay, Lesbian, Bisexual, and Transgender People with Developmental Disabilities and Mental Retardation: Stories of the Rainbow Support Group.* Binghamton, NY: Haworth Press, 2003.

This book, written by the founder of the first support group for GLBT individuals with developmental disabilities, describes the origins of the group, successes, difficulties, and experiences and concerns of group members.

Sexuality Resource Centers

The shops listed below believe in promoting sexual health and pleasure. Beyond quality products, they employ knowledgeable, well-trained staff who can provide individualized or couple support on more advanced sexuality topics like pleasure and human sexual response. Starred stores have staff who are familiar with people with the unique educational needs of individuals with intellectual disabilities.

A Woman's Touch*
200 Jefferson St.
Milwaukee, WI
414 221-0400
or
600 Williamson Street
Madison, WI 53702
608-250-1928
www.awomanstouchonline.com

Babeland
7007 Melrose Ave.
Los Angeles, CA 90038
323-634-9480
ww.babeland.com
or
707 E. Pike St.
Seattle, WA 98122
206-328-2914
or
43 Mercer St.
New York, NY 10013
212-966-2120

Come As You Are*
701 Queen Street West
Toronto, Ontario, Canada
877-858-3160
www.comeasyouare.com

Good Vibrations
308-A Harvard Street
Brookline, MA 02446
617-264-4400
www.goodvibes.com
or
603 Valencia St.
San Francisco, CA 94110
415-522-5460

or
1620 Polk St.
Berkeley, CA 94109
415-345-0400

Software for Creating Visual Teaching Materials

Mayer-Johnson Company
P.O. Box 1579
Solana Beach, CA 92075
858-550-0084
www.mayer-johnson.com

    This company produces a nice collection of Picture Communication Symbols™ and communication boards focusing on issues of sexuality. Topics address masturbation, puberty, sexual abuse prevention, and more.

Silver Lining Multi-Media
P.O. Box 2201
Poughkeepsie, NY 12601
845-462-8714

    This company produces *Picture This* software which includes photos for teaching basic hygiene and menstrual hygiene. Some of the materials illustrated in this book were produced using this software.

Websites

Disability, Abuse, & Personal Rights Project
http://disability-abuse.com

    A comprehensive website focused on sexual abuse prevention and intervention strategies for supporting individuals with developmental disabilities. This site includes many downloadable research articles, helpful information, and publications for parents, professionals, and individuals who have been abused.

Diverse City Press
www.diverse-city.com

    The website of David Hingsburger, world-renowned speaker and advocate for individuals with intellectual disabilities. His resources are designed to help professionals teach and support clients in understanding healthy sexuality.

James Stanfield Publishing Company
www.stanfield.com

    A long-standing company committed to providing resources to meet the educational needs of individuals with developmental disabilities. Some of the most well-known and popular programs can be found here.

SexualHealth.com
www.sexualhealth.com

This website is committed to providing easy access to sexuality information, support, and resources. One of the only sites that addresses sexuality and individuals with developmental disabilities. Well-respected sexuality professionals from the U.S. and Canada are available to answer questions or address concerns submitted to the website.

Index

modeling peers', 48-49
reasons for changes in, 231
threatening, 306
Body
framework for teaching about, 150-51
illustrations of, 270-75
image, 124-25
maps, 51
odor, 68,75, 143
rights, 40-41, 220, 222-23
tracings, 26
Body parts. *See also* Reproduction; Puberty; Self-care
skills; Touching
differences in male/female, 16-17
functions of, 18-23
illustrations of, 276-77, 280-84
private, 31, 32
teaching activities for, 14, 17, 26
teaching names for, 11-16, 222
Boils, 68
Books
about feelings, 156
about personal space, 41
about reproduction, 22-23
about reproductive health, 102
for parents, 312-13
for people with disabilities, 314-16
for professionals, 317-20
for teaching names of body parts, 14
Boundaries. *See* Affection; Personal space; Touching
Boyfriends. *See* Dating
Bras, 72-73
Breaking up, 187
Breast feeding, 13
Breasts
development of, 72-74
discomfort of, during periods, 76, 77
itchy, 73
touching, 73
Bribes, 306
Bruni, Maryanne, 46
Brushing protocols, 46
Cancer
breast, 101
testicular, 65
Celiac disease, 66
Chaining, 24
Chaperoning, 180-82
Chicoine, Brian, 43, 116, 235
Child Protective Services, 232

Childcare
facts and myths about, 208-209
training, 205-207
Children
deciding whether to have, 204-209
of parents with Down syndrome, 201, 202
Chores, 123-24
Circles curriculum, 265
Clothes, taking off in public, 34. *See also* Dressing
Club NDSS, 122
Cognitive disabilities. *See* Disabilities, people with
Commitment ceremonies, 196
Communication. *See also* Behavior; Talking; Terminology
of "no," 184-86
of pain, 97
using touch as, 49, 50
Contraceptives, 98, 99-100, 210-11, 301-303
Counseling
for self-acceptance problems, 122
genetic, 203-204
premarital, 199-200
Count Us In, 122
Couples interviewed, 198
Couric, Katie, 125
Cramps. *See* Menstruation, pain during
Crushes, 170, 171-73
Cryptorchidism, 64
Curtis, Jamie, 125
Dating
breaking up and, 187
chaperoning, 180-82
developmental patterns of, 174-75
finding a compatible partner for, 176-78
handling rejection, 181
readiness for, 175
respecting boundaries and, 182-86
teaching skills for, 176-79
worksheet for planning, 297
Davis, Phyllis, 54
De Becker, Gavin, 219, 223
Decision making, 127-28
Decision clouds, 71, 90, 128, 290
Deodorant. *See* Body odor
Dependency, 215
Depression, 231, 234
Detienne, Andy and Beth, 198, 200
Diabetes, 98
Diaper changes, 13
Diapers, menstruation and, 88
Disabilities, people with
children of, 210

About the Author

Terri Couwenhoven, M.S, is an AASECT certified sexuality educator who specializes in working with people who have intellectual disabilities, their families, and the professionals who support them. She regularly runs workshops for families and individuals of all ages with intellectual disabilities. Previous publications include *Beginnings: A Parent/Child Sexuality Program for Families with Puberty-Aged Children with Developmental Disabilities* and *Teen-to-Teen: A Sexuality and Life Skills Teaching System for Teens.* When she is not teaching, she is Clinic Coordinator for the Down Syndrome Clinic of Wisconsin at Children's Hospital of Wisconsin. Terri is also the mother of two daughters; her oldest has Down syndrome.